Recent Results in Cancer Research 80

Fortschritte der Krebsforschung
Progrès dans les recherches sur le cancer

Adjuvant Therapies of Cancer

Edited by
G. Mathé G. Bonadonna S. Salmon

With 108 Figures and 146 Tables

Springer-Verlag
Berlin Heidelberg New York 1982

Prof. G. Mathé
Institut de Cancérologie et d'Immunogénétique
Hôpital Paul-Brousse, 14-16 Avenue Paul-Vaillant-Couturier
F-94800 Villejuif

Dr. G. Bonadonna
Istituto Nazionale per lo Studio e la Cura dei Tumori
Via Venezian 1, I-20133 Milan

Prof. S. Salmon
The University of Arizona, Health Science Center
Department of Internal Medicine
Section of Hematology and Oncology
Tucson, AZ 85724 (USA)

Sponsored by the Swiss League against Cancer

ISBN-13 : 978-3-642-81687-1 e-ISBN-13 : 978-3-642-81685-7
DOI : 10.1007 / 978-3-642-81685-7

Library of Congress Cataloging in Publication Data. Main entry under title: Adjuvant therapies of cancer. (Recent results in cancer research; 80) Bibliography: p. Includes index. 1. Cancer–Treatment. I. Mathé, Georges, 1922. II. Bonadonna, G., 1934. III. Salmon, S. E. (Sydney E.), 1936. IV. Series. [DNLM: 1. Adjuvants, Immunologic–Therapeutic use. 2. Adjuvants, Pharmaceutic–Therapeutic use. 3. Neoplasms–Drug therapy. W1 RE106P v. 80/QZ 267 A235] RC261.R35 vol. 80 [RC270.8] 616.99'4s 81-9289 [616.99'406] AACR2.

Typesetting and printing: Carl Ritter GmbH & Co. KG, Wiesbaden
Binding: J. Schäffer OHG, Grünstadt

2125/3140–5 4 3 2 1 0

Contents

I. General Considerations 1

1. Metastatic Potential of Metastases, Tumor Cell Heterogeneity, and Therapeutic Implications (F. Spreafico, A. Mantovani, R. Giavazzi, G. Conti, and A. Anaclerio) 1
2. Immune Imbalance and Immune Modulation in Solid Tumor Patients: New Insights (B. Serrou, D. Cupissol, and C. Rosenfeld) 9
3. Markers of Minimal Residual Disease (A. M. Neville) 17
4. Radiotherapy as Adjuvant Local Therapy of Local Tumors (D. Chassagne) 22

II. Hemopoietic and Lymphoid Neoplasias 26

5. Comparison of HLA Phenotypes in Long-Term Survivors with Acute Lymphoblastic Leukemia Treated with Immunotherapy Versus Chemotherapy (T. Tursz, J. Hors, M. Lipinski. J.-L. Amiel, and G. Mathé) 26
6. An Intensive Chemo- or Chemoimmunotherapy Regimen for Patients with Intermediate and Poor-Prognosis Acute Lymphatic Leukemia and Leukemic Lymphoblastic Lymphosarcoma: Preliminary Results with 14-Month Median Follow-Up (J. L. Misset, F. De Vassal, M. Delgado, P. Ribaud, M. Musset, T. Dorval, D. Machover, C. Jasmin, M. Hayat, L. Schwarzenberg, and G. Mathé) 29

7. Poor-Prognosis Acute Lymphoblastic Leukemias (M. Weil, C. Jacquillat, M. F. Auclerc, G. Schaison, C. Chastang, and J. Bernard) 36

8. Therapeutic Effectiveness of Neuraminidase-Treated Allogeneic Myeloblasts as Immunogen in Acute Myelocytic Leukemia (J. G. Bekesi and J. F. Holland) 42

9. Maintenance Chemoimmunotherapy of Nonlymphoblastic Acute Leukemias (R. Favre, G. Sebahoun, D. Bagarry-Liégey, C. Imbert, P. Ciardelli, J. A. Gastaut, G. Meyer, and Y. Carcassonne) 56

10. Possible Mechanisms of Immunotherapy Action in Acute Nonlymphatic Leukemia: Macrophage Production of Colony-Stimulating Activity (P. Reizenstein, B. Andersson, and M. Beran) ... 64

11. The Finnish Leukaemia Group: Levamisole in Maintenance Therapy of Acute Myeloid Leukemia in Adults (M. Lehtinen, P. Ahrenberg, A. Hänninen, E. Ikkala, R. Lahtinen, A. Levanto, I. Palva, A. Rajamäki, S. Rosengard, T. Ruutu, S. Sarna, O. Selroos, T. Timonen, E. Waris, C. Wasastjerna, J. Vilpo, and P. Vuopio) 70

12. Treatment of Acute Leukemia in Remission by Bone Marrow Transplantation (R. Storb) 73

13. Prevention of Blastic Crisis in Ph[1]-Positive Chronic Myeloid Leukemia (J. C. Sharp) 78

14. A Southwest Oncology Group: Chemotherapy Versus Chemotherapy Plus Radiotherapy in Treatment of Stage III Hodgkin's Disease (P. N. Grozea, E. J. De Persio, C. A. Coltman Jr., C. J. Fabian, F. S. Morrison, E. A. Gehan, and S. E. Jones) 83

15. Maintenance Immunotherapy with BCG in Non-Hodgkin's Malignant Lymphomas: A Progress Report of a Randomized Trial (B. Hœrni, M. Durand, H. Eghbali, G. Hœrni-Simon, P. Richaud, and A. de Mascarel) 92

III. Bone Tumors 98

16. Role of Lung Irradiation in the Adjuvant Treatment of Osteosarcoma (E. van der Schueren and K. Breur) 98

17. Adjuvant Interferon Treatment of Human Osteosarcoma (H. Strander, T. Aparisi, H. Blomgren, L. Å. Broström, K. Cantell, S. Einhorn, S. Ingimarsson, U. Nilsonne, and G. Söderberg) . 103

18. A Strategic Adjuvant Therapy of Osteosarcoma (C. Jasmin) 108

19. Ewing's Sarcoma: Treatment with High-Dose Radiation and Adjuvant Chemotherapy (A. Goldman) 115

20. Adjuvant Chemotherapy in Ewing's Sarcoma Patients (M. Gasparini and F. Lombardi) 120

21. Early Results of Combined Modality Therapy of Patients with Ewing's Sarcoma (D. K. Hossfeld, S. Seeber, E. Siemers, C. G. Schmidt, and E. Scherer) 124

22. Ewing's Sarcoma: 5-Year Survival Under Adjuvant Chemotherapy (B. P. Le Mevel) 128

IV. Breast Carcinoma 134

23. Natural History of Breast Cancer (S. Gore, A. Langlands, S. Pocock, and G. Kerr) 134

24. Adjuvant Chemotherapy in Breast Cancer (R. Nissen-Meyer, K. Kjellgren, and B. Mansson) 142

25. Multimodal Therapy with CMF in Resectable Breast Cancer with Positive Axillary Nodes: The Milan Institute Experience (G. Bonadonna, P. Valagussa, A. Rossi, G. Tancini, C. Brambilla, S. Marchini, and U. Veronesi) 149

26. Follow-Up Results from a Randomized Trial for T_3 and T_4 Breast Cancer Patients: Previous BCG Immunotherapy Improves Response to Chemotherapy in the Relapse Patient (B. Serrou, H. Sancho-Garnier, P. Cappelaere, R. Plagne, R. Metz, M. Schneider, P. Chollet, N. Namer, H. Pujol, J. Gary-Bobo, G. Meyer, and G. Mathé) 157

27. Adjuvant Treatment of Node-Positive Breast Cancer with Adriamycin-Cyclophosphamide with or Without Radiation Therapy: Interim Results of an Ongoing Clinical Trial (S. E. Jones, S. E. Salmon, H. Allen, G. F. Giordano, S. Davis, E. Chase, T. E. Moon, and R. S. Heusinkveld) 162

28. A Randomized Trial of Postoperative Five-Versus Three-Drug Chemotherapy After Mastectomy: A Cancer and Leukemia Group B (CALGB) Study (R. Weiss, D. C. Tormey, F. Holland, V. E. Weinberg, G. Lesnick, M. Perloff, G. Falkson, and O. J. Glidewell) 170

29. Adjuvant Chemoimmunotherapy with LMF Plus BCG in Node-Negative and Node-Positive Breast Cancer – Intermediate Report at 4 Years (H. J. Senn, R. Amgwerd, W. F. Jungi, R. Hochuli, J. Ammann, G. Engelhart, C. Heinz, A. Wick, F. Enderlin, G. Creux, B. Simon, R. Lanz, R. Bigler, and S. Seiler) 177

30. Adjuvant Intermittent Chemoimmunotherapy for Primary Breast Cancer: A Prospective Study with Immunologic Follow-Up (M. Betzler, W. Schreml, M. Lang, H. P. Lohrmann, H. D. Flad, P. Schlag, C. Herfarth, and H. Heimpel) 185

31. Short-Term and Long-Term Effects of Chemoimmunotherapy on Granulopoiesis: Adjuvant Therapy of Breast Cancer (H. P. Lohrmann, W. Schreml, and M. Lang) 192

32. A New Adjuvant Treatment with Polyadenylic-Polyuridylic Acid in Operable Breast Cancer (F. Lacour, J. Lacour, A. Spira, M. Michelson, G. Delage, J. Y. Petit, and J. Viguier) 200

V. Lung Carcinoma 207

33. Metastatic CNS Disease in Small Cell Carcinoma of the Bronchus: The Role of Radiotherapy and Chemotherapy (J. M. A. Whitehouse and C. J. Williams) 207

34. Interim Results of EORTC Protocol 08742: Comparison, After Irradiation of Locally Advanced Squamous Cell Bronchial Carcinoma, of Abstention, Immunotherapy, Combination Chemotherapy or Chemoimmunotherapy (L. Israel, A. Depierre, and O. Dalesio) 214

35. Immunologically Defined Prognostic Subgroups as Predictors of Response to BCG Immunotherapy (J. W. Reid, G. B. Cannon, E. Perlin, J. Blom, R. Connor, and R. B. Herberman) 219

36. Intrapleural BCG Immunotherapy of Lung Cancer Patients (C. Maver, H. Kausel, L. Lininger, and M. McKneally) 227

37. Specific Active Immunotherapy in Lung Cancer: The Induction of Long-Lasting Cellular Responses to Tumour-Associated Antigens (T. H. M. Stewart, A. C. Hollinshead, J. E. Harris, and S. Raman) 232

38. Malnutrition in Lung Cancer: Incidence, Prognostic Implications, and Pathogenesis (D. L. Kisner) 240

39. Follow-Up of a Randomized Trial for Oat Cell Carcinoma Evaluating the Efficacy of Peripheral Intravenous Nutrition (PIVN) as Adjunct Treatment (B. Serrou, D. Cupissol, R. Plagne, P. Boutin, P. Chollet, Y. Carcassonne, and F. B. Michel) . . . 246

VI. Melanoma 254

40. Clinical Trials of Chemotherapy and Chemoimmunotherapy in Primary Malignant Melanoma (C. Jacquillat, P. Banzet, and J. Maral) 254

41. Trial 6: Randomized Study of Prolonged Chemotherapy, Immunotherapy, and Chemoimmunotherapy as an Adjuvant to Surgery for Stage I and II Melanoma. A Progress Report (G. Beretta) 259

42. Current Status of Melanoma Chemotherapy and Immunotherapy (B. M. Czarnetzki, E. Macher, H. Behrendt, and F. Lejeune) 264

VII. Testicular Neoplasia 269

43. Adjuvant Therapy of Testicular Carcinoma (C. G. Schmidt) 269

VIII. Gastrointestinal Neoplasms 277

44. Adjuvant 5-Fluorouracil and BCNU Chemotherapy in Gastric Cancer: 3-Year Results (P. Schlag, W. Schreml, W. Gaus, C. Herfarth, M. M. Linder, W. Queisser, and M. Trede) 277

45. Adjuvant Chemotherapy in Colon and Gastric Cancer (J. S. Macdonald, D. G. Haller, and D. L. Kisner) 284

46. Chemotherapy of Metastatic Gastrointestinal Cancers: Prospects for Future Adjuvant Systemic Therapies (D. L. Kisner and J. S. Macdonald) 291

47. Chemotherapy of Carcinomas of the Digestive Tract (C. Gisselbrecht, D. Belpomme, L. Mignot, M. Marty, G. Mathé, and M. Boiron) 296

IX. Conclusions and Prospects 303

48. Clinical Trials on Adjuvant Therapies in Cancer: Short-Term and Long-Term Results (P. Valagussa and G. Bonadonna) 303

49. Long-Term Costs of Adjuvant Radiotherapy (F. Volterrani and D. Sigurtà) 308

50. Long-Term Cost of Combined Radiotherapy and Chemotherapy (M. Weil, C. Jacquillat, G. Auclerc, P. F. Unger, and J. Bernard) 312

51. Studies of Clonogenic Human Tumor Stem Cells (S. E. Salmon) 317

52. Current Status of Clinical Trials of m-AMSA, Dihydroxyanthracenedione, and Deoxycoformycin (J. S. Macdonald, S. Marsoni, S. Bruno, and D. Poster) 323

53. Three New Agents for Immunotherapy Trials: Azimexon, Bestatin, and Tuftsin (G. Mathé, I. Florentin, M. Bruley-Rosset, A. Goutner, and B. Serrou) 331

54. Emerging Immunologic Approaches to Treatment of Neoplastic Diseases (L. Olsson and G. Mathé) 334

55. Cellular Interactions Modulating Host Resistance to Tumours
(R. W. Baldwin, V. S. Byers, D. Hannant, J. A. Jones, M. V. Pimm, and M. R. Price) 338

56. Preliminary Clinical Results with Norgamen (Thioproline) and Revercan (S-Amino-2-Thiazoline): The First Inducers of Reverse Transformation
(A. Brugarolas and M. Gosálvez) 346

57. Biologic Response Modifiers and Adjuvant Chemotherapy: Consideration of Selected Preclinical Investigations in Relation to Clinical Potential
(A. Goldin, M. A. Chirigos, J. S. Macdonald, A. Fefer, and E. Mihich) 351

List of Senior Authors

R. W. Baldwin
Cancer Research Compaign Laboratories, Nottingham, United Kingdom

J. G. Bekesi
The Mount Sinai School of Medicine and Hospital, New York, NY, USA

G. Beretta
Ospedale San Carlo, Milan, Italy

M. Betzler
Universität Ulm, Ulm, Germany

G. Bonadonna
Istituto Nazionale Tumori, Milan, Italy

A. Brugarolas
Hospital General de Asturias, Oviedo, Spain

D. Chassagne
Institut Gustave-Roussy, Villejuif, France

B.M. Czarnetzki
Dermatologische Klinik, Münster, Germany

R. Favre
Institut J. Paoli, I. Calmettes, Marseille, France

M. Gasparini
Istituto Nazionale Tumori, Milan, Italy

C. Gisselbrecht
Hôpital Saint-Louis, Paris, France

A. Goldin
National Cancer Institute, NIH, Bethesda, MD, USA

A. Goldman
Royal Marsden Hospital, London, United Kingdom

S. Gore
MRC Biostatistics Unit, Medical Research Council Center, Cambridge, United Kingdom

P.N. Grozea
Oklahoma Medical Research Foundation, Oklahoma City, OK, USA

B. Hoerni
Foundation Bergonié, Bordeaux, France

D.K. Hossfeld
Medizinische Universitätsklinik, Essen, Germany

L. Israel
Hôpital Avicenne, Bobigny, France

C. Jacquillat
Institut de Recherches sur les Mélanomes Malins, Lariboisière Saint-Louis, Paris, France

C. Jasmin
Hôpital Paul-Brousse, Villejuif, France

S.E. Jones
Arizona Health Sciences Center, Tucson, AZ, USA

D.L. Kisner
National Cancer Institute, Bethesda, MD, USA

F. Lacour
Institut Gustave-Roussy, Villejuif, France

M. Lethinen
Tampere Central Hospital, Tampere, Finland

B.P. Le Mevel
Centre René Gauducheau, Nantes, France

H.P. Lohrmann
Universität Ulm, Ulm, Germany

J.S. Macdonald
National Cancer Institute, Bethesda, MD, USA

G. Mathé
Hôpital Paul-Brousse, Villejuif, France

C. Maver
Albany Medical College, Albany, NY, USA

J.L. Misset
Hôpital Paul-Brousse, Villejuif, France

A.M. Neville
Ludwig Institute for Cancer Research, Sutton, Surrey, United Kingdom

R. Nissen-Meyer
Oslo, Norway

L. Olsson
Hôpital Paul-Brousse, Villejuif, France

J.Y. Petit
Institut Gustave-Roussy, Villejuif, France

J.W. Reid
Naval Regional Medical Center, Portsmouth, VA, USA

P. Reizenstein
Karolinska Hospital, Stockholm, Sweden

S.E. Salmon
University of Arizona, Health Sciences Center, Tucson, AZ, USA

P. Schlag
Universität Ulm, Ulm, Germany

C.G. Schmidt
Innere Universitätsklinik und Poliklinik, Essen, Germany

H.J. Senn
Kantonsspital, St. Gallen, Switzerland

B. Serrou
Hôpital Saint-Eloi, Montpellier, France

J.C. Sharp
King's College Hospital, London, United Kingdom

F. Spreafico
Istituto di Ricerche Farmacologiche 'Mario Negri', Milan, Italy

T.H.M. Stewart
University of Ottawa, Ottawa, Ontario, Canada

R. Storb
Fred Hutchinson Cancer Research Center, Seattle, WA, USA

H. Strander
Karolinska Hospital, Stockholm, Sweden

T. Tursz
Institut Gustave-Roussy, Villejuif, France

P. Valagussa
Istituto Nazionale Tumori, Milan, Italy

E. van der Schueren
Academisch Ziekenhuis St. Rafael, Leuven, Belgium

F. Volterrani
Istituto Nazionale Tumori, Milan, Italy

M. Weil
Institut de Recherches sur les Maladies du Sang,
Hôpital Saint-Louis, Paris, France

B. Weiss
National Cancer Institute, Bethesda, MD, USA

J.M.A. Whitehouse
CRC and Wessex Regional Medical Oncology Unit,
Southampton, United Kingdom

I. General Considerations

*1. Metastatic Potential of Metastases, Tumor Cell Heterogeneity, and Therapeutic Implications**

F. Spreafico, A. Mantovani, R. Giavazzi, G. Conti, and A. Anaclerio

Istituto di Ricerche Farmacologiche 'Mario Negri',
Via Eritrea 62, I-20157 Milan, Italy

Summary

The metastasizing capacity of spontaneous metastases of several murine tumors of different histology, origin, and disseminative pattern was investigated to test the hypothesis that metastases originate from various subpopulations within the primary tumor. Overall, tumor cells from individual metastases did not show greater metastasizing capacity than the cells of the original tumor, although a degree of heterogeneity was seen. Differences in the immunologic profile among metastases of the same tumor were also observed. The possible therapeutic implications of these findings are discussed.

Introduction

Oncologists need not be reminded that the real targets of adjuvant chemotherapy are tumor metastases. Although it can easily be advanced that the formation of metastases is the root of clinical malignancy, our ignorance of metastasis formation, the final result of a complex series of events in which an array of host and tumor factors interact, is still substantial. Yet, to devise more effective and intelligent therapeutic strategies aimed at the prevention and/or treatment of metastatic disease, a more in-depth understanding is needed as to the pathogenesis of invasion, dissemination, and peripheral colonization, and of the properties of metastatic cells vis à vis those of the primary tumor.

The Metastatic Potential of Metastatic Cells

Studies from various groups have recently provided evidence that clones from primary murine neoplasms can differ markedly in various biologic characteristics including their capacity to form secondary tumors [5, 11]. Tumor cell lines could be obtained possessing increased metastasizing capacity or which were capable of homing

* This work was supported by PHS grant R01-CA-12764 from the NCI, USA, and by contract 78.0279.96 from Progetto Finalizzato Controllo Crescita Neoplastica, CNR, Rome, Italy

Recent Results in Cancer Research, Vol. 80

selectively at certain anatomic sites [1, 11, 14]. With this background, the contention has been advanced that the formation of secondary tumors is not the result of the random survival of cells which have disseminated from the primary tumor, but that they derive from the establishment and growth of a specialized subpopulation of cells preexisting within the primary tumor. These cells would be endowed with specific and still largely undefined properties allowing them to more effectively complete a highly complex and very selective process [4, 11]. With regard to the latter point, less than 0.1% neoplastic cells from a primary tumor which have reached the circulation may survive arrest in peripheral organs and, still less, establish and grow into an acutal metastasis. If proven true, the hypothesis of the existence of cell subpopulations with intrinsically greater metastasizing ability could obviously have important implications. It was, therefore, of interest to investigate the metastasizing capacity of cells from spontaneous experimental metastases. In fact, if metastatic cells are the survivors of a highly selective process as the hypothesis implies, it would be expected that metastatic cells are better equipped to undergo the demanding process of metastasization.

In a first series of studies, individual pulmonary metastases of a murine fibrosarcoma (mFS6) were investigated for their capacity to spontaneously metastasize after one s.c. passage in syngeneic animals (protocol A) or immediately after their isolation from the lung (protocol B). Since results obtained with the two protocols were similar, the data from protocol A are shown. Details of experimental conditions can be found elsewhere [7]. Table 1 shows that although all cell lines had comparable growth rates, they were heterogenous in their metastasizing ability; some lines (M4 and M7) being more metastatic, others (M8 and M9) being less metastatic than the primary cells. The majority of cell lines were, however, as metastatic as the primary mFS6 tumor.

Since the B16 melanoma was the tumor first employed to show that clones from the primary tumor can markedly differ in their capacity to give artificial metastases upon i.v. cell inoculation [3], it was of interest to examine the metastatic potential of single spontaneous metastases. Following protocol A, it was found that nine of ten lines from individual pulmonary nodules were as metastatic as the primary tumor in terms of both number of lung lesions and their weight, whereas line B8 had a significantly reduced metastatic capacity (Table 1).

A similar pattern was seen when another murine neoplasm of still different histologic origin and metastases from organs other than the lung were examined. Upon i.m., s.c., or i.p. transplantation the M5076/73 ovarian carcinoma gives secondary tumors only in subdiaphragmatic organs, lung nodules not being observed after i.v. injection [10]. Also, in this condition, the majority of cells lines from individual metastases were not hypermetastatic compared to the primary tumor (Table 2), and equivalent results were seen when protocol B was adopted. This confirms, in this model, the comparability of the two experimental approaches previously observed for the mFS6 tumor. The representative results of Table 2 additionally show that, in the majority, cell lines obtained from single metastasis which originated in a given organ did not appear to preferentially show secondary localizations in organ where they had originally settled. Again, comparable results as regards both the metastatic potential of spontaneous metastases, as well as the general absence of a preferential localization in the site of origin, were seen when the colon 26 carcinoma was studied. Since tumors of relatively long transplantation history had been used for our studies, it was of interest to also investigate a neoplasm of recent origin. For this purpose a second passage, which spontaneously metastasized, methylcholanthrene-induced sarcoma of C57B1/6 mice (MN/MCA 1) was used. Here also a degree of heterogeneity in metastatic potential

Table 1. Spontaneous metastasizing capacity of tumor cell lines derived from individual lung secondary tumors of the mFS6 sarcoma and B16 melanoma

Tumor line	MST (range)[a]	Mice with metastases/ total	Metastases number (± SE)[b]	Metastases weight (mg ± SE)[b]
Primary mFS6[c]	33 (25–50)	17/32	3.3 ± 0.3	18.2 ± 5.4
Cell line from metastasis				
no. M1	38 (25–49)	4/8	5.2 ± 3.2	50.1 ± 0.9
M2	32 (28–55)	6/15	3.2 ± 1.2	7.8 ± 7.0
M3	36 (25–48)	10/16	8.7 ± 3.0	48.9 ± 33.2
M4	36 (30–49)	13/14[e]	16.7 ± 3.6[e]	122.5 ± 38.5[e]
M5	33 (25–41)	10/15	8.7 ± 1.8	45.7 ± 20.0
M6	31 (27–42)	10/15	7.8 ± 2.9	11.3 ± 4.0
M7	44 (33–52)	15/15[e]	13.8 ± 2.6[e]	170.2 ± 12.7[e]
M8	35 (26–27)	1/16[e]	1.0	0.5
M9	38 (30–51)	0/15[e]	–	–
Primary B16[d]	28 (24–33)	11/12	7.11 ± 2.2	4.0 ± 1.1
Cell line from metastasis				
no. B1	28 (24–35)	4/7	7.5 ± 2.5	14.3 ± 3.8
B2	30 (28–37)	4/7	1.7 ± 0.4	2.6 ± 1.7
B3	32 (28–36)	2/6	4.0 ± 1.0	5.7 ± 1.5
B4	31	6/8	8.1 ± 3.0	7.3 ± 3.3
B5	27 (23–32)	2/6	2.5 ± 0.5	1.3 ± 0.9
B6	27 (24–38)	6/9	8.8 ± 3.3	5.8 ± 1.7
B7	32 (29–42)	5/8	3.2 ± 1.1	1.6 ± 0.1
B8	28 (24–37)	1/7[e]	10 ± 0	8.8 ± 0
B9	32 (23–37)	4/5	11.5 ± 4.6	8.7 ± 2.9
B10	35 (26–42)	7/8	10.3 ± 3.9	9.9 ± 3.1

[a] Median survival time in days with range
[b] Number and weight of lung metastases/mouse
[c] Tumor cells (10^4) injected i.m. in C57Bl/6 mice. Metastases counted at death
[d] Tumor cells (10^5) injected i.m. in C57Bl/6 mice. Metastases counted at death
[e] Compared to primary tumor, $P < 0.01$

was seen (Table 3), since the L2 metastatic line was hypermetastatic and lines L5 and L7 were hypometastatic (indeed, not metastasizing) compared to the primary tumor. However, again the majority (10 of 14) of cell lines from metastases produced metastases comparable to the primary in terms of incidence of animals with secondaries, as well as number and weight of lesions per lung.

From the data presented and obtained using a series of murine tumors of different histology, pattern of dissemination, and transplantation history, it appears that cells from spontaneous metastases do not generally possess an enhanced metastasizing capacity in respect to the primary tumor from which they had originated. Although a heterogeneity is clearly recognizable both among metastases and compared to the primary with both hyper- and hypometastatic cells, our findings do not appear to support the general contention that metastases arise from the progeny of cells with

Table 2. Metastasizing capacity of metastases from the M5 ovarian carcinoma. C57Bl/6 female mice were injected s.c. with cells from the primary tumor or individual metastases. Mice were killed 28 days after tumor inoculation. Presence of metastases in various organs was confirmed histologically. As no differences were detected in the number and weight of the lesions, these data are not presented

Tumor line from		Metastatic site[a]					
		Spleen	Kidney	Liver	Lung	Ovary	Uterus
Primary tumor		9/16	7/16	16/16	0/16	12/16	10/16
Metastases from spleen no.[b]	1	0/6	1/6	4/6	0/6	3/6	2/6
	2	1/3	0/3	2/3	0/3	2/3	2/3
	3	0/4 (5/22)[c]	0/4 (5/22)	0/4 (14/22)	0/4 (0/22)	1/4 (12/22)	0/4 (6/22)
	4	4/5	3/5	5/5	0/5	2/5	0/5
	5	0/4	1/4	3/4	0/4	4/4	2/4
Liver no.	1	3/6	2/6	6/6	0/6	3/6	2/6
	2	4/5 (8/16)	3/5 (5/16)	3/5 (11/16)	0/5 (0/16)	3/5 (6/16)	3/5 (5/16)
	3	1/5	0/5	2/5	0/5	0/5	0/5
Ovary no.	1	0/6	1/6	3/6	0/6	2/6	1/6
	2	2/5 (3/16)	1/5 (6/16)	5/5 (12/16)	0/5 (0/16)	3/5 (9/16)	0/5 (4/16)
	3	1/5	4/5	4/5	0/5	4/5	3/5
Kidney no.	1	2/7	0/7	6/7	0/7	2/7	2/7
	2	1/7 (8/22)	1/7 (5/22)	4/7 (16/22)	0/7 (0/22)	2/7 (11/22)	0/7 (5/22)
	3	5/8	4/8	6/8	0/8	7/8	3/8

[a] Mice with metastases/total 28 days after s.c. inoculation with tumor cells

[b] Each tumor line was obtained from an individual nodule after one s.c. passage

[c] Pool of data for metastases from each anatomical site

Table 3. Spontaneous metastases of tumor cell lines derived from lung secondary tumors of MN/MCAl sarcoma

Tumor line[a]	Tumor palpable on day[b]	MST[c]	Mice with metastases/ total	Metastases (number ± SE)[d]	Metastases (mg ± SE)[d]
Primary MN/MCAl	11	39 (27–49)	11/22	2.2 ± 0.5	8.25 ± 3.1
Cell line from Metastasis no.					
L1	13	37 (27–44)	6/7	4.8 ± 1.3	9.06 ± 2.4
L2	13	40 (39–43)	8/9[f]	2.6 ± 0.3	4.11 ± 0.5
L3	12	55 (39–65)[e]	5/8	2.2 ± 0.3	2.40 ± 1.5
L5	12	45 (43–57)	0/6[f]	–	–
L6	10	47 (35–51)	4/6	4.0 ± 1.7	12.79 ± 8.5
L7	10	40 (31–42)	0/4	–	–
L8	12	44 (34–56)	5/8	2.2 ± 0.5	1.04 ± 0.3
L9	13	49 (40–52)	5/8	2.0 ± 0.5	4.49 ± 3.0
L10	15	36 (33–55)	2/5	2.5 ± 1.5	3.01 ± 2.4
L11	10	39 (37–49)	4/6	3.0 ± 1.0	5.23 ± 1.7
L12	11	44 (43–51)	2/4	3.0 ± 0.7	0.78 ± 0.2
L13	11	43 (40–51)	2/4	2.0 ± 1	0.78 ± 0.2
L14	12	44 (33–46)	3/7	3.0 ± 0.1	0.95 ± 0.6
Pool of data for metastases	12	44 (27–57)	46/82	2.8 ± 0.39	4.64 ± 0.8

[a] Tumor cells (10^5) injected i.m. and the metastases were examined at death
[b] Day on which 50% of injected mice showed a palpable tumor
[c] Median survival time in days with range
[d] Number and weight of lung metastases/mouse
[e] Compared to primary MN/MCAl sarcoma, $P < 0.01$
[f] Compared to primary MN/MCAl sarcoma, $P < 0.05$

specialized properties enabling them to survive a strongly selective multisequential process. The possibility, therefore, that metastases are at least to some extent a random representation of the total cell population within the primary tumor cannot at present be discounted.

Immunologic Heterogeneity and Metastases

Much attention is currently centered on immunotherapeutic approaches to metastatic disease. The role of host defenses in the control of metastasis formation, although believed to be significant, is still far from having been satisfactorily clarified. Indeed, certain mechanisms could play opposite roles at the levels of the primary tumor and its secondaries [9]. Also, on the basis of the results obtained in testing the metastatic potential of secondary tumors, it was of interest to investigate possible phenotypic heterogeneity of metastases at the immunogenicity-antigenicity level.

Using the mFS6 fibrosarcoma model, mice were immunized by surgically excising the primary tumor and subsequently challenged with 10^4 cells of lines obtained from

Table 4. Antigenicity of tumor cell lines derived from individual lung metastases of the mFS6 sarcoma

Immunizing tumor	Challenge	No. of takes/total	
		Control	Immune
Primary mFS6	Primary mFS6 (10^4 cells)	20/20	18/38[a]
	M1 (10^4 cells)	15/16	11/17[a]
	M2 (10^4 cells)	12/12	5/13[a]
	M3 (10^4 cells)	12/12	10/11
	M4 (10^4 cells)	25/25	20/31[a]
	M5 (10^4 cells)	15/15	6/15[a]
	M6 (10^4 cells)	20/20	10/23[a]
	M7 (10^4 cells)	12/12	11/20[a]
	M9 (10^4 cells)	15/15	14/17
M3	M3 (10^3 cells)	5/15	5/5
	(10^4 cells)	7/7	7/7
	mFS6 (10^3 cells)	5/5	5/5
	(10^4 cells)	7/7	6/6
M7	M7 (10^4 cells)	6/6	6/12[a]
	mFS6 (10^4 cells)	6/6	6/15[a]
M9	M9 (10^3 cells)	4/4	4/4
	(10^4 cells)	4/4	4/4
	mFS6 (10^3 cells)	4/4	4/4
	(10^4 cells)	4/4	4/4

[a] Versus control mice, $P < 0.05$

individual lung metastases of the same neoplasm. As shown in Table 4, by representative results, whereas cross-protection was seen with seven metastatic lines, immunization with the primary tumor did not protect against two of the nine lines tested. Even when inocula as low as 10^2 cells of the M3 and M9 metastatic cell lines were used, results were superimposable. To obtain indications as to whether the observed absence of cross-protection was attributable to different specificities of metastatic cells or to loss of antigenicity, mice were immunized with the metastatic lines and then challenged either with the immunizing cells or with the primary tumor. Under these conditions, immunization with M3 and M9 not only failed to protect against the primary mFS6 tumor from which these lines were derived, but also failed to protect against challenge with M3 and M9, supporting a loss of antigenicity in these cells. Similar data were obtained when the antigenicity of cell lines from metastases of this tumor was evaluated by concomitant immunity experiments.

Conclusions

Although under these conditions the majority of metastatic cells were found to behave as the primary tumor with regard to their metastatic potential, a degree of heterogeneity among metastases was evident. Although heterogeneity for this specific biologic capacity does not necessarily imply heterogeneity for other cellular characteristics, it could nevertheless be of practical importance. It has been demonstrated that both human and animal neoplasms contain subpopulations of cells having different sensitivities to cytotoxic drugs [6, 8]. A heterogeneity among metastases in their resistance to chemotherapeutic drugs could thus exist, a possibility against which only little protection could be given by the higher drug concentrations, measured in various secondary tumors compared to the primary, as seen in experimental systems [2] and confirmed by observed data in human ovarian cancer (D'Incalci, unpublished work). Direct data on a possible heterogenous "intrinsic" chemosensitivity among metastases are not yet available and experiments to test this possibility are currently in progress. Even if this heterogeneity is shown to involve only a relative minority of cells, as described above, for their metastatic potential, this possibility may have implications in the selection and use of chemotherapeutic drugs for the treatment and prevention of metastatic disease. As discussed elsewhere [12], assays of therapeutic activity on primary tumors may be only partially representative of the sensitivity of metastases to the same or other agents, and assays of therapeutic agents conducted on metastatic cell lines may be more indicative. Similarly, the demonstration of the possibility of an immunologic heterogeneity among metastases, provided above in confirmation of earlier data by others [13], may have implications for specific and possibly nonspecific immunotherapy and calls for a reappraisal of the usefulness of many current experimental approaches to this problem. It is apparent that much more is to be learned about metastasis formation, and of the basis and extent of neoplastic heterogeneity, before our therapeutic approaches to metastatic disease can be considered truly rational.

References

1. Brunson KW, Nicolson GL (1978) Selection and biological properties of malignant variants of a murine lymphosarcoma. J Natl Cancer Inst 61: 1499–1503
2. Donelli MG, Colombo T, Broggini M, Garattini S (1977) Differential distribution of antitumor agents in primary and secondary tumors. Cancer Treat Rep 6: 1319–1324
3. Fidler IJ (1973) Selection of successive tumor lines for metastasis. Nature (London) New Biol 242: 148–149
4. Fidler IJ, Kripke ML (1977) Metastasis results from preexisting variant cells within a malignant tumor. Science 197: 893–895
5. Fidler IJ, Gersten DM, Hart IR (1978) The biology of cancer invasion and metastasis. Adv Cancer Res 28: 149–196
6. Fuji H, Mihich E (1975) Selection for high immunogenicity in drug-resistant sublines of murine lymphomas demonstrated by plaque assay. Cancer Res 35: 946–952
7. Giavazzi R, Alessandri G, Spreafico F, Garattini S, Mantovani A (to be published) Metastasizing capacity of tumor cells from spontaneous metastases of transplanted murine tumors. Br J Cancer
8. Heppner GH, Dexter DL, de Nucci T, Miller FR, Calabresi P (1978) Heterogeneity in drug sensitivity among tumor cell subpopulations of a single mammary tumor. Cancer Res 38: 3758–3763
9. Mantovani A, Giavazzi R, Polentarutti N, Spreafico F, Garattini S (1980) Divergent effects of macrophage toxins on growth of primary tumors and lung metastases in mice. Int J Cancer 25: 617–620
10. Mantovani A, Giavazzi R, Alessandri R, Spreafico F (to be published) The characteristic metastasizing pattern of a murine ovarian carcinoma. Eur J Cancer

11. Poste G, Fidler IJ (1980) The pathogenesis of cancer metastasis. Nature 283: 139–146
12. Spreafico F, Garattini S (1978) Chemotherapy of experimental metastases. In: Baldwin RW (ed) Secondary spread of cancer. Academic Press, New York, pp 101–128
13. Sugarbaker EV, Cohen AM (1972) Altered antigenicity in spontaneous pulmonary metastases from an antigenic murine sarcoma. Surgery 72: 155–162
14. Tao T-W, Matter A, Vogel K, Burger MM (1979) Liver-colonizing melanoma cells selected from B-16 melanoma. Int J Cancer 23: 854–857

2. *Immune Imbalance and Immune Modulation in Solid Tumor Patients: New Insights*

B. Serrou, D. Cupissol, and C. Rosenfeld

Hôpital Saint-Eloi, Centre Paul Lamarque,
Laboratoire d'Immunopharmacologie des Tumeurs,
F-34033 Montpellier Cedex, France

Introduction

Up to now, evaluation of the immune status in tumor patients has been rather disappointing and has not shown clear-cut parameters that can be employed on a day-to-day basis to establish a prognosis, modify treatment, or allow early detection of relapse at the subclinical stage. Part or all these shortcomings can be explained by several findings. To begin with, tumor antigens in man remain poorly defined, making it impossible to precisely evaluate any specific immune response directed against this antigen. In addition, the immune mechanism governing rejection of human tumors remains poorly understood for the following reasons: The role of certain evaluations in vitro are not as evident within an in vivo context, e.g., T-cell cytotoxicity, antibody-dependent cell-mediated cytotoxicity (ADCC), and natural killer (NK) cell activity; different lymphocyte subpopulations are still phenotypically and functionally poorly characterized; and, the role of immune complexes, inflammatory proteins, monocytes and macrophages, as well as leukocytes in antitumor response is still partially speculative.

We would like to focus our attention on some new insights in this field, particularly immune complexes, plasma microviscosity, anti-BCG antibodies, plasma, vitamin A levels, and auto-rosette-forming cells (ARFC). Consideration will also be given to bestatin and retinoic acid derivatives as immune modulators.

Immune Complexes

Numerous recent studies have shown the presence of immune complexes during cancer evolution [8, 13]. These complexes increase with tumor volume, decrease following tumor reduction, and increase during relapse. Carpentier et al. [8] have shown that in acute myeloblastic leukemia, there is a close and significant correlation between the level of immune complexes and the response to treatment. However, presently the study of these immune complexes presents major difficulties. From a methodological viewpoint, no satisfactory techniques exist, since each technique proposed may evaluate different immune complexes. Moreover, the composition of these complexes is poorly elucidated. To begin with, it has not yet been shown that, in the cancer patient, these complexes are of the antigen-antibody type. Phillips et al. [19]

Recent Results in Cancer Research, Vol. 80

Table 1. Immune complexes in cancer patients

DHS	Rheumatoid factor	CIC[a] (mg/dl WHO)[b]		
		IgG	IgM	IgA
+++ (13)	0.0 ± 0	44.9 ± 33.4	9.1 ± 6.5	5.5 ± 2.8
++ (18)	0.5 ± 1.5	39.8 ± 30.9	12.1 ± 7.8	6.4 ± 3.5
+ (25)	0.9 ± 1.9	29.9 ± 21.7	6.9 ± 6.7	5.5 ± 4.0
± (18)	1.4 ± 1.2	25.3 ± 11.4	8.6 ± 7.8	5.4 ± 4.1
0 (9)	1.7 ± 2.5	47.0 ± 26.2	10.4 ± 5.3	8.8 ± 8.0

[a] Circulating immune complexes
[b] World health organisation

recently suggested the presence of two types of complexes in malignant melanoma patients; antigen-antibody complexes, where the antigen is specific for malignant melanoma, and antibody-antibody complexes. Although quite promising, these results still need to be confirmed. Also, the antibody portion of these complexes has yet to be thoroughly studied. Gauci et al. [13] have shown the possible existence of IgM, IgG, and IgA complexes, but this also remains to be confirmed. According to Day et al. [11] and Gauci et al. [13], there appears to be a close relationship between the level of immune complexes and disease evolution. In addition, Gauci et al. [13] showed a strong correlation between the level of these complexes and delayed hypersensitivity (Table 1), whereas we were not able to establish such a correlation for ADCC. Interestingly enough, we observed that a high level of circulating immune complexes (CIC) was correlated with a strongly delayed hypersensitivity reaction and poor prognosis.

The exact role of these immune complexes in the immune response has yet to be defined and little is known on this subject. For example, although suppressor T cells with a receptor for the Fc portion of IgG have been shown, we also observe Tμ-cells presenting suppressor activity [24]. In contrast, the role of T cells is still not clear [20, 23]. Presently, there is an encouraging number of findings which need verification and which could rapidly lead to important practical applications.

Plasma Microviscosity

The plasma membrane lipid bilayer may play an important role in the immune response. Important modifications have been demonstrated in the membrane of leukocytes from acute leukemia patients [18, 21]. Furthermore, these alterations disappear in patients in remission and reappear early in the relapse patient. These results suggest that membrane lipid modifications of leukemic cells are an early event. A parallel decrease in plasma microviscosity was noted.

Similarly, we observed a decrease in plasma microviscosity in solid tumor-bearing patiens [10] during the evolutionary phase (Table 2). Whether this event appears prior to relapse correlating with similar modifications of the lymphocyte membrane is the object of further investigations. Whatever the results, lipids have already been shown to play an important role in lymphocytotoxic responses [14]. Whether the

Table 2. Plasma microviscosity in cancer patients

	Number of patients	Polarization value
1. Healthy donors	31	239.86 ± 27.2
2. Cancer patients	93	256.22 ± 24.15

1 vs. 2, $P < 0.005$

modifications we have observed can be correlated with immune status still remains to be evaluated.

Anti-BCG Antibodies and Plasma Vitamin A

BCG is a widely used immunostimulant agent employed in cancer immunotherapy. However, little is known about the anti-BCG antibodies. We have evaluated these antibodies in three groups of malignant melanoma patients, one treated with interspased chemoimmunotherapy and two other groups included in a randomized study comparing 6 months of chemotherapy followed by 2 years of BCG to 2 years of BCG. The results show that low values of anti-BCG antibodies were significantly related to a poor prognosis and high values to a good prognosis. Furthermore, a 50% decrease in antibody values preceded clinical relapses by 3–6 months. These results suggest that evaluation of anti-BCG antibodies could be of interest in follow-up treatment of cancer patients receiving long-term BCG [28].

Vitamin A has been suggested not only to act on cell differentiation but also to modulate immune response and lengthen survival times in tumor-bearing mice [3]. Recent data have demonstrated that vitamin A may modulate surface antigen expression in much the same manner as neuraminidase [15]. Furthermore, Soukop and Calmann [26] have emphasized the fact that a correlation may exist between the plasma vitamin A levels and the response to chemotherapy. For these reasons, we have investigated plasma vitamin A levels in advanced solid tumor patients. We found a significantly lower level of vitamin A in patients with evolving disease. This finding could be of interest if one considers the fact that vitamin A and its derivatives seem to play a major role in cell differentiation and the expression of immune response [22]. Further studies evaluating not only vitamin A but also its derivatives in the peripheral circulation will have to be undertaken to better appreciate any potential therapeutic applications of these substances.

Auto-Rosette-Forming and Suppressor Cells

ARFC

At least two major classes of T cells which have been characterized are Tμ and Tγ. The first may essentially, but not exclusively, be helper cells, while the second may preferentially correspond to suppressor cells but might also have cytotoxic activity.

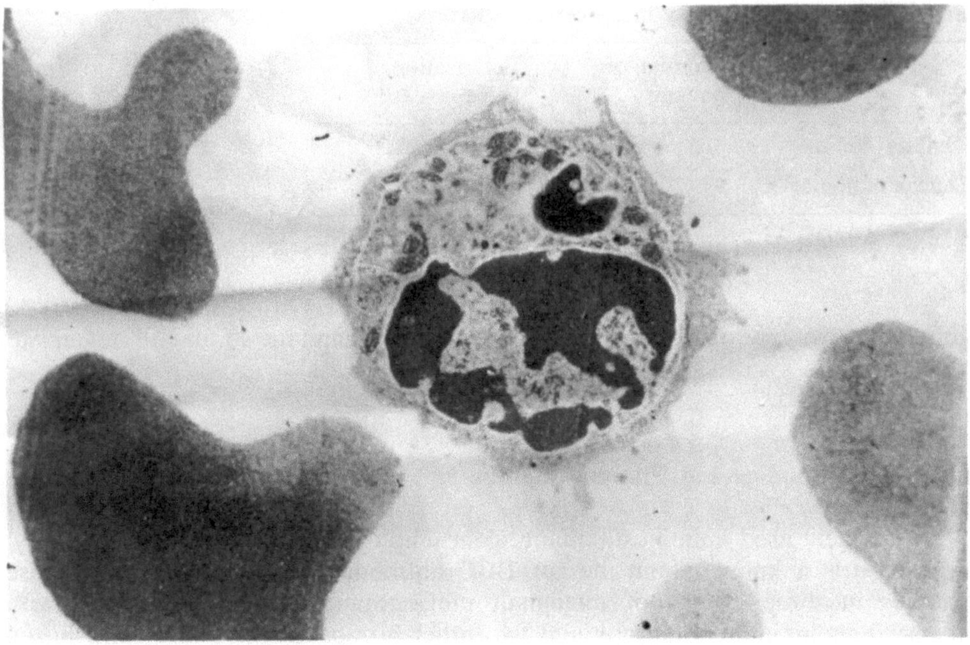

Fig. 1. Electron micrograph of an auto-rosette-forming cell

Table 3. Auto-rosette-forming cells in cancer patients

	Number of patients	Percent
1. Healthy donors	29	25.9 ± 5.65
2. Cancer patients	89	16.5 ± 8.55

1 vs. 2, $P < 0.05$

Others may possess two receptors simultaneously and, by definition, would exhibit those functions relative to these receptors. Modifications of these two subpopulations in the cancer patient have not yet been established. Recently Chretien et al. [9] have shown that, during evolution, patients may show an increase in the Tγ : Tμ ratio and that, in contrast, patients in complete remission have decreased ratios. A T-theophyllin-resistant lymphocyte subpopulation appears to be of great interest in this context. These lymphocytes are responsible for the formation of autologous rosettes. ARFC appear to be a homogeneous population, either slightly activated or detected at an early stage of activation (Fig. 1). They present a very evident Golgi system and endoplasmic reticulum. They are lysosome poor and show low lysosomal enzymatic activity for enzymes such as acid phosphatase and β-glucuronidase. Caraux et al. [5–7] have shown that ARFC significantly decrease in the tumor-bearing patient. In addition there is a significant difference between patients in relapse and those who are not. This decrease in ARFC can sometimes precede relapse by several months. We have just now confirmed these results (Table 3 and Fig. 2). Furthermore,

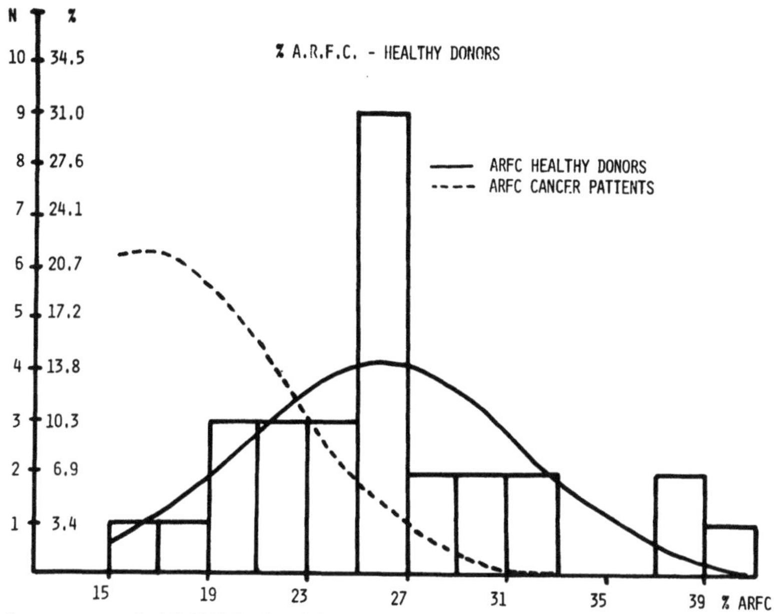

Fig. 2. Comparative frequency of ARFC in healthy donors and cancer patients

these rosettes characteristically are sensitive to thymosin, which can normalize or augment their levels. This must be considered in the light of the clinical results presented by Chretien et al. [9] who showed an improved prognosis for anaplastic lung tumors treated with chemotherapy with thymosin as opposed to the nonthymosin-receiving chemotherapy control group.

A more precise identification of T lymphocyte subpopulations could be of the utmost interest not only from a prognostic point of view or to single out the relapse patient but also, and above all, to adapt treatment and modulate the immune response.

Suppressor Cells

Many recent investigations have made significant advances in the study of suppressor activity in solid tumor patients [24]. This activity can be either macrophage or T lymphocyte-dependent. For macrophages, the role of prostaglandins may be crucial. This activity may be sensitive to antiprostaglandins, particularly indomethacin, therefore leading to possible therapeutic applications. Moreover, macrophage suppressor activity is possibly exacerbated by irradiation, thereby explaining the more or less long-lasting decrease in some immune responses in patients undergoing radiotherapy. A T-dependent suppressor activity has also been demonstrated which may be sensitive to thymosin and levamisole. This could represent far-reaching perspectives for immunologic manipulation. A better understanding of the mechanisms coming into play in the induction of suppressor cells (e.g., immune complexes) should lead to a better modulation of the expression of these cells by cyclophosphamide, corticosteroids, and irradiation, as well as specific antisuppressor-cell antiserum.

Immunomodulation

In vivo cancer patient evaluation of new immunomodulating drugs is still an unsettled topic of discussion. The EORTC Cancer Immunology and Immunotherapy Group (CI2G) has developed a phase 1 trial for evaluation of such drugs in immunodepressed, advanced solid tumor patients (liver metastasis of digestive tract origin, inoperable epidermoid lung tumors, head and neck tumors, and metastatized breast tumors). Evaluation of the immunorestorative potential of a new drug is based on three assays: delayed hypersensitivity skin tests using the Merieux technique; ARFC; and NK activity. We would like to focus on three drugs: bestatin; interferon; and the RO-10 2359 (a retinoic acid derivative). Bestatin is a new drug derived from culture filtrates of *streptomyces olivoreticuli* and prepared by Umezawa et al. [27]. This drug possess antitumoral properties in mice. Bruley-Rosset et al. [4] have shown that bestatin can significantly decrease the number of spontaneous tumors in old mice. We have demonstrated that bestatin given orally (40 mg/m^2) three times a week for 2 weeks can significantly increase delayed hypersensitivity reactions, the number of circulating ARFC, and NK activity [25]. These results confirm those of Blomgren et al. [1] and justify continuation on of this phase I study as well as proposing a randomized study.

Interferon is a subject of much discussion. The results of the first clinical trials are encouraging but not conclusive [2, 12, 16, 17]. For our part, we evaluated the immunomodulating effects of human fibroblast interferon (HFI). We have been able to show that in vivo HFI administration to metastatized breast tumor patients improved the response to delayed hypersensitivity skin tests, NK activity, and the number of ARFC. Two interesting points were noted: We observed a concomitant increase in IgG immune complexes in a responding patient which were not related to the presence of antiinterferon antibodies; and, in vivo, HFI may increase or decrease concanavalin A-induced T-suppressor cell activity depending on the dose used. These results suggest that the natural substance HFI, although only partially purified, cannot only act on tumor cell proliferation but also modulate the immune response in different ways. Relations and comparisons to immune interferon have yet to be established.

Vitamin A and retinoic acid derivatives are known to act on cell differentiation. The effects of RO-109359 on immune functions in immunodepressed cancer patients were evaluated. This drug was given orally at 5 mg/kg/day for 21 and no side effects or tumor effects were noted. Nevertheless during this period, we observed a significantly improved response to skin delayed hypersensitivity antigens as well as an increased number of circulating ARFC. These results suggest that RO-109359 may be a potential immunorestorate drug and should be the object of further investigations [25].

Conclusions

Evaluation of immune status has been disappointing for quite some time, since only skin tests have presented some potential. However, recent significant progress concerning the mechanisms regulating the immune response, as well as the characterization of cells which come into play, have led to many new perspectives. Accordingly, it is possible to foresee in the near future the potential to evaluate the relationship between suppressor and helper activity on one hand, and associated cytotoxic activity on the other. This point is extremely important since immunopharmacology is progressing rapidly and new drugs and means now exist which can selectively act on a given subpopulation (e.g., helper, suppressor, NK). Thus, evaluation of immune status should give rise to better patient surveillance. Adapting and modulating treatment is the first step toward an individual therapy based on a general set of clearly defined principles.

References

1. Blomgren H, Einhorn S, Strander H (to be published) The influence of bestatin on the lymphoid system in the human. In: Umezawa H (ed) Small molecular immunomodulators.
2. Blomgren H, Einhorn S, Strander H (to be published) Modulation of the immune response by interferon in vivo and in vitro. In: Serrou B, Rosenfeld C (eds) New trends in human immunology and cancer immunotherapy. Doin-Saunders., Amsterdam New York
3. Bollag W (1979) Retinoids and cancer. Cancer Chemother Pharmacol 3: 204–215
4. Bruley-Rosset M, Florentin I, Kiger N, Schulz G, Mathé G (1979) Restoration of impaired immune functions of aged animals by chronic bestatin treatment. Immunology 38: 75–83
5. Caraux J, Goldstein AL, Esteve C, Serrou B (1979) Thymosin alpha-1 restores the depressed binding of autologous erythrocytes by T cells from cancer patients. Biomedicine 31: 88
6. Caraux J, Thierry C, Esteve C, Flores G, Lodise R, Serrou B (1979) Human autologous rosettes. I. Mechanism of binding of autologous erytrocytes by T cells. Cell Immunol 45: 36–48
7. Caraux J, Thierry C, Serrou B (1979) Human autologous rosettes. II. Prognostic significance of variations in autologous rosette forming cells in the peripheral blood of cancer patients. J Natl Cancer Inst 63: 593–597
8. Carpentier N, Lambert PH (to be published) Circulating immune complexes in human acute leukemia and lympho-proliferative disease relation to prognosis and study of the composition. In: Serrou B, Rosenfeld C (eds) New trends in human immunology and cancer immunotherapy. Doin-Saunders, Amsterdam, New York
9. Chretien PB, Lipson SD, Makuch R (1979) Effects of thymosin in vitro in cancer patients. Ann NY Acad Sci 332: 135–147
10. Cupissol D, Moscati G, Rosenfeld C, Serrou B (1979) Plasma microviscosity in patients bearing solid tumors: Clinical and prognostic values. Med Oncol 55: 14
11. Day NK, Witkin S, Good RA (to be published) Breast cancer: Circulating immune complexes and humoral antibodies to mouse mammary tumor virus. In: Serrou B, Rosenfeld C (eds) New trends in human immunology and Cancer immunotherapy. Doin-Saunders, Amsterdam, New York
12. Gallagher JG, Louie AC, Sikora K, Levy R, Rosenberg SA, Merigan TC (to be published) The evaluation of human leukocate interferon in patients with non-Hodgkin's lymphoma and Hodgkin's disease: A phase II study. In: Terry WD (ed) Immunotherapy of cancer: Present status of trials in man. Elsevier North-Holland, New York Oxford
13. Gauci L, Caraux J, Serrou B (to be published) Immune complexes in the context of the immune response in cancer patients. In: Serrou B, Rosenfeld C (eds) Immune complexes and peasmapheresis in cancer patients. Human cancer immunology, vol 1. North-Holland Publishing, Amsterdam New York
14. Heiniger HJ, Brunner KT, Cerottini JC (1980) Cholesterol is a critical cellular composent for T-lymphocyte cytotoxicity. Proc Natl Acad Sci USA 75: 5683–5687
15. Hogan-Ryan A, Fennelly JJ (1978) Neuraminidase-like effect of vitamin A on cell surface. Eur J Cancer 14: 113–116

16. Krown S, Stoopler M, Gralla R, Cunningham-Rundles S, Stewart W, Pollack L, Oettgen H (to be published) Phase II trial of human leukocyte interferon (HuLeIF) in non-small cell lung cancer (NSCLC). In: Terry WD (ed) Immunotherapy of cancer: Present status of trials in man. Elsevier North-Holland, New York Oxford
17. Mellstedt H, Aahre A, Bjorkholm M et al. (to be published) Interferon therapy of patients with myeloma. In: Terry WD (ed) Immunotherapy of cancer: Present status of trials in man. Elsevier North-Holland, New York Oxford
18. Petitou M, Tuy F, Rosenfeld C et al. (1978) Decreased microviscosity of membrane lipids in leukemic cells: Two possible mechanisms. Proc Natl Acad Sci USA 75:2306–2310
19. Phillips T, Lewis M, Neefe J, Smith F, Schein P, McDonald JS (to be published) Studies on the composition and significance of immune complexes in cancer patients. In: Serrou B, Rosenfeld C (eds) New trends in human immunology and cancer immunotherapy. Doin-Saunders, Amsterdam New York
20. Reinherz EL, Moretta L, Roper M, Breard JM, Mingari Cooper M, Schlossman SF (1980) Human T lymphocyte subpopulations defined by Fc receptors and monoclonal antibodies. J Exp Med 151:969–974
21. Rosenfeld C, Jasmin C, Mathé G, Inbar M (1979) Dynamic and composition of cellular membranes and serum lipids in malignant disorders. Recent Results Cancer Res 67:63–77
22. Serrou B, Cupissol D (to be published) Phase I evaluation of an aromatic derivative of retinoic acid (RO 109359) in patients with advanced solid tumors. Cancer Treat Rep
23. Serrou B, Rosenfeld C (to be published) New trends in human immunology and cancer immunotherapy. Doin-Saunders, Amsterdam New York
24. Serrou B, Rosenfeld C (to be published) Human suppressor cells in cancer patients. Human Cancer immunology, vol 2. North-Holland Publishing, Amsterdam New York
25. Serrou B, Cupissol D, Flad H et al. (to be published) Phase I evaluation of bestatin in patients bearing advanced solid tumors. In: Terry WD (ed) Immunotherapy of cancer: Present status of trials in man. Elsevier North-Holland, New York
26. Soukop H, Calmann CH (1978) Vitamin A status and chemotherapeutic response in cancer patients. In: Siegenthaler W, Luthy R (eds) Current chemotherapy. Proceedings of the Tenth International Congress of Chemotherapy, vol 2. American Society Microbiology, Washington, pp 1296–1298
27. Umezawa H, Aoyagi T, Suda H, Hamada M, Takeuchi T (1976) Bestatin, a new aminopeptidase B inhibitor produced by actinomycites. J Antibiot (Tokyo) 29:97–99
28. Wile AG, Sparks FC, Morton DL (1977) Monitoring immunotherapy with bacillus Calmette Guerin by antibody titer. Cancer Res 37:2251–2256

3. Markers of Minimal Residual Disease

A. M. Neville

Ludwig Institute for Cancer Research, Royal Marsden Hospital,
Sutton, Surrey SM2 5PX, United Kingdom

Summary

Current methods employing tumour markers to detect small amounts of residual disease are reviewed with respect to human germ cell, colorectal and breast neoplasms. It is concluded that the assay of tumour markers in body fluids has only limited clinical value. Alternative approaches, such as are afforded by radioimmunodetection and immunocytochemistry, are presented and critically appraised.

Introduction

There is an ever-increasing interest in the protean roles which human tumour markers may play in the diagnosis and management of the cancer patient [9]. In recent years, attention has been diverted from a study of their early diagnostic value to their place in the detection of metastases, in particular residual and micrometastatic disease. The need for new methods in this context is readily apparent when it is realised that, all too frequently, physical staging procedures fail at the time of initial presentation to detect extra-organ spread of the primary tumour.

The role of tumour markers in the detection of small amounts of tumour will be reappraised in this paper using germ cell, colorectal and breast neoplasms as illustrative examples.

Germ Cell Tumours

There is now good evidence that human germ cell tumours produce a variety of products, in particular, human chorionic gonadotropin (HCG) or its β-subunit and α-fetoprotein (AFP). The release of HCG by gestational choriocarcinomas appears to have a stoichiometric relationship to tumour cell numbers. Hence its assay in blood or urine has proved of immense value in the detection of small amounts of residual disease, in monitoring and in assessing the duration of therapy [1].

More recently, it has been recognised that so-called testicular embryonal carcinomas (malignant teratoma undifferentiated) may be associated with raised blood levels of β-HCG and AFP despite the absence of classical choriocarcinomatous and yolk sac

Recent Results in Cancer Research, Vol. 80

elements, respectively [9]. The introduction of immunocytochemical techniques to demonstrate β-HCG and AFP in paraffin-embedded sections has enabled the cell types responsible for the formation of these products to be identified. β-HCG-containing cells have been detected, not necessarily forming syncitia characteristic of trophoblast elements, but existing around blood vessels or as isolated single nucleated cells. While AFP is most commonly associated with yolk sac-type differentiation, it may also be found in other types of cells which form solid cords on trabeculae which by conventional microscopy would be regarded simply as embryonal carcinoma.

These structural studies have shown that β-HCG- and AFP-containing cells frequently do not reflect the total population of most embryonal carcinomas. Nonetheless, both plasma β-HCG and AFP levels are useful indexes of residual disease. In patients with AFP-producing tumours, monitoring the half-life of blood AFP after surgery or other therapy has been shown to be of value in predicting whether there is residual disease [8]. When the half-life falls within normal range (5–7 days), then most cases have a good prognosis. When the half-life is greater than 7 days, such patients have residual disease and require further treatment.

Even in patients who exhibit a normal AFP half-life after treatment, it is important to sample subsequently their β-HCG and AFP levels in the blood sequentially. Many studies have shown the value of this approach to detect small amounts of recurrent or metastatic disease above other techniques.

It should be remembered, however, that the cellular and functional heterogeneity of such tumours is considerable and that tumours can be present with no elevated blood marker levels. One recent survey has found this to be the case in 30% of patients with advanced disease [14]. Hence these markers are of significant value in the management of testicular germ cell tumours, although the correlation of marker and tumour presence is not as accurate as in gestational choriocarcinoma.

Colorectal and Breast Carcinoma

Colorectal Carcinoma

The carcinoembryonic antigen (CEA) has been examined intensively for its role in the monitoring and detection of colorectal carcinomas. Current opinion holds that its assay in blood is of value during the follow-up assessment of patients after colorectal surgery to detect residual or metastatic disease (Table 1). Unlike HCG and possibly

Table 1. The role of plasma carcinoembryonic antigens (CEA) in the monitoring of 771 patients with colorectal carcinomas after clinically curative operations. From data of Neville and Cooper 1976 [12]

Clinical condition	Plasma CEA	Number of patients
No evidence of recurrence	Normal	525
	Rising[a]	54
Recurrence	Normal	66
	Synchronous rise[a]	89
	Antecedent rise[a]	37

[a] Rising to > 40 ng/ml with a sustained upward trend in the plasma levels

AFP which reflect tumour load, plasma CEA levels bear little stochiometric relationship to the tumour load. While some patients will develop recurrent and/or metastatic disease in the presence of a normal CEA titre, most will show rising plasma levels, many of which will precede the overt clinical detection of metastases (Table 1) [12]. This lead time is usually of the order of 9–12 months, although periods in excess of 24 months have been found in some patients.

It has been claimed that by estimating the postoperative levels of CEA more frequently and submitting them to analysis by nomogram or computer, a more accurate assessment of the CEA time curves and a readier and earlier detection of metastases can be achieved [10]. This has formed the basis for 'second-look' surgical intervention. The presence of recurrent or metastatic tumour has been confirmed in most but not all cases at second-look surgery. In a certain number (72% in one series) of patients with rising CEA titres, single localised and surgically resectable recurrences were detected [10].

Such operative intervention has been claimed to result in a longer period of subsequent survival, but not all groups agree that this procedure results in the detection of resectable disease [11]. More time will be required to establish the clinical value of operative intervention in the presence of rising CEA titres. Certainly our own experience [13], while not denying that it is possible to detect metastases earlier through the sequential assay of CEA, would tend to support the view that when rising levels of CEA are detected such patients generally have a significant and widespread tumour load.

Breast Carcinoma

There are at present no satisfactory indexes to detect, with precision, residual or metastatic breast cancers [2]. CEA, in association with the enzymes α-glutamyltrans-peptidase and total alkaline phosphatase, have been shown to be of limited assistance. In some patients, rising titres of one or more of these markers develop prior to the detection of overt metastatic disease by other physical or clinical methods, but the lead time is only of the order of 3–4 months [2].

These data from colorectal and breast carcinoma patients serve to emphasise that alternative and new methods are needed to detect residual disease in such cases. Based upon the results gained from the study of HCG, AFP, and germ cell tumours, it would appear to be of potential value if cytoplasmically derived secreted products of breast and colorectal carcinomas could be isolated and then detected in the blood. Until this has been achieved, attempts to detect the tumour cells themselves seem worthy of study.

Alternative Approaches

Radioimmunodetection

On the basis of success in experimental and xenograft systems, Goldenberg et al. [4] have employed methods of radioimmunodetection to localise various human tumours. Using xenogeneic anti-CEA labelled with radioactive iodine, they have demonstrated by scanning techniques that this approach can result in the successful localisation of both primary and metastatic tumours of the colon, rectum, uterus, ovary and breast. Moreover, radioimmunodetection was successful when other physical diagnostic methods did not locate the various lesions [4]. These results have recently been confirmed by other workers [3]. Unfortunately, the limit of radioimmunodetection at present would appear to be a tumour of approximately 2 cm diameter, which represents a significant tumour load.

There are several ways by which this approach might result in the detection of smaller amounts of tumour. These include better scanning techniques, labelling the antibodies with other isotopes more readily detected by present γ-camera techniques and the use of organ or even tumour-specific antibodies. This last aspect may well be attainable through the use of the mouse myeloma hybridoma system [7] for the preparation of monoclonal antibodies. An immunological reagent with apparent colorectal specificity has already been achieved in this manner [5].

Immunocytochemistry

Another approach to detect small amounts of disease may arise from the introduction of immunocytochemical methods, which are able to detect tumour products and antigens at a cellular level in conventionally prepared tissue sections.

An epithelial membrane antigen (EMA) has recently been described and shown to be expressed by both primary and metastatic human breast carcinomas [6]. By immunoperoxidase methods, EMA can be detected in small microscopic foci of breast carcinoma metastases even when occurring as single isolated tumour cells in either the liver or bone marrow biopsies obtained by needle aspiration. A series of bone marrow aspirates from patients considered to be free of micrometastases by conventional light microscopy was re-examined using an immunoperoxidase method to detect EMA (Table 2). While no metastatic foci were seen in 65 patients, in the remaining 11 either by cytology or immunocytochemistry for EMA, micrometastatic foci were detected (Table 2) [15]. All but one of these latter patients have subsequently developed overt osseous metastases.

This approach can be extended to demonstrate a wide variety of other materials shown by human tumours and to antigens detected by monoclonal antibodies. With the knowledge of the commonest sites to which particular tumours may metastasise, the use of immunocytochemical methods on smears made from aspirates or of cell-sorting techniques, may offer an alternative approach to detect residual or micrometastatic

Table 2. Comparison of immunocytochemical staining for epithelial membrane antigen (EMA) and cytology in sections of bone marrow to detect mammary carcinoma metastases. Data of Sloane et al. 1980 [15]

Method	No. of positive results
Conventional histology	5/76
Cytology (smear)	6/76
Immunocytochemistry (EMA)	9/76
Cytology and EMA	11/76

disease which could complement radioimmunodetection and the assay of markers in the body fluids.

References

1. Bagshawe, KD (1973) Recent observations related to the chemotherapy and immunology of gestational choriocarcinoma. Adv Cancer Res 18:231
2. Coombes RC, Gazet JC, Ford HT, Powles TJ, Nash AG, McKinna A, Neville AM (1980) Treatment of malignant disease. Assessment of biochemical tests to screen for metastases in patients with breast cancer. Lancet 1:296–297
3. Dykes PW, Hine KR, Bradwell AR, Blackburn JC, Reeder TA, Drolc Z, Booth SN (1980) Localisation of tumour deposits by external scanning after injection of radiolabelled anti-carcinoembryonic antigen. Br Med J 280:220–222
4. Goldenberg DM, DeLand F, Euishin K, Bennett S, Primus FJ, van Nagell JR, Estes M, DeSimone P (1978) Use of radiolabeled antibodies to carcinoembryonic antigen for the detection and localization of diverse cancers by external photoscanning. N Engl J Med 298:1384–1388
5. Herlyn M, Steplewksi Z, Herlyn D, Koprowski H (1979) Colorectal carcinoma-specific antigen: Detection by means of monoclonal antibodies. Proc Natl Acad Sci USA 76:1438–1442
6. Heyderman E, Steele K, Ormerod MG (1979) A new antigen on the epithelial membrane: Its immunoperoxidase localisation in normal and neoplastic tissue. J Clin Pathol 32:35–39
7. Kohler G, Milstein C (1975) Continuous cultures of fused cells secreting antibody of predefined specificity. Nature 256:495–497
8. Kohn J (1979) The value of apparent half-life assay of alpha-1 fetoprotein in the management of testicular teratoma. In: Lehmann FG (ed) Carcinoembryonic proteins, vol 2. Elsevier/North-Holland Biomedical Press, Amsterdam, p 383
9. Laurence DJR, Neville AM (1980) Biochemical tests in diagnosis and monitoring of cancer. In: Goldberg DM (ed) Annual review of clinical biochemistry, vol 1. Wiley, New York, p 185
10. Martin EW Jr, Cooperman M, King G, Rinker L, Carey LC, Minton JP (1979) A retrospective and prospective study of serial CEA determinations in the early detection of recurrent colon cancer. Am J Surg 137:167–169
11. Moertel CG, Schutt AJ, Go VLW (1978) Carcinoembryonic antigen test for recurrent colorectal carcinoma. JAMA 239:1065–1066
12. Neville AM, Cooper EH (1976) Biochemical monitoring of cancer. Ann Clin Biochem 13:283–305
13. Neville AM, Patel S, Capp M, Laurence DJR, Cooper EH, Turberville C, Coombes RC (1978) Longterm follow-up of colorectal carcinoma patients by repeated CEA radioimmunoassay. Cancer 42:1448–1451
14. Raghavan D, Gibbs J, Nogueira Cost R, Kohn J, Orr AH, Barrett A, Peckham MJ (1980) The interpretation of marker protein assays: A critical appraisal in clinical studies and a xenograft model. Br J Cancer [Suppl 4] 41:191–194
15. Sloane JO, Ormerod MG, Neville AM (to be published) Potential pathological application of immunocytochemical methods to the detection of micrometastases. Cancer Res 40

4. *Radiotherapy as Adjuvant Local Therapy of Local Tumors*

D. Chassagne

Institut Gustave-Roussy, Départment des Radiations, Service de Curietherapie, Rue Camille Desmoulins, F-94800 Villejuif, France

Introduction

We propose to consider radiotherapy as adjuvant when the two following conditions are present: (1) The tumor is not palpable or not visible, therefore the target-volume is a subclinical disease; and (2) the dose delivered to this infraclinical cancer is never higher than 50 Gy (5,000 rad) with the classical time-dose relationship five sessions per week (10 Gy, or 1,000 rad, per week).

In some circumstances the dose can be lower than 50 Gy: when the tumor is very radiosensitive (i.e., testicular seminoma); when the tolerance of critical organs forces a decrease of the delivered dose (i.e., 20 Gy in front of the kidneys for ovarian cancer); and when the dose is delivered with a nonconventional fractionation (i.e., 30 Gy in 2 weeks).

Radiobiologic Basis

It is generally admitted that small tumors require smaller radiotherapeutic doses to be cured than large tumors. Many experimental data have confirmed this clinical experience [1, 2, 6, 8]. The explanations for these facts are numerous: (1) One should never forget that the radiotherapeutic effect is not arithmetically proportional to the dose, but exponentionally proportional to the dose [8, 19]. Due to the tolerance of normal tissue, the dose must be kept under 30–35 Gy in the upper abdomen (such a dose does not destroy macroscopic implants, but can be very effective for microscopic implants). Bush [2, 4] has reported, in stages II and III showing clinical evidence of residual disease following surgery, a 90% 5-year survival rate after abdominal and pelvic radiotherapy and a 50% survival rate after pelvic radiotherapy.

Brachytherapy is a low dose-rate continuous radiation. This type of localized radiation can also be used at a low level as an adjuvant therapy. In adenocarcinomas of uterine corpus the treatment is a total hysterectomy, which shows 15–20% local recurrence in the vaginal cavity. A dose of 50 Gy delivered post- or preoperatively at the upper half of the vaginal cavity decreases the risk of local recurrence to less than 3% [12]. In neurosarcomas of the limbs, there is a very high frequency of recurrence after surgery. By using an after-loading method at the time of surgery we delivered a high dose to the

Recent Results in Cancer Research, Vol. 80

tumor bed and a moderate dose to the whole surgical scar. This therapy was able to prevent local recurrence (Chassagne, unpublished data).

All of the above examples show that a small dose of radiation can destroy small aggregates of cancer cells. In many instances a combination of limited surgery and small-dose radiotherapy gives better results than massive doses of radiation or extensive surgery alone.

With the arrival of new and more effective drugs, one can foresee new combinations which include chemotherapy and radiation (more or less already used with the so-called "iceberg technique" in Hodgkin's disease), chemotherapy followed by surgery, and then radiation (already used in oral cancers), or surgery followed by chemotherapy, and then radiation (as in stage III ovarian cancer). In many instances, if the tumor is not visible or palpable the dose may be decreased to the 50 Gy level without impaired objective results and more desirable subjective results than higher doses.

Fletcher [5], by a careful review of his own data, has shown that 30–35 Gy can eradicate 60–70% of subclinical disease, 40 Gy can eradicate 80–90%, and 50 Gy can eradicate more than 90%. These facts demonstrate the exponential scale of the adjuvant radiotherapy effect.

In head and neck cancers according to the primary site, lesions are best treated by radiotherapy alone or a combination of surgery and radiation either preoperatively or postoperatively. In both circumstances, there are many reports of the outstanding role of adjuvant radiotherapy. For example, in clinically negative nodes in the lymphatic area, Fletcher [7, 11] referred to all the data on squamous cell carcinoma of the upper respiratory and digestive tracts. With a rather small dose of 30–40 Gy in 50 patients, he observed 60–70% eradication and with a dose of 50 Gy in 356 patients, more than 90%. Again, these results fit very well with the potentiality of 50 Gy to eradicate nearly all subclinical diseases.

In soft tissue sarcomas of the extremities, the combination of conservative surgery and postoperative radiation therapy is the best treatment for small- and moderate-size tumors. The local recurrence rate was 22% (24 of 108), comparable to the rate obtained after wide surgery, though the dose delivered by radiotherapy should not exceed 50 Gy so as to avoid damage to the limbs [13, 17].

In ovarian adenocarcinomas, there is considerable discussion concerning radiotherapy. Two basic facts must be recalled: (1) Ovarian carcinoma is a "peritoneal disease", the local implants being widespread through the entire cavity with a higher frequency at the subdiaphragmatic area; and (2) Anoxia, which is the main factor of radioresistance, is shown less in a small aggregate of cancer cells than in a palpable tumor [10, 18, 20]; and (3) The cell kinetics are probably different in small cancer: the growth fraction is higher, the repair of potentially lethal damage is lower [14, 22, 23].

In summary, many experimental data confirm that a dose of 50 Gy is able to completely destroy a subclinical aggregate of 10^5 cancer cells [9, 21].

Clinical Facts

In breast cancer, two classical works are worthwhile to recall: Paterson's [16] clinical trials on postoperative radiotherapy clearly show that a rather small dose can prevent practically all local recurrences in the surgical scar or in the lymphatic areas; and

MacWhirter's [15] reports demonstrate that radiotherapy plus simple mastectomy give the same results as the Halsted operation. These two basic reports also clearly show that the final results are not improved by this adjuvant postoperative radiotherapy, though this is not against the use of radiotherapy. Obviously, the radiation can only destroy cancer cells present within the field of treatment and not outside the target volume, thus, radiotherapy has no effect on distant metastasis.

Nevertheless, these classical facts and also Baclesse's work are the basis of the actual conservative treatment of breast cancer [1, 3, 5]. In T_1 and small $T_2 N_0$, a tumorectomy was performed and was followed shortly after with a dose of 50 Gy to the whole breast, to the potentially involved lymphatic area, and to the chest wall. Results show very few local recurrences, confirming that an adjuvant radiotherapy can eradicate small aggregates of cancer cells, which are present in 30% of the cases, in the remaining part of the breast [3, 5].

References

1. Baclesse F (1965) Five-year results in 431 breast cancers treated solely by roentgen rays. Ann Surg 161: 103–104
2. Bush RS (1979) Malignancies of the ovary, uterus and cervix. II. Malignancies of the ovary. Arnold, London, p 70
3. Calle R, Schlienger P, Vilcoq JR (1977) Place et limite des thérapeutiques à visées conservatrices des épithéliomas mammaires. Résultats à 10 ans. Bull Cancer (Paris) 64: 633–648
4. Chassagne D (1980) Radiotherapy in the treatment of stages III and IV. In: Nijhoff (ed) Therapeutic progress in ovarian cancer, testicular cancer and the sarcomas. The Hague Boerhaave series, vol 16. University Press Leiden, pp 27–40
5. Fletcher GH (1971) Control by irradiation of peripheral lymphatic disease in breast cancer. Am J Roentgenol 111: 115–118
6. Fletcher GH (1972) Clinical dose-response curve of subclinical aggregates of epithelial cells. J Radiol Electrol 53: 201–206
7. Fletcher GH (1972) Elective irradiation of subclinical disease in cancers of the head and neck. Cancer 29: 1450–1454
8. Fletcher GH (1979) Predominant parameters in the planning of radiation therapy of carcinoma of the cervix. Bull Cancer (Paris) 66: 561–572
9. Frindel E, Malaise EP, Alpen E, Tubiana M (1967) Kinetics of cell proliferation of an experimental tumor. Cancer Res 27: 1122–1131
10. Fu KK, Phillips TL, Wharam MD (1976) Radiation response of artificial pulmonary metastases of the EMT-6 tumor. Int J Radiat Oncol Biol Phys 1: 257–260
11. Jesse RH, Lindberg RD (1975) The efficacy of combining radiation therapy with a surgical procedure in patients with cervical metastases from squamous cell cancer of the oropharynx and hypopharynx. Cancer 35: 1163–1166
12. Kagan AR, Nussbaum H, Ziel H, Gordon J (1975) Adenocarcinoma of the endometrium: Vaginal recurrences and mortality. Am J Roentgenol 123: 567–570
13. Lindberg RD, Fletcher GH, Martin RG (1975) The management of soft-tissue sarcomas in adults. Surgery and postoperative radiotherapy. J Radiol Electrol 56: 761–767
14. Little JB, Hahn GM, Frindel E, Tubiana M (1973) Repair of potentially lethal radiation damage in vitro and in vivo. Radiology 106: 689–694
15. McWhirter R (1948) The value of simple mastectomy and radiotherapy in the treatment of cancer of the breast. Br J Radiol 21: 599–610
16. Paterson R, Russell MH (1959) Clinical trials in malignant disease. III. Breast cancer: Evaluation of post-operative radiotherapy. J Fac Radiol (Lond) 10: 175–180

17. Rosenberg SA, Sindelar WF (1980) Surgery and adjuvant radiation-chemoimmunotherapy in soft tissue sarcomas: Result of treatment at the National Cancer Institute. In: Nijhoff (ed) Therapeutic progress in ovarian cancer, testicular cancer and the sarcomas. The Hague Boerhaave series, vol 16. University Press Leiden, pp 397–412
18. Shipley WU, Stanley JA, Courtenay VD, Field SB (1975) Repair of radiation damage in Lewis lung carcinoma cells following in situ treatment with fast neutrons and γ-rays. Cancer Res 35: 932–938
19. Shukovsky LJ, Fletcher GH (1973) Time-dose and tumor volume relationships in the irradiation of squamous cell carcinoma of the tonsillar fossa. Radiology 107: 621–626
20. Suit HD, Maeda M (1967) Hyperbaric oxygen and radiobiology of a C3H mouse mammary carcinoma. J Natl Cancer Inst 39: 639–652
21. Tubiana M (1979) Post-surgical radiotherapy: Rationale and methods. Recent Results Cancer Res 67: 107–114
22. Tubiana M, Frindel E, Malaise EP (1968) The application of radiobiologic knowledge and cellular kinetics to radiation therapy. Am J Roentgenol 102: 822–830
23. Tubiana M, Guichard M, Malaise E (1977) Determinants of cellular kinetics in radiotherapy. In: Drewinko B, Humphrey RM (eds) Growth kinetics and biochemical regulation of normal and malignant cells. Williams & Wilkins, Baltimore, pp 827–842

II. Hemopoietic and Lymphoid Neoplasias

5. Comparison of HLA Phenotypes in Long-Term Survivors with Acute Lymphoblastic Leukemia Treated with Immunotherapy Versus Chemotherapy

T. Tursz, J. Hors, M. Lipinski, J.-L. Amiel, and G. Mathé

Institut Gustave-Roussy, Laboratoire d'Immunologie Clinique,
F-94800 Villejuif, France

Introduction

Experimental data dealing with immunotherapy are usually obtained by studying pure inbred strains, in which all animals carry the same genetic pattern for immune response. In humans, it appears likely that any group of patients includes individuals with the ability to elicit a good immunologic response to a given antigen.

As in animals, most immune-response genes were demonstrated to be linked with the major histocompatibility complex (MHC) [4]. It appeared of interest to see whether HLA phenotype could influence the response to cancer immunotherapy in humans.

In acute lymphoblastic leukemia (ALL), HLA studies have been disappointing [1]. ALL was initially supposed to be a good candidate for HLA-disease association, since in mice the susceptibility to virus-induced leukemia is genetically linked with the I-region of the MHC [3]. Nevertheless, since the pioneer work of Kourilsky in 1968 [2], no clear association could be demonstrated between ALL and any individual HLA antigen.

We report here the HLA phenotypes of children with ALL who are surviving without relapse more than 8 years after immunotherapy.

Patients and Methods

Two comparable groups of patients have been studied, all Caucasians under 20 at diagnosis.

The first group, referred to as chemotherapy group, included 14 patients treated in the Hôpital Saint-Louis, Paris (Prof. J. Bernard), with long-term chemotherapy (4–11 years), without any immunotherapy. These 14 patients are alive in first remission 12–18 years after diagnosis.

The second group (immunotherapy group) included 14 patients treated in the ICIG and the Institut Gustave-Roussy, Villejuif (Prof. G. Mathé). These patients received a short-term remission induction and maintenance chemotherapy. After 6–15 months, the chemotherapy was stopped definitively and immunotherapy was started with BCG (Institut Pasteur) applied weekly on scarifications, together with injections of allogeneic irradiated lymphoblasts. This immunotherapy lasted 4–10 years. No

Recent Results in Cancer Research, Vol. 80

relapse has been observed after 3 years of lasting remission with immunotherapy [5]. These 14 patients are alive with no relapse 9–18 years after diagnosis.
HLA phenotypes were determined by microlymphocytotoxicity assay in microtest plates. Selected monospecific or bispecific antisera, provided by Prof. J. Dausset, allowed testing for 31 HLA-A and B antigens. Frozen rabbit serum was used as the source of complement. Antigen frequencies found in both patient groups were compared with those of 591 healthy individuals tested as controls.

Results and Discussion

HLA-A and B antigens determined in the chemotherapy group patients are listed in Table 1. Antigen frequencies observed in these patients are not different from those found in the healthy control population. Therefore, HLA did not appear of prognostic interest in long-term ALL survivors treated with chemotherapy alone.
Results obtained in the immunotherapy group are shown in Table 2.
As shown in Table 3, a highly significant increase in two HLA antigens was observed (Fisher's exact test and χ^2 comparison with Yate's correction). HLA-B17 was found in 6 of 14 patients and HLA-AW33 in 5 of 14 patients. These results remained significant when corrected for the number of specificities tested. Ten patients possessed at least one of these antigens (71.4% vs. 8% in controls, $P < 0.001$), but only one patient carried both antigens. No patients possessed HLA-B5 antigen (versus 13.2% in controls).
It is noteworthy that no patient carrying HLA-B17 or HLA-AW33 was found in the chemotherapy group.
Our results suggest the existence in man of HLA-linked genes which are related to the response to immunotherapy in ALL.
Besides the theoretical interest, the finding that a good response to immunotherapy in ALL is at least in part genetically determined and HLA-linked could possibly be of

Table 1. Long-term all survivors treated exclusively with chemotherapy

Patient no.	HLA phenotype			
	A locus		B locus	
1	2	3	7	W38
2	11	29	W35	
3	2	11	7	
4	2	11	5	
5	1	9	13	W40
6	1	2	8	12
7	2		12	W41
8	2	19–2	5	W21
9	1	19–2	7	W40
10	9	28	12	W35
11	1	9	8	W15
12	3	W32	8	W35
13	2	28	7	12
14	1	2	W37	W40

Table 2. Long-term all survivors treated with chemotherapy plus immunotherapy

Patient no.	HLA phenotype			
	A locus		B locus	
1	1		14	17
2	3	W33	7	27
3	1	11	17	W18
4	2	W33	7	W15
5	9	W33	8	17
6	3		7	
7	2	W32	17	W40
8	2	3	8	17
9	2	W33	12	
10	9	28	12	14
11	1	29	12	17
12	2	28	W32	W35
13	2	W23	12	
14	3	W33	8	W40

Table 3. HLA antigen frequencies in BCG-treated long-term survivors compared with 591 healthy controls

HLA–B17	42.8%	7.3%	$P<0.01$
HLA–A33	35.7%	1.2%	$P<0.01$
HLA–B17 or A33	71.4%	8.1%	$P<0.001$

clinical relevance. HLA phenotyping would provide an attractive procedure to select those patients with a good chance of cure with immunotherapy or, conversely, those with a poor chance who would require long-term chemotherapy without immunotherapy.

Large prospective immunotherapy trials with HLA-phenotyped patients would be of interest to confirm the validity of this hypothesis.

References

1. Dausset J, Hors J (1975) Some contributions of the HL-A complex to the genetics of human diseases. Transplant Rev 22: 44–74
2. Kourilsky FM, Dausset J, Feingold N, Dupuy JM, Bernard J (1968) Leucocyte groups and acute leukemia. J Natl Cancer Inst 41: 81–87
3. Lilly F, Boyse EA, Old LJ (1964) Genetic basis of susceptibility to viral leukemogenesis. Lancet 2: 1207–1209
4. MacDevitt HO, Benacerraf B (1969) Genetic control of specific immune responses. Adv Immunol 11: 31–74
5. Mathé G, Amiel JL, Schwarzenberg L, Schneider M, Cattan A, Schlumberger JR, Hayat M, de Vassal F (1969) Active immunotherapy for acute lymphoblastic leukaemia. Lancet 1: 697–699

6. *An Intensive Chemo- or Chemoimmunotherapy Regimen for Patients with Intermediate and Poor-Prognosis Acute Lymphatic Leukemia and Leukemic Lymphoblastic Lymphosarcoma: Preliminary Results with 14-Month Median Follow-Up*

J. L. Misset, F. De Vassal, M. Delgado, P. Ribaud, M. Musset, T. Dorval, D. Machover, C. Jasmin, M. Hayat, L. Schwarzenberg, and G. Mathe

Institut de Cancérologie et d'Immunogénétique, (INSERM U-40), Hôpital Paul-Brousse, F-94800 Villejuif, France

Introduction

We previously reported the prognostic factors that can be identified at the onset of acute lymphoid leukemia (ALL) [8]. The factors defining the prognosis are, according to our experience: the WHO Reference Center cytologic types (the "prolymphoblastic" type being always poor, the "microlymphoblastic" type good, and the "macrolymphoblastic" and the "prolymphocytic" intermediate [8]); the T-type is always poor, the null, as they were only characterized in our preceding protocols, intermediate [1]; and, in the cases of those above "intermediate" prognosis types, the volume (V) of the neoplasia plays a prognostic role, i.e., V+ ($\geqslant 10^4$ leukemic cells/mm^3) and/or significant clinical masses suggest a poor prognosis [8].
Applied to a population of 103 children, these criteria enabled us to recognize a subpopulation which accounted for 63% of all ALL patients having a 43% chance of being in first complete remission (CR) at 2 years ("poor prognosis") as opposed to 37% of patients having a 75% chance of being in first CR at 2 years (good prognosis). More or less similar prognosis factors have also been described by other authors, but few of them apply different therapeutic regimens according to prognostic subclasses [13]. For the good-prognosis patients, the problem may be to decrease therapy, especially if we take into account that this population may have a better outcome after a short (9 months) chemotherapy followed by immunotherapy than after a long 21 months) chemotherapy followed by immunotherapy [9].
For the poor-prognosis subpopulation, one is tempted to introduce four changes into our previous protocol 12 [9]: (1) intensifying the remission-induction chemotherapy by adding adriamycin which, when applied alone, can induce CR [7] and does not belong to the series of agents applied in our previous protocols, namely, prednisone, vincristine (VCR), and L-asparaginase [9]; (2) adding a new agent, vindesine (VDN) [10], to the maintenance chemotherapy comprising 6-mercaptopurine (6-MP) and methotrexate (MTX), since VDN resulted in ALL CR even in patients apparently clinically resistant to VCR; (3) applying intense reinforcement combination chemotherapy cycles including cytosine arabinoside [2] in one alternative cycle and cyclophosphamide [6] in the other (the frequency of such cycles being low to avoid the induction of an aplasia which would interrupt the continuous treatment, but as high as possible); and (4) interspersing immunotherapy with chemotherapy, which is the only way to apply it to these patients. In fact, when the protocol proposes immunotherapy

Recent Results in Cancer Research, Vol. 80

following chemotherapy, the patients who relapse during the latter do not receive it. We have chosen a new well-characterized agent, Azimexon (Boehringer Lab.), which stimulates several immune functions in our experimental experience [3, 4] and natural killer (NK) cell activity in our phase I clinical study [5].
This protocol 16 is also applied to the lymphoblastic lymphosarcoma patients who are leukemic at initial presentation and who have so-called leukemic lymphosarcoma (LL) [11].
Although it is too early to evaluate the role of immunotherapy, which is studied in a randomized fashion in this trial, the overall preliminary results can be the object of a preliminary analysis, with a maximal follow-up of 3 years and a median follow-up of 14 months.

Patients and Methods

Protocol 16

The induction period includes prednisone (40 mg/m^2 orally) each day for 28 days, VCR (1.4 mg/m^2 i.v. every week) for 4 weeks, L-asparaginase (*E. Coli*) at 10,000 units/m^2 twice a week i.v. or i.m. for 4 weeks, and adriamycin (20 mg/m^2 i.v. once a week) for 4 weeks (discontinued after 2 weeks if CR is shown).
The CNS prophylaxis period consists of cranial irradiation including C2 at a dosage of 24 Gy delivered over 2.5 weeks and ten fractions, eight intrathecal (i.t.) injections of MTX (10 mg/m^2) during 2–3 weeks. A systemic chemotherapy is applied during this period, including 6-MP (50 mg/m^2 daily), biweekly MTX (10 mg/m^2 i.m. on the same day as the i.t. injections, and bimonthly VDN (2 mg/m^2 i.v. each time bone marrow tolerance allows administration of this drug.
The maintenance therapy includes daily 6-MP (50 mg/m^2 orally), weekly MTX (20 mg/m^2 i.m.), and bimonthly VDN (2 mg/m^2 i.v.). A dose schedule according to peripheral blood cell count is respected.
Every 3 months, a reinforcement course is given in an alternating order. Reinforcement A consists of, on day 1, adriamycin (40 mg/m^2 i.v.), vincristine (1.4 mg/m^2 i.v. on day 2, and on days 3–6, 100 mg/m^2 cytosine arabinoside given by i.v. push of 25 mg/m^2 followed by 12 h infusion of 75 mg/m^2. On days 3–10, prednisone (40 mg/m^2) is given orally. Reinforcement B consists of, on day 1, adriamycin (40 mg/m^2 i.v.), vincristine

Table 1. Distribution of the patients according to sex and age (n = 34)

	No. of patients	Age		Sex		Determination of poor prognosis by		
		< 15 years	> 15 years	M	F	Cytology	Immune markers	Volume of the neoplasia only[a]
ALL	28	19	9	11	17	10	2	16
LL	6	3	3	2	4	1	3	2
Total	34	22	12	13	21	11	5	18

[a] In the case of intermediate-prognosis cytologic types

Table 2. Comparison of the stratification of the main parameters of ALL in protocols 12 and 16 (patients ≤ 15 years of age)

	Patients	Sex		Age			Determination of poor prognosis by		
		M	F	< 3 years	3–12 years	≥ 12 years	Cytology	Immune markers	Volume of the neoplasia only[a]
Protocol 12	40	22	18	9	28	3	7	2	31
Protocol 16	19	10	9	2	15	2	5	2	12
P =		0.39		0.14	0.50	0.50	0.23	0.50	0.47

[a] In the case of intermediate-prognosis cytologic types

(1.4 mg/m^2 i.v.) on day 2, on days 3–6, cyclophosphamide (30 mg/m^2 i.m.), and on days 3–10, prednisone (40 mg/m^2 orally).
Patients are randomized to receive Azimexon or not (130 mg/m^2 orally) on days 20 and 22 after each reinforcement course. Systemic therapy with 6-MP, MTX, and VDS is resumed after reinforcement as soon as bone marrow recovery permits. Any treatment must be interrupted after 3 years of continuous CR.

Patients

This protocol was given to 34 patients whose ages, sex, and diagnoses are presented in Table 1. Twenty-eight had poor-prognosis ALL predicted (19 children and nine adults) and six (three children and three adults) had LL. There were 13 females and 21 males. The main reason for the prediction of poor prognosis is also given in Table 1.
The macrolymphoblastic, prolymphocytic, null, and the cytologically and immunologically unclassified leukemias had to be V+ ($\geq 10^4$ leukemic cells/mm^3) to be included in the protocol (Table 2).

Results

Feasability

Although in many instances drug dosage had to be adapted to hematologic tolerance, the toxicity of the regimen was generally acceptable. No patient died in remission of the 33 patients who entered the maintenance phase; only two could not receive the reinforcements because of permanent cytopenia. Twelve patients of 31 (39%) were able to receive the reinforcements according to the dose and time schedule in the protocol. Seventeen patients had their reinforcements delayed or underdosed because of cytopenia. Two patients have not yet reached the date of first reinforcement. Maintenance therapy dosage was full dose for 12 patients, 50–100% of protocol dosage for 12 patients, and under 50% of the protocol dose for seven patients.

Induction of Remission

One patient with LL failed to respond and died after 3 weeks of induction treatment. A child had to receive 2 weeks of VDN after the standard 4-week induction regimen to achieve CR. The other 32 patients were in CR by the end of the 4-week induction period. The overall CR rate is 97%.

Disease-Free Survival

The actuarial disease-free survival of the 33 patients who achieved CR is shown in Fig. 1; 75% are in first CR with the present follow-up.
Six patients (three LL, three ALL) relapsed and two of them were adults with isolated CNS relapse. Altogether, three of six relapses were isolated CNS relapses and only

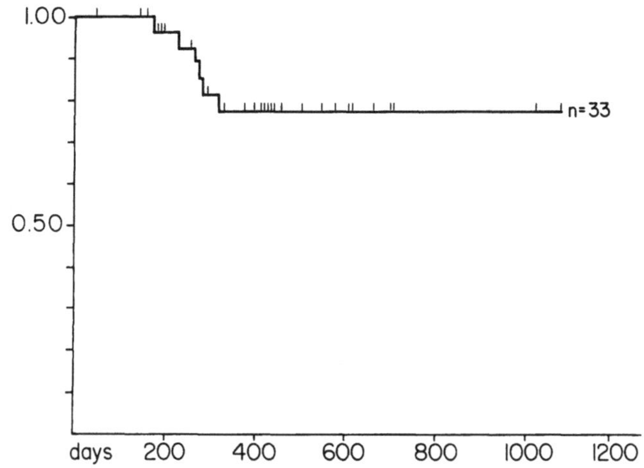

Fig. 1. Actuarial disease-free survival of the poor-prognosis ALL and leukemic lymphosarcoma patients of all ages

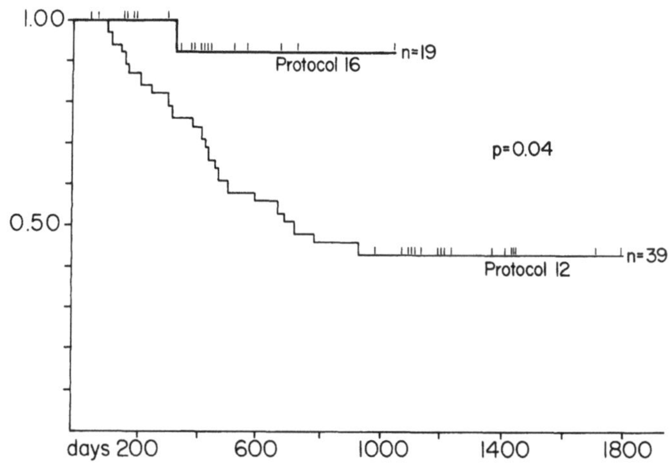

Fig. 2. Compared actuarial disease-free survival curves of the ALL poor-prognosis patients below 15 years of age, according to protocol 12 and protocol 16

1 child of 19 had an isolated bone marrow relapse. We, therefore, confirm our previous work on the relatively poor efficiency of standard CNS prophylaxis regimens in poor prognosis ALL [12].

The 19 children with poor prognosis ALL who submitted to protocol 16 have been compared with the 40 children (39 who achieved CR) with the same disease who submitted to protocol 12. This comparison seems valid because no known variable with prognostic value was significantly different in both groups of patients (Table 2). Fig. 2 shows the disease-free survival curves of the two groups of patients according to these protocols. Although the follow-up is still of short duration and the number of patients small, a difference has already appeared ($P = 0.04$).

In this small group of poor prognosis ALL patients, we did not observe any significant difference between those of whom the age is 15 years or less and those of whom the age is 15 years or more (Fig. 3).

The actuarial survival curves (Figs. 4 and 5) are very similar to those of first disease-free survival, as most patients entered remission.

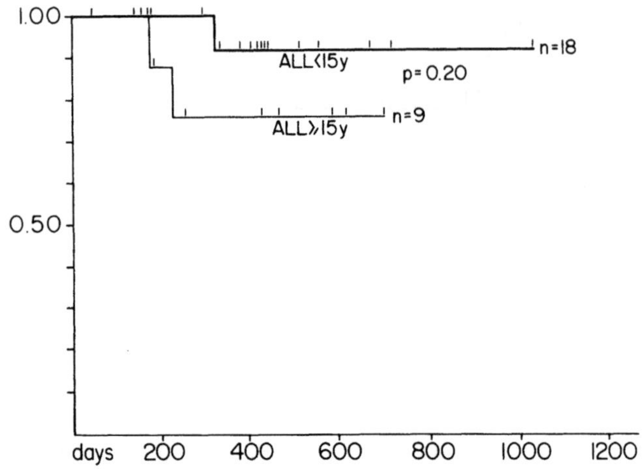

Fig. 3. Actuarial disease-free survival curves of poor prognosis ALL patients who submitted to protocol 16, according to age

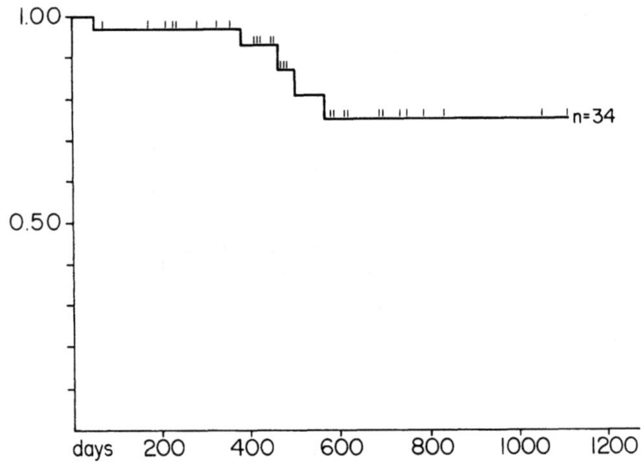

Fig. 4. Actuarial curve of survival of the poor-prognosis ALL and leukemic lymphosarcoma patients of all ages

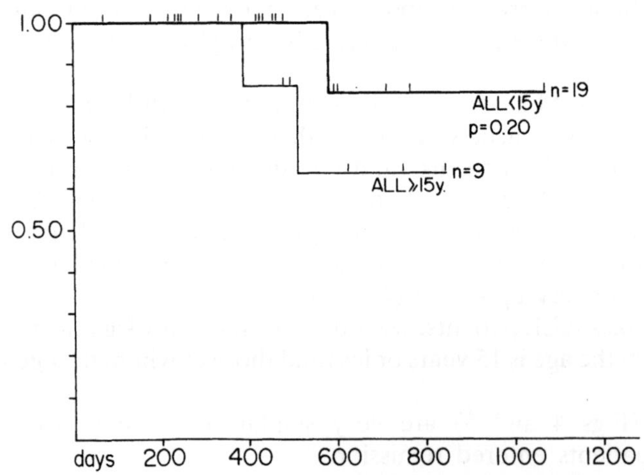

Fig. 5. Actuarial disease-free survival curves of poor-prognosis ALL patients who submitted to protocol 16, according to age

It is too early to analyse the effect of Azimexon. We are only making a preliminary check of the feasability of protocol 16 and of its possible superiority over protocol 12, which had given us mediocre results on a population of ALL patients defined by one of our parameters.
The present preliminary results indicate the applicability of this protocol 16 and its encouraging results in such ALL patients and LL patients. They suggest a superiority over protocol 12 in ALL. As it is a pilot protocol, we cannot attribute this possible superiority to any of the factors introduced.

References

1. Belpomme D, Mathé G, Davies AJS (1977) Clinical significance and prognostic value of the T-B immunological classification of human primary acute lymphoid leukaemias. Lancet 1: 555–558.
2. Bernard J, Boiron M, Jacquillat C, Weil M, Najean Y (1966) Un nouvel agent actif dans le traitement des leucémies aiguës: La cytosine arabinoside. Presse Med 74: 799–802
3. Florentin I, Kiger N, Bruley-Rosset M, Schulz J, Mathé G (1978) Effect of seven immunomodulators on different types of immune responses in mice. In: Serrou B, Rosenfeld C (eds) Human lymphocyte differentiation: Its application to cancer. Elsevier/North-Holland, Biomedical Press, Amsterdam, pp 299–304
4. Florentin I, Schulz J, Bruley-Rosset M, Kiger N, Mathé G (1980) In vivo immunomodulating properties of two synthetic agents: Azimexon and tuftsin. In: Mathé G, Muggia F (eds) Cancer chemo- and immunopharmacology. II. Immunopharmacology, relations and general problems. Springer, Berlin Heidelberg New York
5. Goutner A, Schwarzenberg L, Mathé G (1980) Phase I study of Azimexon in immunodepressed cancer patients. In: Second International Conference: Immunotherapy of cancer, present status of trials in man, Bethesda, April 1980
6. Mathé G, Schweisguth O, Brule G, Schneider M, Amiel JL, Schwarzenberg L, Cattan A (1963) Essai de traitement par la cyclophosphamide de la leucémie lymphoblastique aigue et du lymphoblastosarcome. Presse Med 71: 402–404
7. Mathé G, Amiel JL, Hayat M et al. (1970) Adriamycin in the treatment of acute leukemias. In: Mathé G (ed) Advances in the treatment of acute (blastic) leukemias. Springer, Berlin Heidelberg New York, pp 168–172
8. Mathé G, de Vassal F, Delgado M et al. (1976) 1975 current results of the first 100 cytologically typed acute lymphoid leukemia submitted to BCG active immunotherapy. Cancer Immunol Immunother 1: 77–86
9. Mathé G, de Vassal F, Schwarzenberg L et al. (1978) Preliminary results of three protocols for the treatment of acute lymphoid leukaemia of children: Distinction of two groups of patients according to predictable prognosis. Med Pediatr Oncol 4: 17–27
10. Mathé G, Misset JL, de Vassal F et al. (1978) Phase II clinical trial with vindesine for remission induction in acute leukemia, blastic crisis of chronic myeloid leukemia, lymphosarcoma and Hodgkin's disease: Absence of crossresistance with vincristine. Cancer Treat Rep 62: 805–809
11. Mathé G, Misset JL, Gil-Delgado M, Delgado M, de Vassal F (1978) Leukemic (or stage V) lymphosarcoma. In: Mathé G, Seligmann M, Tubiana M (eds) Lymphoid neoplasias II: Clinical and therapeutic aspects. Springer, Berlin Heidelberg New York, pp 88–107
12. Misset JL, de Vassal F, Jasmin C, Mathé G (to be published) Neuroprophylaxis in acute lymphoblastic leukemia. Correlation of neurological risk and efficacy of prevention with other prognostic factors. Eur J Cancer
13. Schaison G, Harousseau JL, Jacquillat C, Weil M, Bernard J (1979) Phase I treatment protocol for children with increased risk acute lymphocytic leukemia (IRALL). Proc Am Assoc Cancer Res 20: 104

7. *Poor-Prognosis Acute Lymphoblastic Leukemias*

M. Weil, C. Jacquillat, M. F. Auclerc, G. Schaison, C. Chastang, and J. Bernard*

Unité de Chimiothérapie, Institut de Recherches sur les Maladies du Sang, Hôpital Saint-Louis, 2 Place du Docteur Fournier, F-75475 Paris Cedex 10, France

Summary

Burkitt's-type leukemias have specific cytologic, immunologic, and cytogenetic characteristics. Initial symptomatology frequently includes abdominal tumors and initial CNS involvement. Despite intensive treatment including high-dose cyclophosphamide, prognosis remains poor in most patients because of failures to achieve complete remission (CR) or because of early relapses, especially CNS relapses. Class III acute lymphoblastic leukemia in children is defined by the presence of two or more unfavorable parameters and recent progress has been achieved by intensive therapy. Cox's multifactorial analysis allows improved discrimination. A phase I protocol for increased-risk leukemias, including testis preventive irradiation and monthly reinductions without continuous maintenance for the first 6 months of CR, seems promising.

Introduction

Three categories of patients may be considered as increased-risk acute lymphoblastic leukemia (ALL); adults, Burkitt's-type, and class III childhood ALL. We shall discuss the two last categories.

Burkitt's-Type Leukemia

Burkitt's-type ALL are distinctly described: cytologically as L_3, according to FAB classification, with large homogeneous cells with prominent nuclei, deep cytoplasmic basophilia, and prominent cytoplasmic vacuoles; the differentiation markers are surface bound immunoglobulins [3]; and cytogenetics, the $T_{8,14}$ translocation is present [2]. We have gathered the records of 15 children and seven adults with Burkitt's-type

* This research was carried out with the aid of Contrat INSERM, Commission 8; Subvention du Comité Franco-Américain de Recherche sur le Cancer (INSERM); USPHS Research Grant, CA 13239-05 from the National Cancer Institute; Caisse Régionale d'Assurances Maladies de Paris; and Formation de Recherche Associé n° 42 INSERM

Table 1. Clinical symptoms in Burkitt's-type leukemias (22 patients)

Hepatomegaly	15
Splenomegaly	16
Peripheral adenomegaly	12
Abdominal tumors	8
Maxillary tumors	2
Bone involvement	2
Testis	1
Pleural	2
Tonsils	2
Breasts	1
Skin	1
Gums	1
CNS	8 (CSF 7)
No tumor	5

Table 2. Evolution of Burkitt's-type leukemias

Failures	10
CR	12 (55%)
Relapses	9 (CNS 3, bone marrow + CNS 4, bone marrow 2)
Death in CR	1
Lost	1
Alive	1

leukemia (five females and 17 males). The clinical symptoms (Table 1) show an unusual frequency of abdominal tumors and initial CNS involvement. Despite drug combinations, including high-dose cyclophosphamide evolution is characterized by a relatively low rate of complete remission (CR) and by early relapses, especially in the CNS (Table 2). We must admit that we have not yet found an effective treatment for this variety, which fortunately represents only about 1% of ALL cases.

Class III Childhood Leukemias

The definition of class III ALL is empiric. In 1973, the retrospective analysis of 650 cases of ALL. Led us to take into consideration five unfavorable parameters: age of 15 years, or older, white blood cell count of 35,000 or more, lymphnode enlargement of 3 cm, and liver and/or spleen enlargement of 6 cm. If none of these parameters is present, patients belong to class I, if one is present they belong to class II, if more than one is present they belong to class III. Class III patients have a poor prognosis since the median duration of CR is less than 12 months and less than 25% are in CR at 2 years. When this stratification is applied to 797 children treated during 1964–1976 [6], we observe that the incidence of CR is already different between class III and the other classes (Table 3).

Table 3. Induction results in 797 children 20 years of age or less

	Class I	Class II	Class III
1964–1973	96% (67)	92% (127)	75% (98)
1974–1976	96% (146)	80% (158)	80% (101)

Table 4. Percentage of global remission at 3 years according to year of diagnosis and to prognostic class

	Class I	Class III
1964–1968	28%	5%
1969–1973	58%	18%
1974–1976	61%	39%

However, differences between the three prognostic class are more evident when durations of CR are reported, Table 4 confirms the existence of an increased risk group. It indicates also that this group should not be considered static, but as a group of patients who deserve intensive therapy. Namely, the marked improvement observed during 1974–1976 was achieved in children treated by protocol 08 LA 74 [6]. One of the objectives of this protocol was to reduce prognostic handicap by adjusting doses to prognosis. Despite this quantitative adjustment and despite the obvious progress that was achieved, significant differences persist between the three groups. Among the prognostic factors which are implicated in these differences (Table 5), the most important is sex. It may be related to the higher frequency of T phenotype in boys but also to the high rate of testis relapses in this protocol (33 primary relapses of 211 boys). The empiric stratification that was used prospectively in this protocol does not take into consideration the variable importance of individual parameters and their interaction, the Cox method which we applied retrospectively achieves a much better discrimination as shown in Fig. 1.

Thus, in 1977, the following conclusions could be drawn. It is possible to identify increased-risk ALL. This group benefits from intensive treatment and is at high risk of testis relapse. Results of 08 LA 74 under estimate the significance of thymic enlargement. Immunologic markers must be incorporated into prognostic stratification of ALL.

These propositions constitute the basis for a phase I protocol for very increased-risk ALL. We have defined very increased-risk children's ALL (VIRCALL) as: presence of T markers, and/or more than 200,000 WBC/mm^3, and/or patients with thymic enlargement. Patients of these categories before 1974 had a rate of CR at 1 year of 21% for patients with more than 200,000 WBC (mm^3) and 23% for patients with thymic enlargement.

The objectives of this VIRCALL protocol were to increase CR duration in VIRCALL, to prevent testis relapses and to study whether this factor effects survival times, and to prevent pneumolystis pneumonia and CMV by Bactrim and anti-CMV gamma globulin.

Table 5. Analysis of duration of hematologic remissions (HR) as a function of clinical and hematologic factors as well as of prognostic classes

Factor studied	Categories		No. of initial	Actuarial percent and no. HR after	
				3 years	4 years
Sex ($P = 0.02$)	Male		211	47% (59)	35% (21)
	Female		152	60% (54)	56% (22)
Age	< 2		22	43% (3)	29% (1)
	≥ 2	< 8	218	55% (71)	44% (23)
	≥ 8	< 12	57	45% (15)	42% (9)
	≥ 12	< 15	35	43% (9)	43% (4)
	≥ 15	< 20	31	67% (15)	62% (7)
Initial WBC count	< 5		90	58% (26)	44% (9)
(in thousands) ($P = 0.04$)	≥ 5	< 15	114	57% (38)	42% (13)
	≥ 15	< 35	65	59% (24)	54% (8)
	≥ 35	< 100	46	41% (11)	35% (3)
		≥ 100	48	37% (14)	37% (10)
Initial platelet		< 20	109	46% (34)	37% (11)
count ($P = 0.07$)	≥ 20	< 50	113	54% (36)	48% (16)
	≥ 50	< 100	56	44% (10)	33% (16)
		≥ 100	85	63% (33)	52% (13)
Peripheral lymph nodes	No palpable		78	60% (27)	50% (12)
($P = 0.03$)		< 1	188	51% (60)	40% (21)
	≥ 1	< 3	83	52% (24)	49% (10)
		≥ 3	11	22% (1)	22% (1)
Mediastinal lymph-	Yes		27	41% (8)	41% (4)
adenopathies ($P = 0.05$)	No		330	54% (105)	44% (39)
Number of courses		1	246	53% (75)	41% (24)
required ($P = 0.06$)		2	99	54% (34)	51% (18)
		3	18	35% (4)	35% (1)
Prognostic class		1	140	59% (47)	52% (20)
		2	142	52% (45)	37% (12)
		3	81	41% (21)	39% (11)

The induction phase consists in the combination of vincristine (VCR) (2 mg/m^2 on day 1), cyclophosphamide (600 mg/m^2 on day 2), daunorubicin (DNR) (80 mg/m^2 on days 2 and 4), and L-asparaginase (1,000 IU/kg from day 5 for 10 days).
Consolidation combines one intermediate dose of methotrexate (MTX) (500 mg/m^2) with one IT dose of MTX (12 mg/m^2), followed 6 days later by one dose of VCR (2 mg/m^2) and cyclophosphamide (600 mg/m^2). Then prophylactic radiotherapy is used on the skull (3,500 rad) and the testis (2,400 rad). The first six patients received thymic irradiation (2,400 rad), but thereafter we stopped this practice since it increases the cardiac risk of DNR and cyclophosphamide.
Maintenance is characterized by the absence of continuous treatment for the 6 first months. However, monthly courses are given alternating a treatment of DNR (40

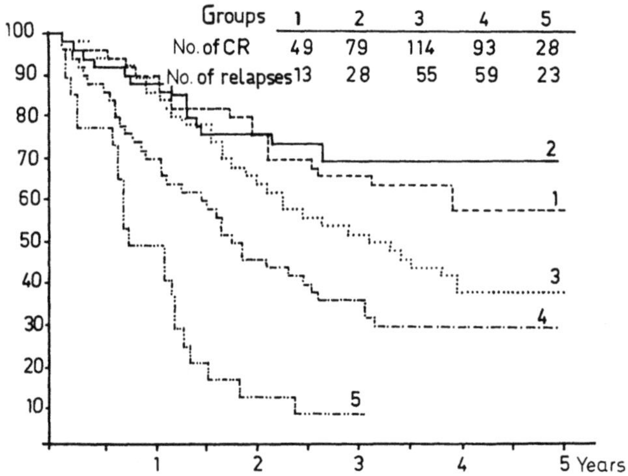

Fig. 1. Global remission in groups at various risk according to Cox method

mg/m² on days 1 and 3), cyclophosphamide (600 mg/m² on day 1), Ara C (100 mg/m² from day 1 for 5 days), and L-asparaginase (1,000 IU/kg from day 6 for 5 days) and the same combination where DNR is replaced by vincristine (2 mg/m²). The repetition of L-asparaginase courses is justified by the observation of Onnuma and Holland [9] on the specificity of this enzyme for T lymphoblasts. After 6 months 6-mercaptopurine and MTX are used, with reinduction by prednisone VCR every 3 months.

Supportive treatment includes hyperhydration, urate oxydase and allopurinol to prevent hyperuricemic nephropathy and during remission, and bactrim to prevent interstitial pneumonia.

Among the 33 children who entered this protocol, 24 were boys, 21 had E-rosettes, 22 had thymic enlargement, and 19 had more than 200,000 blasts/mm³. Twenty-nine achieved CR, four died during induction from sepsis, four died during remission (among them, two cardiac failures in children who had thymic irradiation), and six relapsed. Nineteen (70%) of these children are in CR after a follow-up of more than 18 months in 18 patients. With the very severe presumed prognosis of these patients, these results are very encouraging.

Conclusion

For poor-prognosis ALL we have no effective treatment. Burkitt's-type leukemias belong to this category. For the other poor-risk ALL, especially for T-cell leukemias, significant progress has been made by the intensification of therapy. However, despite our progress, our predictions are far from satisfactory. Unexpected failures are seen as well may be observed as, fortunately, unexpected successes. Parameters such as the sensitivity to drugs and the reserves of normal stem cells are poorly appreciated. It is hoped that progress in prediction and management will further reduce the number of poor-prognosis ALL cases.

References

1. Bennett JM, Catovsky D, Daniel MT, Flandrin G, Galton DA, Gralnick HR, Sultan C (1976) Proposals for the classification of the acute leukemias (FAB cooperation group). Br J Haematol 33: 451–458
2. Berger R, Bernheim A, Brouet JC, Daniel MT, Flandrin G (1979) (8; 14) Translocation in a Burkitt's type of lymphoblastic leukemia (L_3). Br J Haematol 43: 87–90
3. Brouet JC, Preud'homme JL, Seligmann M (1975) The use of B and T membrane markers in the classification of human leukemias with special reference to acute lymphoblastic leukemia. Blood Cells 1: 81–90
4. Harousseau JL, Tobelem G, Schaison G, Chastang C, Auclerc MF, Weil M, Jacquillat Cl, Bernard J (1978) High-risk acute lymphocytic leukemia. A study of 141 cases with high blast counts. Abstracts 17th Int Congr Hematol (Paris) 1: 252
5. Jacquillat C, Le Gall E, Schaison G, Auclerc MF, Chastang C, Flandrin G (1978) Les leucémies aigües avec localisation thymique. Actual Hematol 44: 52
6. Jacquillat C, Weil M, Schaison G, Chastang C, Bernard J (1980) Results of protocol 08 LA 74 in childhood acute lymphoblastic leukemias. Proc Am Assoc Cancer Res 490: 122
7. Ravidranath Y, Kaplan J, Zuelzer NN (1975) Significance of mediastinal mass in acute lymphoblastic leukemia. Pediatrics 55: 889–893
8. Schaison G, Harvusseau JL, Jacquillat C, Weil M, Bernard J (1979) Phase I treatment protocol for children with increased-risk acute lymphocytic leukemia. Proc Am Assoc Cancer Res 419: 104
9. Sen L, Borella L (1975) Clinical importance of lymphoblastes with markers in childhood acute leukemia. N Engl J Med 292: 828–832
10. Simone JV, Verzosa MS, Rudy JA (1975) Initial features and prognosis in 363 children with acute lymphoblastic leukemia. Cancer 36: 2099–2108

8. *Therapeutic Effectiveness of Neuraminidase-Treated Allogeneic Myeloblasts as Immunogen in Acute Myelocytic Leukemia**

J. G. Bekesi and J. F. Holland

City University of New York, The Mount Sinai School of Medicine and Hospital, Department of Neoplastic Diseases, New York, NY 10029, USA

Summary

Our chemoimmunotherapy study shows significantly longer remission and survival in acute myelocytic leukemia (AML) patients who have been immunized with neuraminidase-treated allogeneic myeloblasts as compared to patients who received chemotherapy alone or neuraminidase-treated myeloblasts plus MER. MER impairs the immunotherapeutic effectiveness of neuraminidase-treated allogeneic myeloblasts in AML patients. The in vivo and in vitro immunologic status in each arm of the protocol correlate well with the duration of remission and survival of the patient.

Introduction

Based on a wealth of experimental observations that immunization with X-irradiated, chemically, or enzymatically modified tumor cells with or without BCG or MER leads to a significant increase in the life span of tumor-bearing animals, immunotherapy has become an important tool in the treatment of human leukemias. Mathé demonstrated the therapeutic value of irradiated allogeneic myeloblasts in combination with BCG in treating childhood lymphoblastic leukemia [14]. Similar studies were conducted by Powles [15] and Gutterman [9] in patients with acute myelocytic leukemia (AML) involving chemotherapy with or without irradiated allogeneic myeloblasts and BCG.

Glycoproteins are an integral part of the surface structure of normal and neoplastic cells and play a significant role in blood group antigens, histocompability, and tumor antigens. Treatment with neuraminidase (N'ase) causes several changes in the

* This work was supported in part by grant and contracts CA-1-5936-02, CA-5834, NCI Cancer Virus Program 1-CB-43879 and NCI Immunotherapy Program 1-CO-43225, and the T. J. Martell Memorial Fund for Leukemia Research. We express our appreciation to the Behring Institute, Behringwerk AG, Marburg, Federal Republic of Germany, for supplying the highly purified neuraminidase for this study. We also thank Patricia Mason, Svetlana Perova, and Khanitha Tangnavarad for the excellent assistance in performing the immunotherapeutic manipulations and Rogena Brown for secretarial assistance

physical, biologic, and immunologic properties of normal and neoplastic cells. Enzymatic removal of plasma membrane-bound N-acetylneuraminic acid reduces the negative surface charge which facilitates cell-to-cell interaction, increases the susceptibility of the treated cells to phagocytosis, and enchances macrophage cytotoxicity [12, 17, 19]. Lymphocytes treated with N'ase form a significantly higher percent of rosettes with sheep-red blood cells and give a higher value with sheep erythrocyte-antibody-complement complex (EAC)-rosetting. The change in surface marker properties following the treatment of lymphocytes with N'ase appears to indicate that the penultimate sugar residue D-galactose may be the immunodeterminant in the T-antigen of the mammalian lymphocytes. N'ase-treated lymphocytes also show increased blastogenic response to specific T and B cell mitogens, such as phytohemagglutinin (PHA), ConA, or pokeweed mitogen (PWM) [18, 19].

N'ase of *Vibrio cholerae* origin has been successfully used in inducing increased tumor immunogenicity of various experimental tumors, which can be attributed almost exclusively to the enzymatic release of N-acetylneuraminic acid from the surface of tumor cells [1–5, 8, 11, 16, 18, 19]. Increased immunogenicity of autochthonous methylcholanthrene-induced tumors after treatment with N'ase has also resulted in immunospecific rejection of established solid tumors. In a DBA/2 leukemia L1210 system, a single leukemic cell is capable of producing leukemia and ultimate death of the host. On the other hand, mice which were immunized with N'ase-treated leukemia L1210 cells remain protected against a challenge of 100,000 untreated leukemia cells [1–6, 21, 22].

Using chemotherapy plus N'ase-treated leukemic cells, administered in a sequence preserving the host's immunobiologically competent lymphocytes, resulted in the cure of a significant portion of immunized mice [3, 6, 8]. The immunity induced by N'ase-treated leukemic cells was specific for the particular tumor and could be transferred by sera or splenic lymphocytes into nonimmunized syngeneic mice [3, 6, 8, 22].

N'ase-modified spontaneous and transplantable tumors as immunogen in immunoprophylactic and chemoimmunotherapeutic experiments in syngeneic mice, as well as pilot clinical studies, was effective [5–7, 10, 18, 19]. We have repeatedly demonstrated that N'ase-treated E_2G leukemic cells, which are gross-virus induced (cf. AKR leukemia), were as effective as syngeneic leukemic cells in prolonging survival of AKR leukemic mice [6, 7, 18, 19]. This suggested the existence of a cross-reacting common viral membrane antigen and may suggest that if a similar etiology existed for human acute leukemia, it would not be essential to use autologous leukemic cells for immunization. These data provided the basis for the human immunotherapeutic investigation, the results of which are presented in this paper [4–7, 10, 18].

Immunotherapy

Collection of Allogeneic Myeloblasts

Myeloblasts were collected from patients after satisfying the following criteria: negative HA-A as determined by radioimmunoassay; total WBC higher than 24,000/ml; and higher than 75% myeloblasts in the peripheral blood. The separation of myeloblasts is achieved by leukophoresis, which commenced immediately after clinical diagnosis. In the last 5 years, we collected leukemic myeloblasts from 84 patients (14–72 years of age). There were no important side effects due to the procedure. After leukophoresis, the myeloblasts were separated from contaminating RBC and were mixed with a special freezing medium containing autologous or normal AB plasma and 10% dimethyl sulfoxide (DMSO). Myeloblasts were frozen by program freezing and stored in the vapor phase of liquid nitrogen.

Determination of Neuraminidase-Susceptible and Total N-Acetylneuraminic Acid Content

A selected ion-monitoring technique was developed by us for the quantification of N'ase-susceptible and total cellular N-acetylneuraminic acid content of myeloblasts used as immunogen in the immunotherapy of patients with AML. Total N-acetylneuraminic acid content of myeloblasts is 0.3–0.6 μmol/10^9 leukemic cells. Under optimum conditions, using about 10–15-fold excess of N'ase in proportion to the receptor sites, 68–75% of the bound N-acetylneuraminic acid was cleaved by the enzyme. Studies are in progress to determine the existence of a direct relationship between the total sialic acid content of the myeloblasts and the magnitude of the delayed hypersensitivity reaction in patients immunized with the modified allogeneic myeloblasts.

Preselection of Antigenic Myeloblasts

To avoid using nonantigeneic myeloblasts for immunotherapy, we ran a battery of tests designated to pretest their antigenicity. Fresh myeloblasts from all donors who were leukophoresed were tested in a mixed leukocyte culture against remission lymphocytes of AML patients randomized to receive N'ase-treated cells. Simultaneously, we tested the delayed-type hypersensitivity response to the N'ase-modified myeloblasts in designated AML recipients. Table 1 shows representative data obtained from such a study. Myeloblasts obtained from donor M-74 gave poor results with remission lymphocytes as well as poor DCH response. Consequently, these myeloblasts were not used for immunization.

Immunotherapy with Neuraminidase-Treated Myeloblasts and MER

Myeloblasts were thawed and washed twice with mixed salt and glucose media at 4° C and purified on a 22% human albumin gradient, layered over 45% sucrose for separation of viable blast cells. After purification, myeloblasts were washed and incubated with N'ase at a concentration of 20 units of enzyme/5 × 10^7 myeloblasts/ml in sodium acetate buffer for 60 min at 37° C. The cells were then washed and resuspended in physiological saline and used as immunogen within 30 min.

Immunization with N'ase-treated allogeneic myeloblasts was performed by interdermal injections. To get maximum exposure to the immunogen, sites were widely spread in the supraclavicular, infraclavicular, arm, forearm, parasternal, thoracic, suprainguinal, and femoral regions draining to major node-bearing areas.

Table 1. Pretest antigenicity of myeloblasts in vivo and in vitro against designated recipients (cpm × 10^3)

AML patients in CR (designated recipients)	M-71		M-72		M-73		M-74	
	MLTC[a]	DCH[b]	MLTC[a]	DCH[b]	MLTC[a]	DCH[b]	MLTC[a]	DCH[b]
1	19.7	13.0	ND[c]	ND	21.0	11.0	7.5	8.4
2	21.4	15.3	ND	ND	ND	ND	ND	ND
3	ND	ND	22.3	14.0	ND	ND	2.8	3.0
4	9.6	10.2	18.3	10.2	ND	ND	3.5	5.6
5	14.5	12.5	12.0	11.9	19.6	16.4	4.7	3.8
6	24.5	16.0	27.3	19.0	36.5	18.0	2.6	4.0
7	ND	ND	10.0	12.0	8.6	10.5	ND	ND
8	29.5	18.0	14.6	10.5	13.5	16.4	6.1	4.7

[a] Ratio of donor myeloblasts to responding lymphocytes (2 : 1)
[b] Mean induration in mm obtained from interdermal injection of 2 × 10^8 N'ase-treated myeloblasts
[c] ND, not determined

Table 2. Effect of MER on the DCH response to neuraminidase-treated allogeneic myeloblasts in AML patients. DCH was measured 48 h after injection

Immunization cycles	Immunotherapy			
	Cells[a]	Cells[a]	+	MER[b]
1	13.2 ± 3.5	9.3 ± 2.7		10.3 ± 3.0
3	16.9 ± 4.1	10.4 ± 2.0		13.9 ± 3.4
6	18.7 ± 4.6	7.1 ± 2.3		21.8 ± 5.1
12	21.6 ± 5.1	6.8 ± 1.7		26.7 ± 5.9
Patients tested	4		5	

[a] Mean induration ± SD in mm obtained from 48 sites injected with neuraminidase-treated myeloblasts using the same donor's myeloblasts
[b] Mean induration ± SD in mm obtained from ten sites injected with 100 μg MER per site

A dose-dependent cellular titration was performed with each immunization with 0.5, 1.5, 2.0 × 10^8, and 0 cells. The total immunization load was about 10^{10} N'ase-treated allogeneic myeloblasts at 48 body sites. In addition, as control injection, heat-denatured N'ase, X-irradiated myeloblasts, and supernatant of the incubation fluid were also injected. Reaction was measured by induration at 48 h. The injections of N'ase-treated myeloblasts produced no local lesions other than the delayed-type hypersensitivity reaction. No patients developed chills, fever, or adenopathy. No hypersensitivity reaction was apparent at the site of injection of physiological saline, heat-denatured N'ase, or the supernatant of cell incubation media. In patients randomized to receive MER, we used ten intradermal sites of 10 mg/0.1 ml each (total 1,000 mg MER). In patients receiving N'ase-treated allogeneic myeloblasts plus MER, the DCH reaction to the specific immunogen was reduced rather than increased, due to the intradermal injection of the nonspecific immunoadjuvant MER, when compared to the induration in patients immunized with neuraminidase-N'ase-treated myeloblasts alone from the same donor (Table 2).

Effect of Immunotherapy on Remission and Survival

Results of the interim analysis are presented below. Computer analysis of remission and survival data were carried out using the Kaplan and Meier method (J. Analytical-Statistical Analysis 53 : 547, 1968). Remission and survival curves were also compared using Breslow's extension of Gehan's generalized Wilcoxon test, the log rank procedure, and the Cox regression analysis.

The study originally consisted of a protocol of induction chemotherapy and maintenance with or without neuraminidase-treated cells. The chemotherapy consisted of 7 days cytosine arabinoside continuous infusion at 100 mg/m²/day and 3 days daunorubicin at 45 mg/m². All patients received cyclical maintenance chemotherapy every 4 weeks. The maintenance consisted of rotational cycles of cytosine arabinoside (100/mg/m² every 12 h i.v. × ten doses) and thioguanine (10 mg/m² every 12 h orally × 10), cytosine arabinoside as above and cyclophosphamide

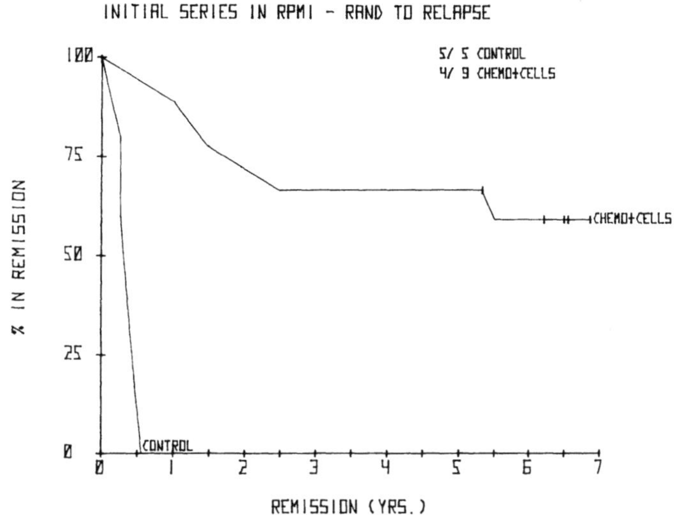

Fig. 1. Remission duration of patients with acute myelocytic leukemia immunized with neuraminidase-treated allogeneic myeloblasts. Remission duration is calculated from day of randomization

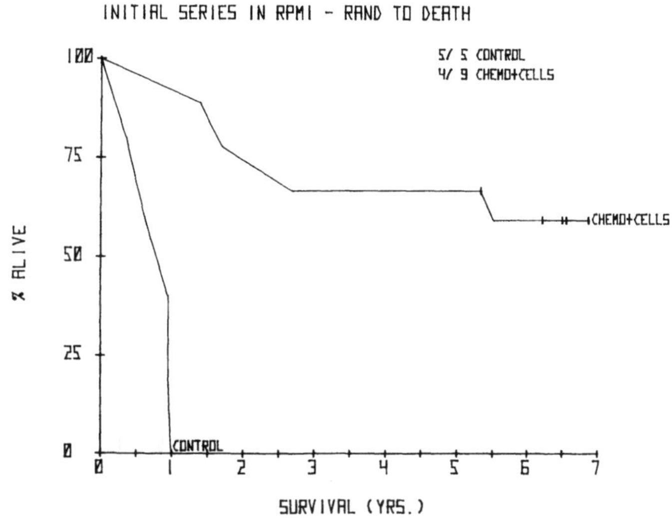

Fig. 2. Impact of immunotherapy on the survival of patients with acute myelocytic leukemia. Survival time is calculated from day of randomization

(1,000/m^2 i.v. $\times$ 1), and cytosine arabinoside as above and daunorubicin (45 mg/m^2 $\times$ 2). Beginning on day 8, after the first sustaining course of chemotherapy, and on day 15 of each cycle thereafter, patients were randomly allocated to receive chemotherapy alone or chemotherapy plus N'ase-treated myeloblasts.

Figs. 1 and 2 show the remission and survival curves of AML patients randomly allocated in our initial study. Four patients treated with chemotherapy plus N'ase-treated myeloblasts are still in their first remission in excess of 6 years. One immunized patient died of myocardial infarction in clinical remission on day 1941. All patients treated with chemotherapy alone relapsed within the first 12 months. The difference between the two remission curves is highly significant ($P < 0.0001$).

In the second series of patients, designated as New York Study 1, identical chemotherapy was used except that an additional maintenance cycle of cytosine

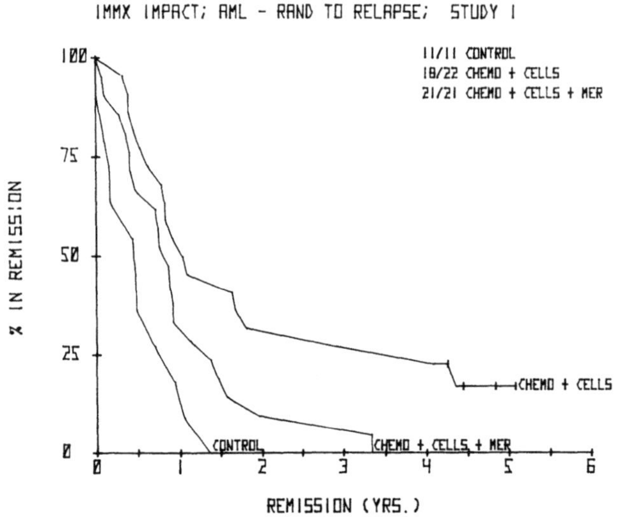

Fig. 3. Comparison of the effect of immunization with neuraminidase-treated allogeneic myeloblasts versus neuraminidase-treated allogeneic myeloblasts plus MER on the remission duration in patients with AML

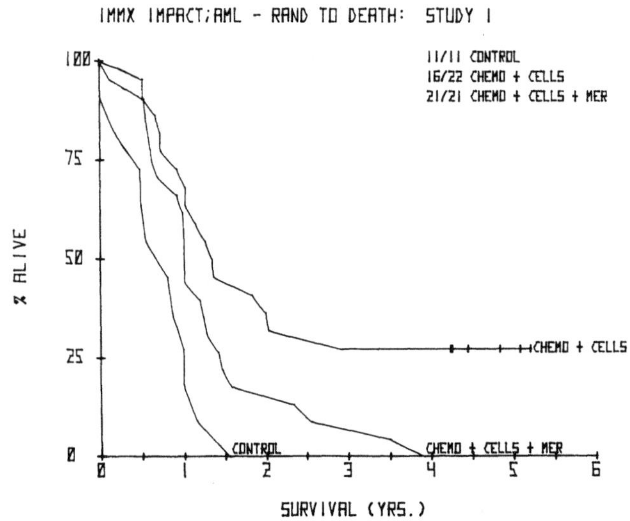

Fig. 4. Duration of survival in AML patients who received chemotherapy alone or specific or combination of specific plus adjuvant immunotherapy

arabinoside and CCNU was added. Three arms of randomization were used: chemotherapy alone; chemotherapy plus N'ase-treated myeloblasts as immunogen; and chemotherapy plus N'ase-modified allogeneic myeloblasts and MER, the methanol retraction residue of BCG. Data presented in Figs. 3 and 4 summarize the impact of specific immunotherapy and specific immunotherapy plus MER on the remission and survival of patients with AML as compared to the patients maintained on chemotherapy alone.

Comparison of the three groups' remission and survival times shows a difference of $P < 0.001$ (specific immunotherapy versus specific immunotherapy plus MER, $P = 0.004$). Four of 22 patients from the groups treated with N'ase-treated myeloblasts are still in their first remission and six are alive in excess of 4 years after randomization. Combination of specific plus adjuvant immunotherapy with MER did not act synergistically in the treatment of AML patients. Patients immunized with N'ase-treated myeloblasts plus the full prescribed dose of MER had a mean remission duration of 318 days and mean survival time of 416 days. All patients treated with a combination of N'ase-treated myeloblasts plus MER therapy relapsed and died by 3.5 years after the onset of therapy. Despite the poor performance of the patients who received this mode of immunotherapy, the difference between the control versus specific immunotherapy plus specific immunotherapy plus MER is still significant ($P = 0.04$).

Immunological Status of AML Patients in the Immunotherapy Study

In Vivo Skin Test with Recall Antigens

The in vivo immunologic status of each AML patient entered in the immunotherapy protocol was measured by DCH response to five antigens: tuberculin purified protein (PPD); mumps; Candida; Varidase (Lederle); and dermatophytin. In both immunotherapy studies, the initial skin testing was performed at the time of randomization. The skin tests were considered positive if the perpendicular bisector diameters of induration exceeded 5 mm when measured at 48 h.

Data obtained from study 1 are presented in Table 3. They show that initially there was considerable improvement in the response of AML patients receiving N'ase-treated myeloblasts or N'ase-treated myeloblasts plus MER, but not in patients treated with chemotherapy alone. There was continued improvement in the response to recall antigens in patients receiving N'ase-treated myeloblasts. However, the group treated with N'ase-treated cells plus MER showed a gradual decline. The decline or complete loss in response to recall antigens preceded subsequent relapse of those patients who had been receiving MER plus N'ase-treated myeloblasts. It is interesting to note that none of the patients treated with cells plus MER converted from PPD(−) to PPD(+) as was originally anticipated.

Partial Restoration of Percent and Absolute Number of T and B Lymphocytes

Quantification of the total mononuclear cells and E and EAC rosette-forming lymphocytes from patients in the chemoimmunotherapy study were routinely performed. Table 4 shows three test periods for each of the studies: the initial T and B lymphocytes and total mononuclear cells at the time of randomization; the impact of immunotherapy at 12 months; and after 24 months of chemoimmunotherapy. The median value for normal total mononuclear cells is 2,589; E-rosetting PBL is 74.4%, with 1,986 as the absolute number of T lymphocytes; EAC-rosetting PBL is 22.1%, with 251 as the number of absolute B lymphocytes. Patients at the time of randomization, still in recovery from induction and consolidation chemotherapy, showed a significantly lower number of mononuclear cells (range 837−981); T lymphocytes, a percentage of 49.2−53% and an absolute number of 412−519; and B lymphocytes, a percentage of 18.2−19.8% and an absolute number of 152−180. Patients receiving immunotherapy, specifically those immunized with N'ase-treated myeloblasts alone, showed continuous improvement in number of mononuclear cells,

Table 3. Delayed hypersensitivity response to the recall antigens in AML patients in the New York Study 1

Antigens	Percent of patients positive to skin test antigens[a]											
	At randomization			Month 12			Month 24			Month 36		
	Chemotherapy	Chemotherapy + cells	Chemotherapy + cells + MER	Chemotherapy	Chemotherapy + cells	Chemotherapy + cells + MER	Chemotherapy	Chemotherapy + cells	Chemotherapy + cells + MER	Chemotherapy	Chemotherapy + cells	Chemotherapy + cells + MER
PPD	9	13	10	0	0	8		7	33		0	0
Mumps	36	48	25	50	61	0		57	66		57	50
Candida	54	70	40	50	94	25		79	100		100	100
Varidase	54	65	55	75	94	50		100	100		100	100
Dermatophytin	27	22	15	25	50	0		29	33		43	50
No. of Patients tested	11	21	20	4	14	7	0[b]	11	3	0[b]	7	2

[a] Skin test diameter at 48 h ≧ 5 mm
[b] All control patients relapsed prior to chemotherapy cycle 24

Table 4. Lymphocyte subpopulations in AML patients in the chemoimmunotherapy study (mean ± SD)

	Treatment groups								
	Chemotherapy			Chemotherapy + N'ase cells			Chemotherapy + N'ase + MER		
	At randomization	At 12 months	At 24 months	At randomization	At 12 months	At 24 months	At randomization	At 12 months	At 23 months
Total mononuclear cells (number/mm)	981 ± 78	1,153 ± 128		837 ± 72	1,283 ± 91	1,601 ± 129[a]	941 ± 112	1,297 ± 89	1,307 ± 102
T cells									
Percentage	53	65.2		49.2	69.3	70.1	51.7	70.1	72.3
Absolute number	519 ± 47	752 ± 63		412 ± 35	889 ± 95[a]	1,122 ± 129[a]	487 ± 45	909 ± 101[a]	945 ± 93[a]
B cells									
Percentage	18.3	21.9		18.2	21.6	21.2	19.8	22.3	20.3
Absolute number	180 ± 21	253 ± 25		152 ± 13	277 ± 41	337 ± 35[a]	146 ± 17	289 ± 13	263 ± 28
Patients tested	11	4	0[b]	23	14	11	20	7	3

[a] Statistical significance between absolute E- or EAC-rosetting lymphocytes at the time of randomization vs. during therapy of AML ($P < 0.0001$)
[b] All control group patients relapsed in this study prior to course 24 of chemotherapy treatment

Table 5. Comparison of PHA-induced lymphoblastogenesis of AML patients immunized with neuraminidase-treated cells with or without MER

Status	Randomization			After course 12			After course 24		
	No. patients	cpm $10^3 \pm$ SEM	SI[c]	No. patients	cpm $10^3 \pm$ SEM	SI[c]	No. patients	cpm $10^3 \pm$ SEM	SI[c]
	Maximum stimulation induced by PHA[a]								
Normal donor	79	102.2 ± 8.7	257						
Chemotherapy alone	11	39.3 ± 4.3	87	4	56.9 ± 5.3	145			***
Chemotherapy + N'ase myeloblasts	23	37.12 ± 4.38	90	14	76.5 ± 7.3 $P = 0.0004$	233	11	88.5 ± 9.2 $P = 0.0001$	244
Chemotherapy + N'ase myeloblasts + MER	21	38.3 ± 5.4	85	7	51.2 ± 6.4 $P = 0.42$	113	3	69.9 ± 7.1 $P = 0.0008$	196
	Maximum stimulation induced by PWM[b]								
Normal donor	79	95.13 ± 6.4	194						
Chemotherapy alone	11	36.3 ± 4.9	66	4	53.7 ± 6.1	92			***
Chemotherapy + N'ase myeloblasts	23	35.8 ± 6.4	73	14	73.1 ± 6.9 $P = 0.0005$	145	11	83.2 ± 11.6 $P = 0.0001$	162
Chemotherapy + N'ase myeloblasts + MER	24	38.1 ± 4.9	79	7	46.60 ± 6.1 NS	68	3	61.7 ± 6.3 $P = 0.001$	139

[a] Maximum stimulation was attained with 30 μg PW mitogen per well or 0.30 μg/well with PHA
[b] Statistical significance in maximum stimulation at time of randomization vs. during therapy of AML patients
[c] Stimulation index = cpm of maximum stimulation/cpm of unstimulated lymphocytes

percentages, and absolute numbers of T and B lymphocytes as compared to values at the time of randomization or to patients treated with chemotherapy alone.

Lymphocyte Function

Lymphocyte blastogenesis for the peripheral blood lymphocytes (PBL) was determined by selected mitogens (PHA) and PWM. After isolation of PBL by the Ficoll-Hypaque gradient method, 100,000 PBL were cultured in each of the five replicate wells of Falcon microplates with RMPM 1630 medium supplemented with 20% autologous plasma in the presence of high-purity PHA and PWM. Maximum stimulation occurred at 0.15–0.03 μg per well for PHA and 30 μg per well for PWM from normal donors, as well as for the remission lymphocytes from patients randomized into the studies. Lymphocyte blastogenesis was determined by measuring the level of DNA synthesis upon addition of 1 μCi ^{3}H-thymidine to each well 18 h prior to termination of the culture. The data are represented as mean ± SE. The calculation of the stimulation index is based on cpm maximum stimulation/cpm unstimulated lymphocytes.

Table 5 summarizes the maximum lymphocyte stimulation induced by selective mitogens. A progressive restoration of lymphocyte function as measured by response to synthetic mitogens is apparent in PBL obtained from AML patients immunized with N'ase-treated myeloblasts as immunogen. The lymphocyte response to mitogens approached the normal range by 12 months after the start of vaccination with N'ase-modified myeloblasts (Table 5). However, there was no appreciable improvement in lymphocyte response to mitogens in AML patients who received chemotherapy alone.

Change of Lymphocyte Function in AML Patients Immunized with Neuraminidase-Treated Allogeneic Myeloblasts plus MER

We also compared the PHA and PWM stimulation of remission lymphocytes from patients immunized with N'ase-treated myeloblasts plus MER (Table 5). It was observed that during the first 6 months of immunotherapy in this group of patients there was an increase in PHA, and to a lesser degree in PWM-induced lymphoblastogenesis, followed by a gradual decline. As shown in Table 4, the decrease of blastogenesis is not attributable to any change in the T lymphocyte subpopulation of patients receiving cells plus MER as compared to those who were treated with cells alone. However, there was a marked change in response among the lymphocytes which formed stable rosettes at 4° with SRBC. The clinical and laboratory data obtained on patients treated with N'ase-treated myeloblasts plus MER are summarized in Fig. 5. Blastogenesis with PHA and DCH response were both in the normal range in patient M. K. through seven monthly cycles of MER (100 μg) in ten sites each. A sharp decline in both blastogenic transformation and DCH was recognized and at the next cycle MER was omitted. There was a prompt recovery in both the DCH and PHA blastogenesis and therefore MER was reinstituted at an attenuated dose. This was followed by further decline in the immunologic parameters and by relapse soon thereafter.

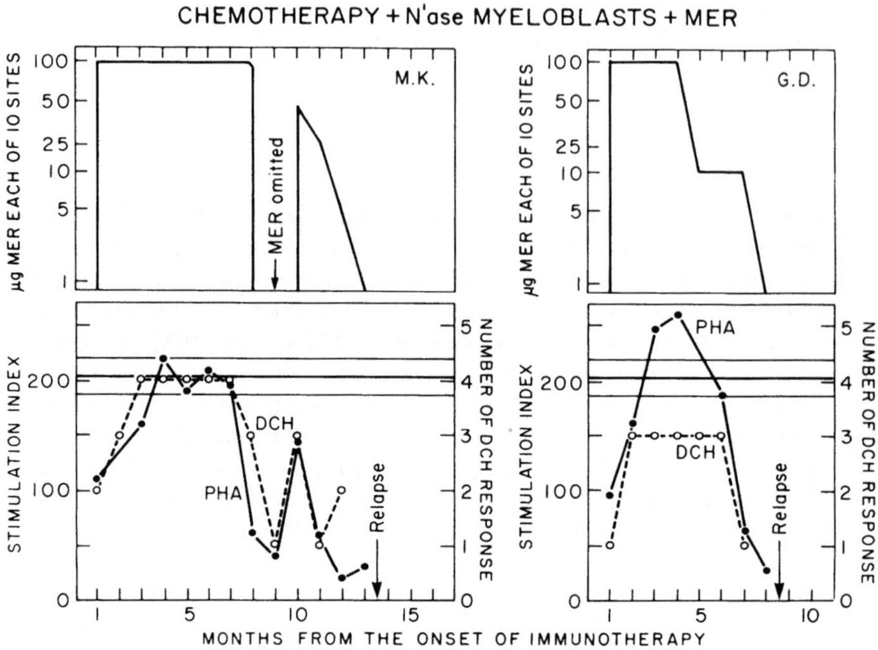

Fig. 5. Impact of neuraminidase-treated myeloblasts plus MER on various immunologic parameters in AML patients

In the case of patient G. D. a similar decline from high normal levels of PHA blastogenesis and DCH was encountered during MER plus in N'ase-treated cells. Reduction in MER dose from 1,000 μg was practiced nonetheless, accompanied by continued decline in in vivo and in vitro lymphocyte function.

The fact that AML patients treated with N'ase-treated myeloblasts plus MER appear to be similar to patients treated with cells alone in their level of percentage and absolute number of E-rosetting PBL, but have decreased in vitro and in vivo lymphocyte function, raised the possibility that the T cells might exhibit normal function when separated from inhibitory mononuclear cells. Indeed, enriched T cell fractions from AML patients immunized with N'ase-treated cells plus MER who exhibited a declining in vitro and in vivo immunologic response, gave three- to five-times greater thymidine incorporation in response to PHA than did unseparated PBL. The response of enriched T cells was, however, strongly inhibited by addition of autologous adherent cells. In contrast, the nonadherent nonrosetting autologous lymphocytes, or addition of normal adherent cells, did not alter the T cell function. These findings suggest that depression of cell-mediated immunity seen in most of the tested AML patients who received N'ase-treated myeloblasts plus MER, but not N'ase-treated myeloblasts alone, may be due to the suppression of T cell functions by circulating monocytes.

It is apparent that MER can impair the therapeutic activity of N'ase-treated myeloblasts. The time of appearance of apparent suppressor cell activity was different from patient to patient. Based on our observations, it is suggested that the nonspecific immunostimulation of MER is not advantageous in the presence of N'ase-modified myeloblasts.

References

1. Bagshawe KD, Currie GA (1968) Immunogenicity of L1210 murine leukemia cells after treatment with neuraminidase. Nature 218: 1254
2. Bekesi JG, St Arneault G, Holland JF (1971) Increase of leukemia L1210 immunogenicity by *Vibrio cholerae* neuraminidase treatment. Cancer Res 31: 2130
3. Bekesi JG, St Arneault G, Walter L, Holland JG (1972) Immunogenicity of leukemia L1210 cells after neuraminidase treatment. J Natl Cancer Inst 41: 107
4. Bekesi JG, Roboz JP, Walter L, Holland JF (1974) Stimulation of specific immunity against cancer by neuraminidase-treated tumor cells. Behring Inst Mitt 55: 309
5. Bekesi JG, Holland JF, Fleminger R, et al. (1977) Immunotherapeutic efficacy of neuraminidase-treated allogeneic myeloblasts in patients with acute myelocytic leukemia. In: Chirigos MA (ed) Control of neoplasia by modulation of the immune system. Raven Press, New York, p 573
6. Bekesi JG, Roboz JP, Holland JF (1976) Therapeutic effectiveness of neuraminidase-treated tumor cells as an immunogen in man and experimental animals with leukemia. Ann NY Acad Sci 277: 313
7. Bekesi JG, Holland JF (1979) Impact of specific immunotherapy in acute myelocytic leukemia. In: Neth R (ed) Modern trends in human leukemia III. Springer, Berlin Heidelberg New York, p 79
8. Currie GA, Bagshawe KD (1969) Tumor-specific immunogenicity of methylcholanthrene-induced sarcoma cells after incubation in neuraminidase. Br J Cancer 23: 141
9. Gutterman JU, Rodriquez V, Mavligit G, Burgess MA, Geham E, Hersh EM, McCredie KB, Reed R, Smith T, Bodey GP, Freireich EJ (1974) Chemoimmunotherapy of adult acute leukemia: Prolongation of remission in myeloblastic leukemia with BCG. Lancet 2: 1405
10. Holland JF, Bekesi JG (1976) Immunotherapy of human leukemia with neuraminidase-modified cells. Med Clin North Am 60: 539
11. Hughes RC, Sanford BH, Jeanloz RW (1972) Regeneration of the surface glycoproteins of a transplantable mouse tumor cells after treatment with neuraminidase. Proc Natl Acad Sci USA 69: 942
12. Lee A (1968) Effect of neuraminidase on the phagocytosis of heterologous red cells by mouse peripheral macrophages. Proc Soc Exp Biol Med 128: 891
13. Lindenmann J, Klein PA (1967) Immunological aspects of viral oncolysis. Recent Adv Cancer Res 9: 66
14. Mathe G (1972) Immunological approaches to the treatment of acute leukemia. Clin Haematol 1: 165
15. Powles RL, Crowther D, Bateman CJ, Beard ME, McElwain TJ, Russell J (1973) Immunotherapy for acute myelogenous leukemia. 28: 365
16. Sanford BH (1967) An alteration in tumor histocompatability induced by neuraminidase. Transplantation 5: 1273
17. Schmidtke JR, Simmons RL (1975) Augmented uptake of neuraminidase-treated sheep red blood cells: Participation of opsome factors. J Natl Cancer Inst 54: 1379
18. Sedlacek HH, Seiler FR (1978) Immunotherapy of neoplastic diseases with neuraminidase: Contradictions, new aspects, and revised concepts. Cancer Immunol Immunother 5: 153
19. Sedlacek HH, Seiler FR, Schwick HG (1977) Neuraminidase and tumor immunotherapy. Klin Wochenschr 55: 199
20. Sethi KK, Brandis H (1973) Neuraminidase-induced loss in the transplantability of murine leukemia L1210 induction of immunoprotection and the transfer of induced immunity to normal DBA/2 mice by serum and peritoneal cells. Br J Cancer 27: 106
21. Sethi KK, Frandis H (1973) Synergistic cytotoxic effect of macrophages and normal mouse serum on neuraminidase-treated murine leukemia cells. Eur J Cancer 9: 809
22. Sethi KK, Teschner M (1974) Neuraminidase-induced immunospecific destruction of transplantable experimental tumors. Postepy Hig Med Dosw 28: 103

9. *Maintenance Chemoimmunotherapy of Nonlymphoblastic Acute Leukemias*

R. Favre, G. Sebahoun, D. Bagarry-Liégey, C. Imbert,
P. Ciardelli, J. A. Gastaut, G. Meyer, and Y. Carcassonne*

Institut J. Paoli, I. Calmettes, 232 Boulevard de Ste. Marguerite, F-13009 Marseille, France

Summary

A trial of maintenance chemotherapy of nonlymphoblastic acute leukemia led to a comparison of two groups of patients in complete remission. Group 1 (14 patients) received only monthly reinduction chemotherapy. Group 2 (17 patients) received identical chemotherapy together with weekly immunotherapy combining BCG and irradiated leukemic cells. While the duration of the first complete remission was unmodified, the overall survival time and, above all, survival after the first relapse were prolonged in group 2 chemoimmunotherapy. These results were all the more marked when a homogeneous group of patients having received the same induction chemotherapy were considered.

Introduction

Chemotherapy has improved the prognosis of nonlymphoblastic acute leukemias (NLAL). However, long remissions are not common [7] and complete remissions (CR) are usually short [6]. According to Hamilton Fairley [10, 11], we added immunotherapy to maintenance treatment of NLAL patients in CR. We compared two groups of patients; one treated with chemoimmunotherapy and the other with chemotherapy alone. This trial was started in 1973, and 31 patients with NLAL achieved CR and entered the trial up to June, 1977. We reported our results 3 years ago, i.e., 7 years after starting the trial.

Patients and Methods

Chemotherapies used to induce CR were as follows: for 19 patients, daunorubicin (2 mg/kg/day from day 1–3) plus ara C (3 mg/kg from day 1–7) (protocol A); for seven patients, ara C (3 mg/kg from day 1–7) plus thioguanine (3 mg/kg from day 1–7) (protocol B); and for five patients, rubidazone (4 mg/kg from day 1–3) plus

* We wish to thank Mrs. M. Mouren for efficient technical help and J. Ingrand for illustrations

Recent Results in Cancer Research, Vol. 80

thioguanine (3 mg/kg from day 1–7). When CR was achieved, maintenance therapy consisted of monthly inductions using ara C (3 mg/kg from day 1–5) and/or thioguanine (given ID) plus daunorubicin (1 mg/kg on days 1 and 2). Fourteen patients were given chemotherapy alone (group 1) and 17 others were given chemoimmunotherapy (group 2).

Immunotherapy was 1×10^9 allogenic irradiated leukemic myeloblasts weekly and BCG (Pasteur F) using a Sterneedle (Heaf gun) at a dose of 75 mg crude BCG. Allogeneic cells were chosen because of immunologic purposes, solving the difficulty of collecting large numbers of cells for immunotherapy from every patient. The cells were preserved less than 6 months at −90° C and irradiated (100 GY) before decongelation thawing).

The statistical analysis of results was made by actuarial methods [12]. There was no real randomization of patients, although their distribution into the two groups was determined by their place of residence, i.e., those who lived far away from the hospital were not given immunotherapy which needed hospitalization.

Results

Table 1 shows patient distribution according to sex, age, and blast cell type. There are more women in group 2 and patients are younger. Table 2 gives more details concerning group 1, including some of the usual prognotic data, such as white blood cell count (WBC) and blast cells in blood and bone marrow. Table 3 gives the same information concerning group 2, showing no significant difference between the two groups, especially concerning WBC and blast cell count.

Table 4 shows that in group 1, four patients are still alive and three remain in CR. The 11 others relapsed: One is in his fourth relapse and ten have died. Table 5 shows that in groups 2, four patients are still in CR and the 13 others have died.

We made statistical analyses of actuarial curves of survival times since diagnosis (Fig. 1), of first CR (Fig. 2), and of survival time since first relapse (Fig. 3). The duration of survival is slightly longer for group 2, but the difference is not significant.

Table 1. Distribution of patients

	Total	Group 1 (chemotherapy)	Group 2 (immunotherapy)
No. of patients	31	14	17
Sex (males/females)	17/14	11/3	6/11
Age (years)	15–66	24–66 (mean 43.8)	15–64 (mean 36.4)
Cytology			
AML	21	9	12
AMML	6	3	3
APL	3	1	2
AMonoL	1	1	0

AML, Acute myeloblastic leukaemia; AMML, Acute myelomonocytic leukaemia; APL, Acute promyelocytic leukaemia; AMonoL, Acute monoblastic leukaemia

Table 2. Fourteen patients treated with chemotherapy alone

Patient	Cytology	Age (years)	Sex	WBC/mm³	Blast cells (%)		Protocol
					Blood	Bone marrow	
1	AMML	30	F	10,700	98	68	A
2	AMML	43	F	2,900	34	50	A
3	AML	37	F	30,000	80	80	A
4	AMML	55	M	36,000	57	79	B
5	AMonoL	52	M	87,000	92	90	A
6	APL	58	M	2,200	16	95	C
7	AML	27	M	73,000	85	95	B
8	AML	54	M	42,000	91	67	A
9	AML	24	M	22,600	94	88	B
10	AML	57	M	8,300	37	70	A
11	AML	27	M	15,300	36	30	A
12	AML	66	M	32,000	98	86	C
13	AML	36	M	15,400	5	45	A
14	AML	47	M	4,900	0	22	C

AML, Acute myeloblastic leukaemia; AMML, Acute myelomonocytic leukaemia; APL, Acute promyelocytic leukaemia; AMonoL, Acute monoblastic leukaemia

Table 3. Seventeen patients treated with chemoimmunotherapy

Patient	Cytology	Age (years)	Sex	WBC/mm³	Blast cells (%)		Protocol
					Blood	Bone marrow	
1	AMML	49	F	100,000	100	100	A
2	AMML	22	F	2,700	17	83	C
3	APL	16	F	102,000	22	74	C
4	APL	15	F	8,900	78	85	A
5	AML	56	F	5,200	73	25	A
6	AML	24	F	2,500	13	54	B
7	AML	26	F	53,000	75	66	A
8	AML	56	F	7,100	48	80	B
9	AML	33	F	34,000	93	71	A
10	AML	36	F	39,000	92	95	B
11	AML	19	F	14,600	60	70	A
12	AMML	53	M	35,000	85	60	A
13	AML	46	M	18,000	27	66	B
14	AML	24	M	6,200	82	57	A
15	AML	37	M	11,000	52	80	A
16	AML	43	M	6,100	25	60	A
17	AML	64	M	110,000	98	91	A

AML, Acute myeloblastic leukaemia; AMML, Acute myelomonocytic leukaemia; APL, Acute promyelocytic leukaemia

Table 4. Results in patients treated with chemotherapy alone (in days)

Patient	Cytology	Duration of CR 1	Duration of CR 2	Duration of CR 3	
1	AMML	553	178	127	Relapse 4
2	AMML	769	–	–	Died (relapse 1)
3	AML	609	–	–	Died (relapse 1)
4	AMML	1,957	–	–	CR 1
5	AMonoL	115	–	–	Died (relapse 1)
6	APL	76	978	–	CR 2
7	AML	30	–	–	Died (relapse 1)
8	AML	300	–	–	Died (relapse 1)
9	AML	386	69	–	Died (relapse 2)
10	AML	187	–	–	Died (relapse 1)
11	AML	672	–	–	Died (relapse 1)
12	AML	313	–	–	Died (relapse 1)
13	AML	632	–	–	CR 1
14	AML	287	130	–	Died (relapse 2)

Median (months) 11
AML, Acute myeloblastic leukaemia; AMML, Acute myelomonocytic leukaemia; APL, Acute promyelocytic leukaemia; AMonoL, Acute monoblastic leukaemia

Table 5. Results in patients treated with chemoimmunotherapy (in days)

Patient	Cytology	Duration of CR 1	Duration of CR 2	Duration of CR 3	
1	AMML	194	–	–	Died (CR 1)[a]
2	AMML	1,889	–	–	CR 1
3	APL	128	–	–	Died (relapse 1)
4	APL	377	181	57	Died (relapse 3)
5	AML	718	150	–	Died (relapse 2)
6	AML	196	42	–	Died (relapse 2)
7	AML	251	158	–	Died (relapse 2)
8	AML	49	–	–	Died (relapse 1)
9	AML	317	–	–	Died (relapse 1)
10	AML	151	–	–	Died (relapse 1)
11	AML	198	–	–	Died (relapse 1)
12	AMML	342	424	1,100	CR 3
13	AML	225	163	–	Died (relapse 2)
14	AML	1,251	573	725	CR 3
15	AML	31	76	17	Died (CR 3)[a]
16	AML	2,163	–	–	CR 1
17	AML	304	–	–	Died (relapse 1)

Median (months) 11
[a] Daunorubicin accident
AML, Acute myeloblastic leukaemia; AMML, Acute myelomonocytic leukaemia; APL, Acute promyelocytic leukaemia

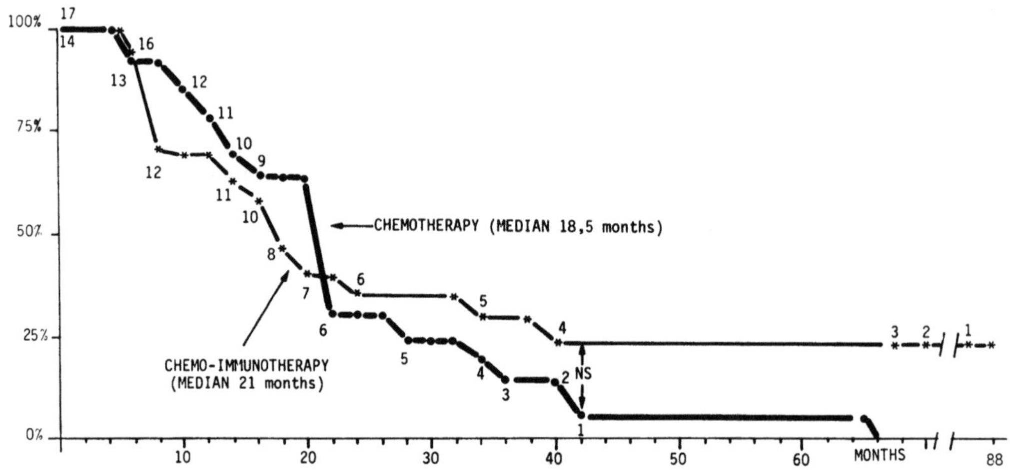

Fig. 1. Actuarial curve of survival time from diagnosis

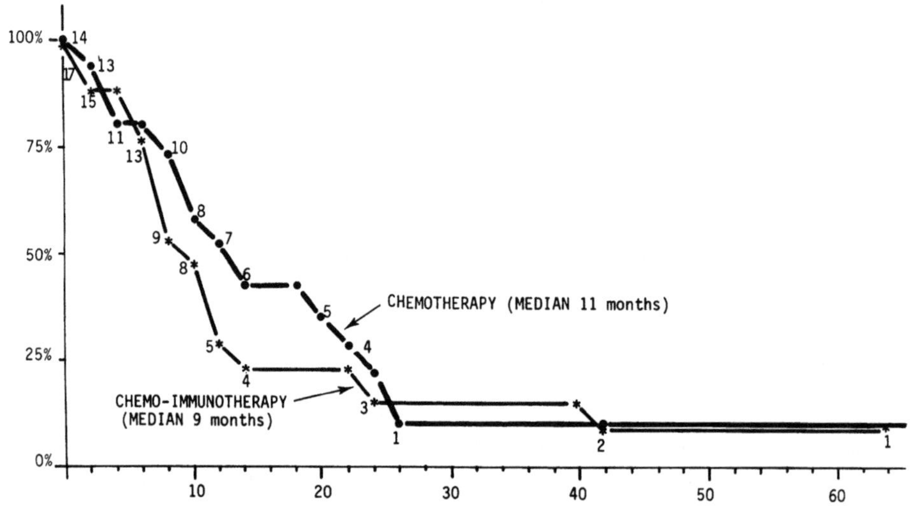

Fig. 2. Actuarial curve of duration of first complete remission

We analysed separately the results of the 19 patients who had the same induction chemotherapy (group 1). Table 6 shows the distribution of patients treated with protocol A.

Actuarial curve of duration of first CR (Fig. 4) shows a better result for group 2, but the difference is not significant. However, actuarial curve of survival time since diagnosis (Fig. 5) shows a significant difference for group 2, (chemoimmunotherapy) after month 40. A significant difference is also observed for group 2, after the sixteenth month, on the actuarial curve of survival time since first relapse (Fig. 6).

We found, as have others [5, 15], that second and even third remissions were relatively easy to obtain for our immunotherapy patients.

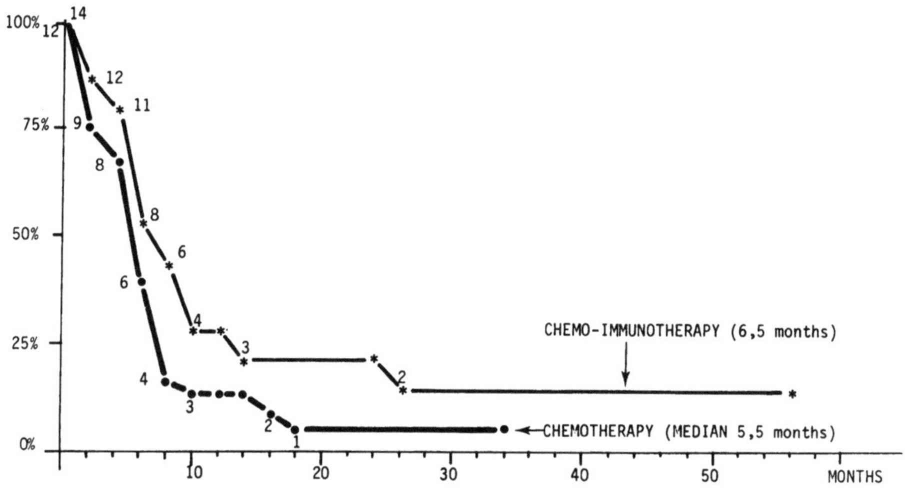

Fig. 3. Actuarial curve of survival time from first relapse

Table 6. Distribution of patients treated with protocol A

No. of patients	Total 19	Chemotherapy 8	Chemoimmunotherapy 11
Sex (male/female)	10/9	5/3	5/6
Age (years)	15–64	27–57 (mean 42)	15–64 (mean 39.5)
Cytology			
AML	15	5	8
AMML	4	2	2
APL	1	0	1
AMonoL	1	1	0

Median (months) 11
AML, Acute myeloblastic leukaemia; AMML, Acute myelomonocytic leukaemia; APL, Acute promyelocytic leukaemia; AMonoL, Acute monoblastic leukaemia

Discussion

Our study has shown increased survival times but no modification in first-remission duration, and Whittaker [15] also found a significant increase in survival time after relapse, which explains the increased total survival. Much research has been done on this subject since the first trial of Mathé in acute lymphoblastic leukemia. A great variety of immunotherapeutic agents have been examined; BCG alone (Glaxo, Pasteur, etc.) [1, 3, 13], BCG plus allogeneic cells with or without maintenance chemotherapy [7, 8], allogeneic cells plus MER, MER alone, and allogeneic cells plus *parvum* or *Pseudomonas* vaccine [14]. The results show a longer total survival time [1, 8, 14] but not a longer first CR. We found no correlation with the occasional infections

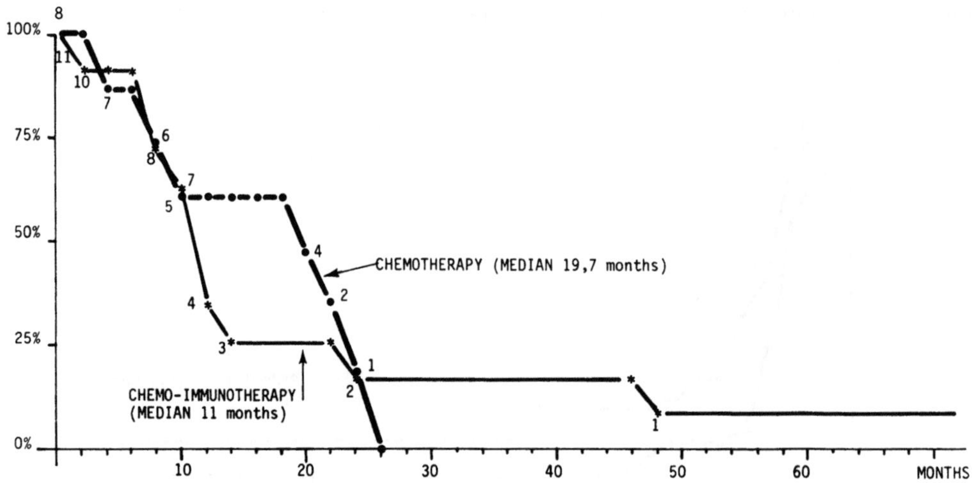

Fig. 4. Actuarial curve of group A. Duration of first complete remission

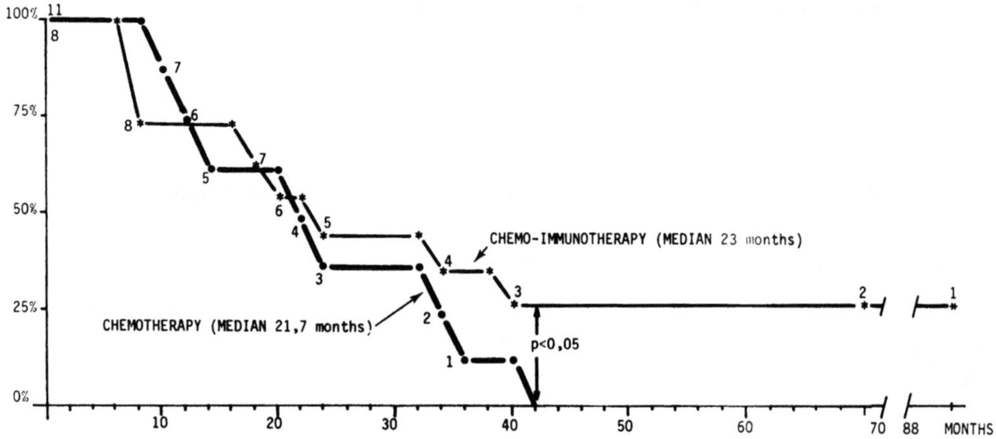

Fig. 5. Actuarial curve group A. Survival time from diagnosis

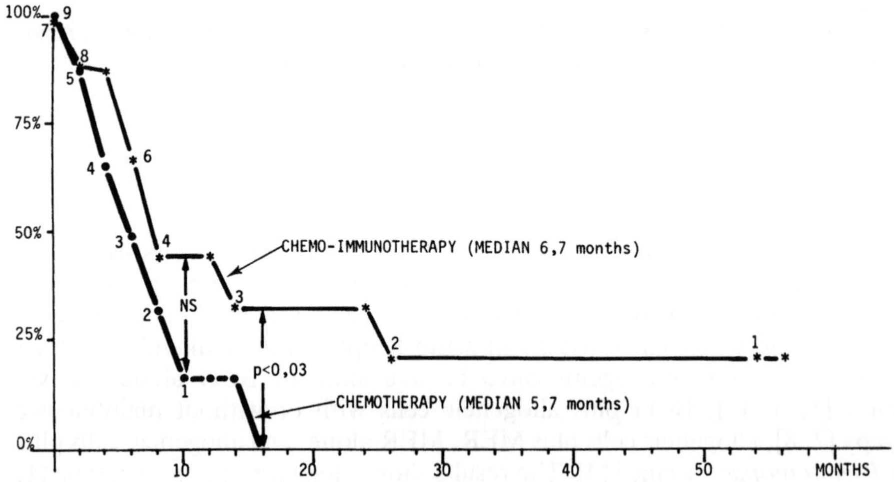

Fig. 6. Actuarial curve group A. Survival time from first relapse

in such patients, which would have suggested increased nonspecific antigerm immunity [5].

It is likely that immunotherapy has little influence on leukemia itself, but increases bone marrow defense against chemotherapy.

The results of immunotherapy in acute nonlymphoblastic leukemias could be improved by the use of more specific immunostimulating agents and by the modification of leukemic cell surface to allow better recognition of antigens.

References

1. Alexander P, Powles R (1978) Immunotherapy of human acute leukaemia. Clin Haematol 7: 275–294
2. Eppinger-Helft M, Pavlowsky S, Hidalgo G, Muriel FS, Suarez A, Garay G, Russo C, Santos M, Macchi A, Lein J (1980) Chemoimmunotherapy with *Corynebacterium parvum* in acute myelocitic leukemia. Cancer 45: 280–284
3. Ezaki K, Hersh EM, Keating M, Dyre S, Hollinshead A, McCredie KB, Mavlight GM, Guterman JV (1978) Active specific immunisation with allogenic leukemia associated antigens or irradiated allogenic leukemia cells in acute leukemia. Cancer 41: 70–83
4. Gale RP (1979) Advances in the treatment of acute myelogenous leukemia. N Engl J Med 300: 1189–1199
5. Galton DA (1979) Can remission duration be prolonged in acute myeloid leukaemia? Recent Results Cancer Res 69: JJ–62
6. Gunz FW, Vincent PC (1977) Towards a cure of acute granulocytic leukaemia? Leuk Res 1: 51–66
7. Harris R, Zuhrie SR, Freeman CB, Taylor GM, McIver JE, Geary CG, Delamore IW, Hull PJ, Tooth JA (1978) Active immunotherapy in acute myelogenous leukaemia and the induction of second and subsequent remissions. Br J Cancer 37: 282–288
8. Holland JF, Bekesi JG, Cuttner J (1978) Immunotherapy of human cancer. Raven Press, New York, pp 237–244
9. Jacquillat C, Weil M, Gemon MF, Izrael V, Schaison G, Auclerc G, Ablin AR, Flandrin G, Tanzer J, Bussel A, Weisgerber C, Dresh C, Najean Y, Goudemand M, Seligman M, Boiron M, Bernard J (1973) Evaluation of 216 four-year survivors of acute leukemia. Cancer 32: 286–293
10. Powles RL (1979) The application of immunotherapy to the treatment of cancer. Pharmacol Ther 4: 281–306
11. Powles RL, Crowther D, Bateman CJT, Beard MEI, Mc Elwain JJ, Russell J, Lister TA, Whitehouse JMA, Wrigley PFM, Pike M, Alexander P, Hamilton Fairley G (1973) Immunotherapy for acute myelogenous leukaemia. Br J Cancer 28: 365–372
12. Schwartz D, Flamant R, Lellouch J (1970) L'essai therapeutique chez l'homme. Flammarion, Paris
13. Vogler WR, Chan VK (1974) Prolonging remission in myeloblastic leukaemia by Tice-strain bacillus Calmette-Guérin. Lancet 2: 128–131
14. Whiteside MG, Gauchi MN, Paton C, Stone JJ (1976) Chemoimmunotherapy for maintenance in acute myeloblastic leukemia. Cancer 38: 1581–1586
15. Whittaker JA (1980) Immunotherapy in the treatment of acute leukaemia. Br J Haematol 45: 187–193

10. *Possible Mechanisms of Immunotherapy Action in Acute Nonlymphatic Leukemia: Macrophage Production of Colony-Stimulating Activity**

P. Reizenstein, B. Andersson, and M. Beran

Karolinska Hospital, Division of Hematology, Department of Medicine, S-104 01 Stockholm, Sweden

Summary

Earlier studies show that immunotherapy (IT) improves prognosis in acute nonlymphatic leukemia (ANLL), and that ANLL cells probably have tumor-associated antigens, for autologous lymphocytes can react to them. Also, IT seems to immunize against allogeneic ANLL cells, but there is no cross-immunity to autologous ones. Moreover, patients immunized against their ANLL cells have no better prognosis than patients not having lymphocytes reacting to their ANLL cells.
It has also been suggested that IT causes nonspecific immunostimulation, but IT patients' lymphocytes actually react less than those of patients not given IT. The current hypothesis is macrophage activation: Lymphocyte suppression in IT could be explained by suppressor macrophages. Colony-stimulating activity, produced by bone marrow macrophages, decreases during remission in patients not given IT, but not in IT patients. Numerically, blood cells from patients given IT form more colonies than those from patients not given IT. Three of eight patients given IT had more colonies than the upper normal limit.

Introduction

Immunotherapy (IT) with BCG and/or leukemic cells has been reported to prolong the duration of first remission [10], the frequency of second remission [3], and survival [11] in most, but not all reported studies. The mechanism of IT action is unknown and the following hypothetical mechanisms will be considered: (1) Immunization against tumor-specific group antigens, followed by immune surveillance and immune defense; (2) nonspecific immunostimulation; and/or (3) macrophage activation.
In a series of studies we tried to examine these three hypotheses. It has been shown earlier [5] and could be confirmed [2, 14] that human ANLL cells do probably have tumor-associated antigens. Moreover, at least relative to the immunity to allogeneic lymphocytes, some immunity to allogeneic ANLL cells seems to develop in the later part of remission during IT [12]. However, IT with allogeneic cells does not seem to produce more frequent or more intense reactivity against autologous cells [9].

* Supported by grant 699 : B80 from the Swedish Cancer Research Foundation

Recent Results in Cancer Research, Vol. 80

Moreover, even in the patients whose remission lymphocytes do react with their own ANLL cells, prognosis is no better [8, 9]. For these reasons, hypothesis 1 seems unlikely.

Hypothesis 2 also seems unlikely to be true, since, if it were, lymphocytes from IT patients would be expected to react more than those of patients not given IT, while they actually react less [12]. Therefore, hypothesis 3 was studied, since it was recently shown in a murine system that BCG injections caused an elevation in serum colony-stimulating activity (CSA) values [14]. The first of the macrophage functions studied was phagocytosis and killing of *Candida albicans* [6], but no difference was found between patients given and those not given IT. Therefore, a second macrophage function, namely, production of CSA, was studied.

Patients and Methods

In vitro cultures of bone marrow and peripheral mononuclear white blood cells (MWBC) were performed in nine patients (29–59 years of age) with ANLL in remission, maintained with chemotherapy (CT) plus IT with BCG plus viable allogeneic ANLL cells [15], and in seven patients (22–64 years of age) given only CT.

The culture method has been previously described [1]. Briefly, 10^5 buffy-coat bone marrow cells (BCBM) and 5×10^5 MWBC were mixed with 1 ml modified McCoy's 5A medium with 0.3% agar (w/v) and 15% FCS and plated in 35 mm Petri dishes. Conditioned medium from MWBC served as a source of CSA. The CSA was incorporated as a feeder layer in a concentration giving a maximal number of colonies, as tested with normal human bone marrow cells as target. The fraction of granulocyte-monocyte-colony forming cells (GM-CFC) in S-phase was determined by the ^{3}H-TdR technique.

To assay the CSA-producing capacity, 5×10^5 and 10^6 BCBM cells were incorporated as a feeder layer prepared as above but with 0.5% agar. There was always a parallel control with conditioned medium in the feeder layer. As target cells, 10^5 normal BCBM cells were obtained from a healthy donor.

The cultures were incubated for 6 days in a fully humidified atmosphere of 5% CO_2 in air. At the end of the culture period, clones of 8–50 cells were scored as clusters and clones of more than 50 cells as colonies by the use of a Zeiss inverted phase contrast microscope. Repeated assays were performed in 13 of 16 patients and a total of 35 assays were performed.

Results

No significant difference was found between CT plus IT and CT patients regarding the colony and cluster formation in bone marrow and peripheral MWBC. Numerically, the CT plus IT patients' MWBC formed more colonies that the CT patients' (Table 1). The colony formation of bone marrow cells was higher than the upper normal limit in three of eight CT plus IT and one of seven CT patients. The fraction of GM-CFG in S-phase is shown in Table 1. CSA production was numerically somewhat higher in the CT plus IT than in the CT group (Table 2). The gradual reduction in granulo-

Table 1. Bone marrow and blood cell cloning capacity. Weighted means ± SD

	Bone marrow cells					Blood cells (MWBC)		
	No. subjects	No. tests	Colonies per 10^5 cells	Clusters per 10^5 cells	GM-CFC in S-phase (%)	No. tests	Colonies per 10^6 cells	Clusters per 10^6 cells
CT + IT	8	18	148.2 ± 46.9	158.6 ± 24.7	36.8 ± 9.1	19	13.0 ± 18.3	28.7 ± 36.6
CT	7	12	145 ± 45.1	161.2 ± 34.2	44.7 ± 15.3	11	6.5 ± 4.6	21.4 ± 15.4
Normal range [1]	13	13	88 ± 51[a]	103 ± 52[a]	ND	13	43 ± 47	31 ± 19

[a] $P < 0.05$

Table 2. Bone marrow production of colony-stimulating activity (CSA) in percent of normal standard assayed simultaneously. Weighted means ± SD

	No. subjects	No. tests	CSA (% ± SD)	No. of subjects with a gradual decrease of > 20% in CSA of initial value in patients where more than one assay was done
CT + IT	8	17	96.5 ± 27.7	0/7
CT	7	13	85.5 ± 36.4	3/5
			Not significant	$P < 0.05$

cyte-monocyte-colony stimulating factor (GM-CSF) seen in most CT patients was not found in CT plus IT and this difference may be significant (Table 2).

Discussion

Published results of IT with BCG plus viable leukemic cells show slightly, though significantly, prolonged first remission duration, frequency of second remission, and survival [3, 4, 10–12]. The three hypothetical mechanisms outlined initially will be considered here.

There may in fact be leukemia-associated antigens, for leukemic relapse marrow stimulates autologous lymphocytes significantly more than remission marrow, and one of four patients have circulating blast cells capable of stimulating their own lymphocytes [9]. It also seems possible to immunize with IT against allogeneic leukemia cells [12], since the reaction of lymphocytes to allogeneic leukemic blasts was significantly higher in relation to that against allogeneic lymphocytes, in patients given IT plus CT than in patients given only CT. This was true both in vitro and in vivo. No evidence was found that these antigens are cross-reactive, since the lymphocyte reaction to autologous blast cells was not stronger or more frequent in the patients given IT plus CT than those given only CT [9]. No evidence for immune surveillance or immune defense was found, since prognoses in patients with lymphocytes stimulated by autologous leukemic cells was no better than in patients without this autoimmunity to blast cells [8, 9]. Preliminary results did not indicate better prognoses in patients given IT with BCG plus leukemic cells than those given IT with BCG alone [11]. Therefore, the mechanism is not believed to be surveillance and rejection of cells with tumor-specific antigens.

Nonspecific immunostimulation is not likely to be the mechanism. During the later part of remission, the lymphocyte reactivity to nonspecific stimulators like phytohemagglutinen (PHA) and allogeneic lymphocytes in the patients given IT plus CT was not higher than that in the patients given CT only. Had this been the case, one might have suggested that IT results in nonspecific immunostimulation. However, the IT plus CT reactivity was significantly lower [12] than that in the CT patients. Thus, IT actually results in nonspecific immunosuppression.

Some preliminary evidence for macrophage activation is being found. While the phagocytic and fungicidal activity of individual macrophages, as well as the monocyte number, was the same in CT plus IT and CT [6], there were significantly fewer patients in the CT plus IT group, compared to the CT group, whose CSA activity decreased during late remission. This may suggest a stimulation of the macrophage CSA production. The immune suppression in the CT plus IT groups could be a result of IT stimulation of suppressor macrophages.

There is appreciable support in experimental systems for the long-lasting inhibition by maintenance cytostatics of suppressor cells [16] and of the activation by BCG of both the chemotactic [7], CSA-producing [2], and cytotoxic macrophage effects. If this rather nonspecific maintenance, by BCG and despite cytostatics, of the macrophage suppressor and CSA-producing functions is really the mechanism of It action, this would also explain the slight and temporary effect of IT. However, once in vitro methods become available to measure IT activity, more efficient schedules may perhaps be devised. For instance, ANLL subclasses could be designated where IT is more active than others. Some studies [10] suggest that the subgroup of acute myeloblastic leukemia showing remission most easily may respond, while those patients who are more difficult to bring into remission may be refractory to IT. In ALL, there are indications that HLA-BW17 patients may respond better than others (Tursz, in preparation). In ANLL, HLA-B12 patients show remission more easily than others [4]. It is therefore possible that an IT-sensitive subgroup of patients with ANLL can be defined.

References

1. Beran M, Reizenstein P, Udén A-M (1980) Response to treatment in acute non-lymphatic leukemia: Prognostic value of colony-forming and colony-stimulating capacities of bone marrow and blood cells compared to other parameters. Br J Haematol 44: 39–50
2. Butler N (1978) Colony-stimulating activity after BCG stimulation. Proc Natl Acad Sci USA 75: 289–296
3. Galton D, Kay H, Reizenstein P, Penchansky M, Vogler W, Whittaker J (1977) Infection and second-remission rates in patients having immunotherapy for acute myeloid leukemia. Lancet 2: 973
4. Harris R, Zuhrie A, Read C, Freeman C, Melver JE, Geary CG, Delamore IW, Tooth N (to be published) Randomised trial of immunotherapy alone versus no maintenance treatment in adult AML. In: Terry W (ed) Immunotherapy of cancer. Raven Press, New York
5. Hollinshead AC (1978) Active-specific immunotherapy. Immunotherapy of human cancer. Raven Press, New York, pp 213–232
6. Miale T, Stenke L, Penschansky M, Lehtinen T, Reizenstein P (1979) The role of macrophages in phagocytosis and mixed leukocyte reactivity in human acute myeloid leukemia. Immunol Commun 8: 279
7. Norris D, Weston W, Tuberger D, Rose B, Odom L (1979) Immunotherapy as therapeutic regimen. Cancer Immunol Immunother 7: 15–18
8. Ohno R, Yamada K, Ezaki K (1979) Response of remission lymphocytes to autochthonous leukemic cells, no correlation with the prognosis. Abstr Int Congr Haematol Paris p 165
9. Pauli C, Vanky F, Hast R, Lindemalm C, Udén A-M, Reizenstein P (1978) Cell-mediated immunity in human acute myeloblastic leukemia. Cancer Immunol Immunother 5: 1–10
10. Reizenstein P (to be published) BCG plus leukemic cell-therapy of patients with acute myeloid leukemia. In: Terry E (ed) Immunotherapy of cancer: Present status of trials in man. Raven Press, New York, p 25

11. Reizenstein P, Miale T (1978) Immunotherapy of acute myeloid leukemia in man. In: Rainer A (ed) Immunotherapy of malignant diseases. Schattauer, Stuttgart New York, pp 441–460
12. Reizenstein P, Ogier C, Sjögren A-M (to be published) Immunotherapy versus chemotherapy of AML. Response to PHA, allogeneic lymphocytes and leukemic myeloblasts of remission lymphocytes from leukemic patients. 1979 EORTC plenary meeting. In: Mathé G, Muggia FM (eds) Cancer chemo- and immunopharmacology II. Recent results in cancer research, vol 75. Springer, Berlin Heidelberg New York, pp 29–36
13. Schorlemmer H, Opitz W, Etschenberg E, Haddunger N (1979) Macrophage-mediated cytotoxicity. Abstr Physiol Chem 360: 1193
14. Singer I, Bernstein I (1978) Granulopoietic increase by BCG in mice. Exp Hematol 6: 760–766
15. Udén A-M, Lindemalm Ch, Pauli C, Vanky F, Reizenstein P (1978) Effects of immunotherapy and chemotherapy on immunocompetence. A study of patients with acute myeloblastic leukemia in remission. Cancer Immunol Immunother 4: 239–245
16. Zigelbhom I (1979) Deficiency of antibody-dependent cytotoxicity and mitogen-induced cellular cytotoxicity effector cell function in patients with AML in remission. Cancer Res 39: 3357–3362

11. The Finnish Leukaemia Group: Levamisole in Maintenance Therapy of Acute Myeloid Leukemia in Adults

M. Lehtinen, P. Ahrenberg, A. Hänninen, E. Ikkala, R. Lahtinen, A. Levanto, I. Palva, A. Rajamäki, S. Rosengard, T. Ruutu, S. Sarna, O. Selroos, T. Timonen, E. Waris, C. Wasastjerna, J. Vilpo, and P. Vuopio

Tampere Central Hospital, SF-33520 Tampere 52, Finland

Summary

The Finnish Leukaemia Group has carried out a randomized, multicenter trial to study the effect of levamisole on the remission maintained with 6-mercaptopurine and methotrexate in acute myeloid leukaemia in adults. Levamisole was given on 3 consecutive days every 2 weeks. Twenty-five patients received only chemotherapy, while 26 patients received levamisole as well. The patients receiving levamisole showed significantly better remission duration than those given only chemotherapy ($P = 0.033$, Mantel's summary χ^2-test). There are four long term survivors in the levamisole group versus none in the chemotherapy group. The remissions have lasted 48–75 months.

Introduction

Levamisole, S-(2,3,5,6 tetrahydro-6-phenylimidazo[2,1 b]-thiazole) hydrochloride, has two different clinical activities. It is a known anthelminthic agent, but it also acts as an immunostimulator in individuals whose immune defences are impaired. Levamisole restores cell-mediated immune reactions in the compromised host, but it does not stimulate normal cellular reactivity.

Levamisole has been used extensively as adjuvant therapy in the treatment of several malignancies. There are, however, very few reports on levamisole in the treatment of acute myeloid leukemia (AML) in adults [1, 4, 7] and the results are contradictory. The Finnish Leukaemia Group (FLG) has carried out a randomized multicenter trial to study the effect of levamisole on the remission maintained with 6-mercaptopurine (6-MP) and methotrexate (MTX). The trial was started in December, 1973, and closed in August, 1976. The whole series comprises all adult (more than 15 years of age) patients with untreated acute leukemia and will be reported separately [8]. This report concerns adult patients with AML who were entered into the trial. As of June, 1980, they have been followed-up for at least 4 years.

Patients and Methods

Fifty-one adult patients with AML who showed complete remission are included in this report. As induction treatment the patients received either daunorubicin, cytosine

Recent Results in Cancer Research, Vol. 80

arabinoside, and prednisone (RAP) or daunorubicin, cytosine arabinoside, prednisone, and thioguanine (RAP + T). The remission rates were the same with both combinations. A detailed report of this comparison has been published [3]. In defining remission, the criteria of the Midwest Cooperative Chemotherapy Group [2] were used. During remission, after one additional consolidation course the patients were randomized to receive only chemotherapy (25 patients) or chemotherapy with levamisole (26 patients). The maintenance chemotherapy consisted of daily 6-MP and weekly MTX. Levamisole was given on 3 consecutive days every 2 weeks (standard daily dose, 150 mg). All maintenance therapy was given orally.

Results

The chemotherapy and chemotherapy-levamisole groups were similar with regard to age of the patients, to type of leukemia, and also to the amount of cytostatic agents given during induction and consolidation. The medians of the remission durations (197 and 243 days, respectively) did not differ significantly, but statistical analysis of the whole curves by the summary χ^2-test [5] revealed that patients who received levamisole showed significantly better remission duration than patients treated with chemotherapy only ($P = 0.033$).

When all chemotherapy patients had relapsed, there were five levamisole patients still in their first complete hematologic remission. One patient with acute promyelocytic leukemia died from pulmonary fibrosis during remission, which had lasted 41 months. As of June, 1980, the remissions of four long-term survivors have lasted 48, 58, 62, and 75 months. Their median age is the same as that in the whole series (45 years) as is the age range (22–72 years). They required the same amount of cytostatics as all other responders to show a remission. At diagnosis their hemoglobin level and platelet count were essentially the same as in the total series of 194 patients, but their white blood cell count was slightly lower ($1.4-31 \times 10^9$/l, median 3.9×10^9/l) than in the whole series ($0.4-418 \times 10^9$/l, median 8.8×10^9/l).

During this trial, no serious side effects attributable to levamisole were reported.

Discussion

Reports on levamisole in the treatment of AML are conflicting. In the Danish study [7], levamisole was found to have no effect on remission maintained with intermittent high-dose chemotherapy. Also, in the study carried out at NCI-Baltimore Cancer Research Center [1], levamisole showed no additional benefit to patients when given from week 2 of induction throughout remission, which was maintained with escalating doses of MTX combined with leucovorin rescue. There is, however, one positive result as well. The Argentine Acute Leukemia Group [6] has used levamisole as adjuvant of maintenance chemotherapy in acute lymphoblastic leukemia. They conclude from their study that levamisole, used as immunotherapy in combination with maintenance chemotherapy, prolongs duration of complete remission in patients with acute lymphoblastic leukemia. Increased positivity of DNCB (2,4-dinitrochlorobenzene) skin test was established during administration of levamisole. These results warrant further investigations with levamisole in the treatment of acute leukemia. In 1978, FLG started a new trial using levamisole in combination with thioguanine and cytosine arabinoside.

References

1. Chang P, Wiernik PH, Lichenfeld JL, Schiffer CA (1978) Levamisole (L), cytosine arabinoside (Ara-C), and daunorubicin (DNR) induction therapy of adult acute nonlymphocytic leukaemia (ANLL) In: Proc Am Assoc Cancer Res Am Soc Clin Oncol, vol 19. Waverly Press, Inc. Baltimore, p 370
2. Hewlett JS, Battle JD Jr, Bishop RC, Fowler WM, Schwarz SO, Hagen PS, Louis J (1964) Phase II study of A-8103 (NSC-25154) in acute leukaemia in adults. Cancer Chemother Rep 42: 25–28
3. Ikkala E, Ahrenberg P, Hänninen A et al. (1979) The effect of thioguanine on a combination of daunorubicine, cytarabine, and prednisone in the treatment of acute leukaemia in adults. Scand J Haematol 23: 124–128
4. Lehtinen M, Ahrenberg P, Hänninen A, Ikkala E, Levanto A, Palva I, Rajamäki A, Rosengård S, Saarni M, Selroos O, Timonen T, Waris E, Wasastjerna C, Vuopio P (1978) Levamisole as immunotherapy in acute non-lymphocytic leukaemia. In: Abstracts XVII Cong Int Soc Hematol, vol I. Imp. Amelot, Brionne, p 469
5. Mantel N (1966) Evaluation of survival data and two new rank order statistics arising in its consideration. Cancer Chemother Rep 50: 163–70
6. Pavlovsky S, Garay G, Giraudo C, Sackmann F, Hayes A, Svarch E (1978) Chemoimmunotherapy with levamisole in acute lymphocytic leukemia. Proc Am Assoc Cancer Res Am Soc Clin Oncol 19: 204
7. Thorling K, Brincker H, Björn Jensen K (1978) Chemoimmunotherapy of acute myeloid leukaemia with levamisole and nine cytostatics (Abstr). In: XVII Cong. Int. Soc. Hematol. Paris, vol I. Amelot, Brionne, p 471
8. Vuopio P, Ahrenberg P, Hänninen A et al. (to be published) Levamisole in the maintenance treatment of acute leukaemia in adults

*12. Treatment of Acute Leukemia in Remission by Bone Marrow Transplantation**

R. Storb

Fred Hutchinson Cancer Research Center, Division of Oncology, 1124 Columbia Street, Seattle, WA 98104, USA

Summary

Before 1975 only patients with chemotherapy-refractory acute leukemia were treated by marrow transplantation. The preparative regimen developed in Seattle consisted of cyclophosphamide (60 mg/kg on each of 2 successive days) followed 2–3 days later by 1,000 rad total body irradiation from two opposing cobalt sources and a marrow transplant from an HLA-identical sibling. Of the first 100 patients, 13 are alive in unmaintained remission 5.5–10 years after transplantation with functioning marrow grafts. In this initial series of patients leukemic recurrence was one of the major problems. Attempts to reduce recurrent leukemia by the use of more aggressive antileukemic regimens before transplantation were unsuccessful. However, the fact that a number of "end-stage" patients had apparently been cured of their disease encouraged the Seattle team to begin a study in early 1976 of acute leukemia patients transplanted in remission. Twenty-two patients with acute lymphoblastic leukemia were transplanted in second, third, or subsequent remission and eight (35%) are now in unmaintained remission 2.5–4.5 years later. Recurrent leukemia was the cause of death for 11 patients in the acute lymphoblastic leukemia group. Twelve of the first 19 patients with acute nonlymphoblastic leukemia grafted in first remission are now alive and well in unmaintained remission 2–4 years after transplantation. At present 48 patients have been included in the study and 31 (65%) are living in remission. Only one of the 48 patients has had a recurrence of leukemia. The principal causes of death were graft-versus-host disease and interstitial pneumonia.

Marrow transplantation for patients with chronic myelogenous leukemia in blast crisis has resulted in one unmaintained remission surviving now, at 4.5 years, among six patients with syngeneic grafts and four long-term survivors (8, 15, 27, and 31 months) among 22 patients with allogeneic grafts. Three of four patients with chronic myelogenous leukemia in chronic phase given syngeneic transplants are now in remission with lack of Philadelphia chromosome at 3–4 years, while one had reappearance of the Philadelphia chromosome at 2.5 years and is now surviving in the chronic phase.

---

* This investigation was supported by grant numbers CA 18029, CA 15704, and CA 18221, awarded by the National Cancer Institute, DHEW

Introduction

Transplantation of syngeneic (donor is a monozygous twin) or allogeneic (donor is an HLA-identical sibling) marrow provides the opportunity for aggressive antileukemic therapy without regard to marrow toxicity. Until 1975, marrow transplantation was carried out only after failure of all other therapy. Consequently, most patients were in advanced relapse. Six of 16 recipients of syngeneic marrow and 13 of 100 recipients of allogeneic marrow are still in remission after 5.5–10 years [3, 7]. An actuarial survival curve of the first 100 patients grafted in Seattle after conditioning with cyclophosphamide (60 mg/kg on each of 2 successive days) and total body irradiation (1,000 rad) showed three periods of interest: (1) The first 4 months showed a rapid loss of patients associated with advanced illness, graft-versus-host disease, infections (in particular interstitial pneumonias), and recurrent leukemia; (2) from 4 months to 2 years, the curve showed a much slower rate of decline attributable primarily to recurrent leukemia; and (3) from 2–10 years, the curve was almost flat with a negligible loss of patients and no recurrent leukemia. This flat portion of the curve corresponded to 13% of the patients and indicates a strong probability that the majority of these survivors are cured of their disease [8].

Attempts at reducing the incidence of leukemic relapse after transplantation were made by a number of marrow transplant groups by added chemotherapy. In general, this approach proved to be toxic, increased the time of maximum panytopenia, and recurrent leukemia continued to be seen. Ultimate survival after these various regimens proved not to be different from that of the cyclophosphamide-total body irradiation regimen used in Seattle.

Current efforts for reducing leukemic relapse and increasing long-term survival in patients with acute leukemia transplanted in the end stage of their disease involve the use of higher doses of total body irradiation by means of fractionating the radiation. Perhaps these efforts are misdirected, since, in an exponential killing process, it is difficult to kill the last leukemic cell. Some of the apparent cures may have occurred because of destruction of leukemic cells by immunologic mechanisms involving non-HLA antigens and/or leukemia-associated antigens. Such a possibility is suggested by the observation of a graft-versus-leukemia effect in man [11].

As has been true with other agents and regimens used in the therapy of acute leukemia, the demonstration that a treatment is effective in the otherwise refractory end-stage patient constitutes a rational basis for its application earlier in the course of the disease. Accordingly, in early 1976, the Seattle group initiated a study of treating patients with acute nonlymphoblastic leukemia by marrow transplantation in first or subsequent remission and those with acute lymphoblastic leukemia in second or subsequent remission using the same conditioning regimen of cyclophosphamide and total body irradiation which previously had been shown to be well-tolerated. The assumption was that patients with acute leukemia in remission would be more readily cured since the body burden of leukemic cells could be expected to be minimal and the residual leukemic cell population should not have become resistant to therapy. Moreover, our earlier study showed that patients in good clinical condition had a much better chance of surviving the transplantation procedure. Hence, by transplanting while the patients were in remission with good hematologic values, they could be expected to have a better chance of surviving the critical first weeks after transplantation.

Transplantation of Allogeneic Marrow for Treatment of Acute Lymphoblastic Leukemia in Second or Subsequent Remission

Approximately 50% of patients with acute lymphoblastic leukemia, particularly children in the "good risk" category can be cured by combination chemotherapy. However, once marrow relapse has occurred only 5% of the patients are alive at 2 years after relapse with conventional chemotherapy [2]. It seemed, therefore, reasonable to use transplantation in patients with this disease in second or subsequent remission. The risk of losing some of these patients early after transplantation due to graf-versus-host disease and/or infections seemed acceptable if others could be "cured" of their disease.

The first 22 patients were transplanted between April, 1976, and December, 1977, using the customary cyclophosphamide-total body irradiation regimen [9]. Three patients died of interstitial pneumonia during the first 3 months after transplantation. Eleven patients died of recurrent leukemia. The latest relapse was at 27 months in the CNS of a patient who had active CNS leukemia at the time of transplantation. The median survival was 1 year compared to the 6–8 months median survival usually observed after combination chemotherapy. The eight surviving patients now show, 32–41 months after transplantation, continued remission without any therapy since the time of transplantation. Seven of the eight are without problems while one has moderately severe, chronic graft-versus-host disease with a Karnofsky performance score of 70%. It is clear from these observations that recurrent leukemia was the major problem in patients with acute lymphoblastic leukemia transplanted in second or subsequent remission. These recurrences were exclusively in cells of host type, indicating that the conditioning regimen was ineffective in eradicating the residual leukemic cell population in approximately half of the patients. Further improvement in survival rates will depend on the development of new preparative regimens.

Transplantation of Allogeneic Marrow for Treatment of Acute Nonlymphoblastic Leukemia in Remission

Patients with acute nonlymphoblastic leukemia are known to have a poor prognosis. The median duration of the first chemotherapy-induced remission in most reported series is approximately 1 year and only 15–20% of patients are alive 3 years after initial chemotherapy. A Kaplan-Meier plot of duration of survival with a logarithmic ordinate for the fraction surviving usually shows no evidence of a plateau [6]. Our past observation that, even among end-stage refractory patients, marrow transplantation could lead to an operational cure of a fraction of the patients made it ethically acceptable to consider marrow transplantation for acute nonlymphoblastic leukemia in first remission. The first 19 consecutive patients were transplanted between March, 1976, and March 1978 [10]. Transplantation was carried out at a median of 4 months following initial treatment or 10 weeks following the achievement of the first complete remission. Twelve of the first 19 patients are alive, showing continued remission with a functioning marrow graft 27–48 months after transplantation. Nine of these patients are entirely well while three have mild chronic graft-versus-host disease with Karnofsky scores of 80–90%. A Kaplan-Meier plot of the probability of survival shows a plateau at 65% with the long-term survivors very far out on the plateau and presumably cured of their disease.

Of particular interest is the fact that only one of these 19 patients has had a recurrence of leukemia. Forthy-eight patients have now been included in the study and, again, recurrence has been limited to one single patient. Evidently the preparative chemo-radiotherapy regimen is capable of eradicating the leukemic cell population in most of these patients. Six of the first 19 patients died from graft-versus-host disease and/or interstitial pneumonia.

More recently the Seattle results have been confirmed by reports from the marrow transplant teams at the City of Hope in Duarte, California, USA [1], and at the Royal Marsden Hospital in Sutton, Surrey, England [5].

Marrow Transplantation for Treatment of Chronic Myelogenous Leukemia

The Seattle team has carried out six marrow transplants for chronic myelogenous leukemia in blast crisis using marrow grafts from monozygous twin donors and one of these patients continues to be in remission, with disappearance of the Philadelphia chromosome, 53 months after transplantation. Similarly, only four of 22 patients with chronic myelogenous leukemia in blast crisis given marrow grafts from HLA-identical sibling donors are alive in unmaintained remission 8, 15, 27, and 31 months after grafting while the remainder of the patients died either of transplantation-associated complications or recurrent leukemia.

In an effort to improve the results in patients with chronic myelogenous leukemia, a study was initiated during the chronic phase of the disease for those patients who had a monozygous twin as marrow donor [4]. The objective was to eradicate the Philadelphia chromosome positive clone by the conditioning regimen consisting of chemotherapy and total body irradiation and, thus, to prevent transformation into blast crisis and to cure the disease. An initial group of patients was treated with a combination of dimethylbusulfan, cyclophosphamide, and total body irradiation followed by marrow infusion. Complete hematologic and cytogenetic remissions were induced in all four patients. One patient has relapsed 30 months after transplantation and is now back in the original state of chronic myelogeous leukemia. The other three patients are clinically, hematologically, and cytogenetically normal at 36, 39, and 44 months after transplantation. It appears that the Philadelphia chromosome-positive clone has been eradicated in these patients. Obviously, a longer follow-up of these three patients and of seven similar patients transplanted since the initial report is in order.

References

1. Blume KG, Beutler E, Bross KJ et al. (1980) Bone-marrow ablation and allogeneic marrow transplantation in acute leukemia. N Engl. J Med 302: 1041–1046
2. Chessels JM, Cornbleet M (1979) Combination chemotherapy for bone marrow relapse in childhood lymphoblastic leukemia (ALL). Med Pediatr Oncol 6: 359–365
3. Fefer A, Buckner CD, Thomas ED et al. (1977) Cure of hematologic neoplasia with transplantation of marrow from identical twins. N Engl J Med 297: 146–148
4. Fefer A, Cheever MA, Thomas ED et al. (1979) Disappearance of Ph^1-positive cells in four patients with chronic granulocytic leukemia after chemotherapy, irradiation and marrow transplantation from an identical twin. N Engl J Med 27: 227–230
5. Powles RL, Morgenstern G, Clink HM et al. (1980) The place of bone-marrow transplantation in acute myelogenous leukaemia. Lancet 1: 1047–1050

6. Powles RL, Palu G, Raghavan D (1980) The curability of acute leukemia. In: Roath S (ed) Topical reviews in haematology. Wright, London, pp 186–219
7. Thomas ED, Buckner CD, Banaji M et al. (1977) One hundred patients with acute leukemia treated by chemotherapy, total body irradiation, and allogeneic marrow transplantation. Blood 49:511–533
8. Thomas ED, Flournoy N, Buckner CD, Clift RA, Fefer A, Neiman PE, Storb R (1977) Cure of leukemia by marrow transplantation. Leuk Res 1:67–70
9. Thomas ED, Sanders JE, Flournoy N et al. (1979) Marrow transplantation for patients with acute lymphoblastic leukemia in remission. Blood 54:468–476
10. Thomas ED, Buckner CD, Clift RA et al. (1979) Marrow transplantation for acute nonlymphoblastic leukemia in first remission. N Engl J Med 301:597–599
11. Weiden PL, Flournoy N, Thomas ED, Prentice R, Fefer A, Buckner CD, Storb R (1979) Antileukemic effect of graft-versus-host disease in human recipients of allogeneic marrow grafts. N Engl J Med 300:1068–1073

13. Prevention of Blastic Crisis in Ph^1-Positive Chronic Myeloid Leukemia

J. C. Sharp

King's College Hospital, Department of Haematology,
Denmark Hill, London SE5 9RS, United Kingdom

Summary

Fourteen untreated patients with Ph^1-positive chronic myeloid leukaemia received combination chemotherapy consisting of blocks of doxorubicin, vincristine, cytosine arabinoside and 6-thioguanine. Significant karyotypic conversion occurred in six patients, the percentage of Ph^1-positive cells in the bone marrow falling by at least 50%. Maintenance therapy comprised vincristine, busulphan, hydroxyurea, 6-mercaptopurine and dibromannitol in rotation. Reinduction therapy was administered when Ph^1 positivity reverted to 100%. Karyotypic reconversion was achieved in three of four patients. After induction, chromosme analysis of the bone marrow was performed every 3–6 months to detect the appearance of aneuploid clones, the intention being to intensify therapy at that stage.

Introduction

Transformation to an accelerated malignancy in Ph^1-positive chronic myeloid leukaemia (Ph^1+ CML) is the direct cause of death in most patients. Transformation may take various forms, from a slowly evolving acceleration to a rapidly developing acute leukaemia (acute blast crisis) which is poorly responsive to chemotherapy. Karyotypic mosaicism with Ph^1+ and chromosomally normal cells, either at presentation [8] or during the disease especially where there has been bone marrow hypoplasia (usually with busulphan therapy) [1, 4, 6, 7], has been associated with longer survival.

In an effort to achieve a more consistent reduction of Ph^1+ cells, a combination of anti-myeloid drugs comprising day 1 doxorubicin and vincristine and days 1–7 cytosine arabinoside (ara-C) and 6-thioguanine (6TG) have been used. Initially, the aim was to give six blocks at approximately 3-week intervals. This was later reduced to three blocks.

Rotational chemotherapy with drugs having an established part in the management of Ph^1+ CML might logically be expected to delay the development of abnormal clones and transformation. Maintenance therapy was based on this rationale. Reinduction therapy, when Ph^1 positivity reverted to 100%, was presumed likely to reduce the

Recent Results in Cancer Research. Vol. 80

percentage of Ph^1+ cells. Day 1 vincristine with days 1–5 ara-C and 6TG were chosen for this purpose.
The early detection of marrow transformation on the appearance of clones with chromosomal abnormalities additional to the Ph^1 [10] justified intensification of chemotherapy to eliminate the abnormal clone.

Patients and Methods

Fourteen patients, thirteen under the age of 60 years, were accepted for treatment (Table 1). No patient had received prior chemotherapy. Treatment comprised day 1 doxorubicin, initially 30 mg/m^2 i.v., which was increased to 60 mg/m^2 i.v. after experience wth patients 1 and 2; vincristine, 1.5 mg/m^2 i.v. (maximum 2 mg); days 1–7 ara-C, initially in patients 1 and 2 30 mg/m^2 as a 12-h infusion, then increased to 50 mg/m^2, and with patients 11–14 thereafter 100 mg/m^2; days 1–7 6TG 80 mg/m^2 orally but from patient 11, increased to 80 mg/m^2 orally twice daily. Six blocks were given to patients 1–12. Patients 13 and 14 had three blocks.
Patients 6 and 14 had transformed disease at presentation. Both had 30% myeloblasts in the bone marrow and patient 14 had a major clone of 48 Ph^1+ 8 + 8.
Patients 7 and 8 received, in addition on day 7, daunorubicin (60 mg/m^2 i.v.) and vincristine (1.5 mg/m^2 i.v.) in the first course. Patient 7 received no further anthracycline. Patient 8 completed five further courses of the standard induction regime. Splenectomy was performed on patient 7 at the end of the induction phase because of persisting splenomegaly.
Patient 5 defaulted after one course but returned for two further courses before defaulting again. He was seen at another hospital 14 months after presentation and was reported to have had a normal blood count and no splenomegaly.

Table 1. Presenting features

Patient	Sex, age (years)	Spleen (cm)	Hemoglobin (g/dl)	WBC ($\times 10^9$/l)	Platelets ($\times 10^9$/l)	Percent Ph^1+ metaphases[b]
1	M, 56	12	7.2	451	340	100
2	F, 44	20	8.7	520	650	100
3	F, 49	3	13.5	76	428	100
4	M, 37	15	10	223	831	100
5	M, 55	5	14.6	54.5	712	100
6	M, 47	20	6.1	111	193	100
7	F, 52	20	7.5	240	380	50
8	F, 56	10	9.2	185	422	100
9	M, 47	0[a]	14.7	40.9	332	100
10	M, 64	15	12.1	120	308	100
11	M, 56	0	12.2	37	227	95
12	M, 26	17	11.5	109	445	100
13	M, 35	20	4.8	360	300	100
14	M, 41	18	12.6	166	92	100

[a] Enlarged radiographically
[b] 25 Metaphases were examined in all patients except 7 (30) and 11 (40)

Maintenance therapy consisted of a rotating sequence of drugs, initially of 11 weeks but later converted to 22 weeks. The drugs initially used were day 1, vincristine (1.5 mg i.v.); days 1–21, busulphan (4 mg); days 28–48, hydroxyurea (1 g) and 6-mercaptopurine (50 mg); days 55–75, dibromannitol (250 mg). Later, all surviving patients were converted to day 1, vincristine (1.5 mg); days 1–42, hydroxyurea (1 g) and 6-mercaptopurine (50 mg); days 48–89, busulphan (4 mg); days 95–136, dibromannitol (250 mg). Reinduction therapy with day 1 vincristine and days 1–5 bolus ara-C and twice-daily 6TG was given to patient 3 in months 24 and 36; to patient 4 in month 7; to patient 7 in month 30; and to patient 11 in month 14.
Bone marrow examination and chromosome analysis were performed before each intensive block and at the beginning of each maintenance cycle. Chromosome preparations were obtained by a direct harvesting technique. At least 25 metaphases were examined. Chromosome banding was by Seabright's trypsinisation technique [9].

Results

Banding showed that the Ph^1 in all patients was the result of a 9 : 22 translocation. The percentage Ph^1 positivity fell in 7 of 14 patients during the intensive treatment phase (Tabelle 2). The fall was considered to be significant (at least 50%) in six patients. In patient 6, with transformed disease, a transient fall to 77% was achieved before total acute blast crisis developed. The 48-cell clone in patient 14 was abolished, only to be replaced with a 47 cell line (47 Ph^1 + Ph^1).
Initial experience with patients 1 and 2 and the failure to induce hypoplasia and karyotypic conversion suggested the increased doses of doxorubicin and ara-C.

Table 2. Response to combination chemotherapy. Figures in parentheses indicate number of courses of chemotherapy given before results were obtained. At least 30 metaphases were analysed

Patient	Nadir of blood count		Lowest percent Ph^1 positively	Comments
	Leukocytes ($\times 10^9$/l)	Platelets ($\times 10^9$/l)		
1	5.8 (4)	164 (1)	100	Died
2	2.2 (6)	125 (6)	100	Died
3	3 (4)	14 (3)	7 (4)	Alive
4	2.5 (4)	99 (2)	4 (4)	Died
5	0.7 (3)	9 (3)	10 (3)	
6	1.9 (1)	59 (2)	77 (2)	Died
7	0.3 (1)	13 (1)	0 (4)	Alive
8	0.6 (1)	19 (1)	100	Alive
9	1.4 (3)	18 (3)	100	Alive
10	1.3 (4)	23 (3)	100	Alive
11	1.7 (1)	19 (2)	7 (2)	Alive
12	1.8 (1)	30 (1)	50 (2)	Alive
13	2.2 (2)	194 (2)	100	Alive
14	2.8 (1)	22 (1)	100	Alive

Patients 1 and 2 died of transformed disease 25 and 27 months after presentation respectively. Patient 13 developed transformed disease after 12 months but remains alive at 14 months.

Conversion occurred in patients 3–5, 7, 11, and 12. Reversion to 100% took place in 3, 4, 7, 11, and 12 during maintenance treatment. Reconversion was achieved in patient 3 (at 24 months and again at 36 months); in patient 4 (at 7 months) but transformation then ensued and he died in month 17; and in patient 11 (at 14 months). Two blocks of reinduction therapy were given to patient 7. Each was followed by hypoplasia but not reconversion and such treatment was abandoned.

Karyotypic conversion and reconversion has been associated with normal marrow morphology and a normal or reversed leukocyte:erythrocyte ratio. During maintenance therapy, patients 5 and 7 had sepsis which required intensive antibiotic therapy and white cell concentrates. There was minimal bleeding in patients 3, 5–7, 9–12, and 14 in induction phase and associated with thrombocytopenia; they were given platelet support. Patients 3 and 7–10 became thrombocytopenic during maintenance treatment. This resulted at various phases of treatment but particularly during or immediately after dibromannitol. Transfusions of red cells were given to all patients during the induction phase.

While patient 5 was ill with septicaemia, he had an episode of frequent extrasystoles. At the time, he also had hypokalaemia.

Discussion

In an effort to prevent or, more likely, postpone transformation in Ph^1+ CML, three discrete studies have been conceived. The number of patients studied is, to date, small and the duration of the study too short to provide meaningful data on survival. In the second study, fairly conventional drugs in rotation have been administered to patients at the end of the induction phase (first study) and to others who, on the grounds of age or additional disease, were considered unfit to receive intensive chemotherapy. In the latter group, Ph^1 status has remained unchanged. In the former, where karyotypic conversion had taken place, reversion to 100% Ph^1 positivity occurred. Such therapy is, therefore, incapable of maintaining conversion. This experience resembles that of Cunningham et al. [2] although their maintenance regime was different. The third study proposes routine monitoring of marrow chromosomes during chronic phase. Although transformation may present in different ways, an early manifestation of this may be the appearance of cells with chromosome abnormalities additional to the Ph^1 [10]. Fuscaldo et al. [5] have shown that such intensification treatment will not only eliminate the transformed clone but may improve survival. Thus far, we have achieved success only in the first study, namely that karyotypic conversion with combination chemotherapy is possible if CML is treated in this way from the outset. Six of twelve patients with chronic-phase disease have achieved such conversion; One of these (patient 4) died despite this after 17 months. The others are at present alive, 19–40 months after starting treatment. Furthermore, although Ph^1 positivity reverted to 100%, in all converters, reinduction therapy regularly brought about a further reduction. In the first CML schedule, it was intended that converters would receive intensive treatment during maintenance, but no patient actually received this on a regular basis. In an updated schedule, this will be incorporated as a feature. There must be an end point to intensive maintenance treatment and we propose to give such treatment for 2 years. This part of the regime will consist of a 7-week rotating schedule with initially a 5-day block of day 1, daunorubicin (60 mg/m^2 i.v.) (total dose of anthracyclines to be limited to 500 mg/m^2) and vincristine (1.5 mg/m^2 i.v.); days 1–5, bolus ara-C (100 mg/m^2 i.v.) and 6TG (80 mg/m^2 orally twice daily). This will be followed by oral hydroxyurea and 6-mercaptopurine.

Although improved survival seems to be a possibility with the various approaches discussed here, it is unlikely that cure can be shown with chemotherapy alone. The most promising results to date are those of Fefer et al. [3] who treated four patients with chemoradiotherapy and syngeneic bone marrow rescue. All these were alive with normal marrow karyotypes 15–24 months after transplantation. A similar approach with allogeneic transplantation is now being undertaken.

References

1. Brandt L, Mitelman F, Panani A, Lenner HC (1976) Extremely long duration of chronic myeloid leukaemia with Ph^1x-negative and Ph^1-positive bone marrow cells. Scand J Haematol 16: 321–325
2. Cunningham I, Gee T. Dowling M et al. (1979) Results of treatment of Ph^1+ chronic myelogenous leukaemia with an intensive treatment regimen (L-5 protocol). Blood 53: 375–395
3. Fefer A, Cheever M, Thomas ED et al. (1979) Disappearance of Ph^1-positive cells in four patients with chronic granulocytic leukaemia after chemotherapy, irradiation and marrow transplantation from an identical twin. N Engl J Med 300: 333–335
4. Finney R, McDonald GA, Baikie AG, Douglas AS (1972) Chronic granulocytic leukaemia with Ph^1-negative cells in bone marrow and a ten-year remission after busulphan. Br J Haematol 23: 282–288
5. Fuscaldo KE, Brodsky I, Kahn SB, Conroy JF (1977) C.G.L.: Effect of sequential chromosomal analysis, splenectomy, and intensive chemotherapy of survival. Proc Am Soc Clin Oncol 18: 294
6. Galton DAG (1972) Radical therapy for chronic granulocytic leukaemia. Proceedings at 11th Padua Seminar on Clinical Oncology, October 1972, pp 95–96
7. Golde DW, Bersch NL, Sparkes RS (1976) Chromosomal mosaicism associated with prolonged remission in chronic myelogenous leukaemia. Cancer 37: 1849–1852
8. Sakurai M, Hayata I, Sandberg AA (1976) Prognostic value of chromosomal findings in Ph^1-positive chronic myelocytic leukaemia. Cancer Res 36: 313–318
9. Seabright M (1971) A rapid banding technique for human chromosomes. Lancet 2: 971–972
10. Sharp JC, Potter AM, Wood JK (1976) Non-random and random chromosomal abnormalities in transformed chronic granulocytic leukaemia. Scand J Haematol 16: 5–12

14. A Southwest Oncology Group: Chemotherapy Versus Chemotherapy Plus Radiotherapy in Treatment of Stage III Hodgkin's Disease*

P. N. Grozea, E. J. De Persio, C. A. Coltman, Jr., C. J. Fabian, F. S. Morrison, E. A. Gehan, and S. E. Jones

Oklahoma Medical Research Foundation, University of Oklahoma, College of Medicine, Department of Medicine, 825 N.E. 13th Street, Oklahoma City, OK 73104, USA

Summary

The Southwest Oncology Group (SWOG) performed a randomized study (SWOG 7518, CAR 2) of chemotherapy using ten courses of nitrogen mustard, vincristine, procarbazine, and prednisone (MOPP) plus low-dose bleomycin (LDB), versus three courses of combined therapy, MOPP + LDB plus radiotherapy (XRT) from October, 1974, to April 1980, in pathologic stage III Hodgkin's disease. The present report includes data on 136 registered patients, of whom 112 are fully or partially evaluable. At this preliminary analysis, complete remission rates are 82% for chemotherapy alone and 82% for combined treatment. There are no statistically significant differences in survival or relapse-free survival between the two treatment programs, and no specific trends for stage IIIA versus IIIB. The estimated 3-year survival rate for all patients was 82%. Toxicities are comparable when considering the highest grades. There was one case of acute myeloblastic leukemia on combined treatment. Preliminary evidence suggests that patients with nodular sclerosis histologic type are more likely to relapse on chemotherapy alone than on combined treatment.

Introduction

It is generally accepted that radical radiation therapy is the treatment of choice for localized Hodgkin's disease [8, 11]. In the early 1970s, however, the relapse-free survival (RFS) rate for stage III disease treated by conventional total nodal irradiation (TNI) alone was rather low [9]. The development of successful combination chemotherapy [nitrogen mustard (Mustargen), vincristine (Oncovin), procarbazine, and prednisone] (MOPP) by National Cancer Institute workers [4] led SWOG in 1971 to devise a single limb study (SWOG 160, CAR 1) consisting of three MOPP cycles followed by TNI in pathologic stages IIB, IIIA, and IIIB Hodgkin's disease cases. This

* This investigation was supported in part by the following grant numbers awarded by The National Cancer Institute, HEW: CA 16957, CA 12644, CA 16385, CA 22411, CA 13612, CA 64919, CA 03096, CA 04920, CA 13238, CA 04915, CA 21116, CA 10379, CA 20319, CA 14028, CA 13392, CA 26766, CA 11233, CA 03389, CA 22433, CA 12014, and CA 16943

trial, completed in 1975, accumulated 145 evaluable patients and achieved a complete remission (CR) rate of 88% (80% for stage IIB, 91% for IIIA, and 88% for IIIB) and an actuarial 5-year survival and RFS of 78% and 68%, respectively. Toxicity was acceptable [2]. These results were superior to those obtained by previous workers [7] using non-MOPP combinations with TNI.

Another protocol (SWOG 774-75, MOPP 4), completed in 1974, showed that when low-dose bleomycin (LDB) (2 mg/m^2) was added to MOPP and compared with MOPP alone for advanced Hodgkin's disease (stages IIIB and IV) the CR rate was raised from 70–84% ($P = 0.076$). The complete and partial response (PR) rate of 96% for MOPP plus LDB was significantly higher than the CR plus PR of MOPP (84%, $P = 0.03$). Furthermore, there was suggestive evidence that survival was better with MOPP plus LDB than on MOPP alone ($P = 0.06$) [1]. These findings prompted SWOG to initiate, in October, 1975, a randomized trial of chemotherapy alone compared to the previous combined modalities of chemotherapy plus TNI for stages IIIA and IIIB Hodgkin's disease with LDB added to the chemotherapy regimen (SWOG 7517, CAR 2) [3, 6] (Fig. 1 and Table 1).

Patients and Methods

Eligibility included all patients with exploratory laparotomy-established pathologic diagnosis of stages IIIA or IIIB Hodgkin's disease with no prior chemotherapy or

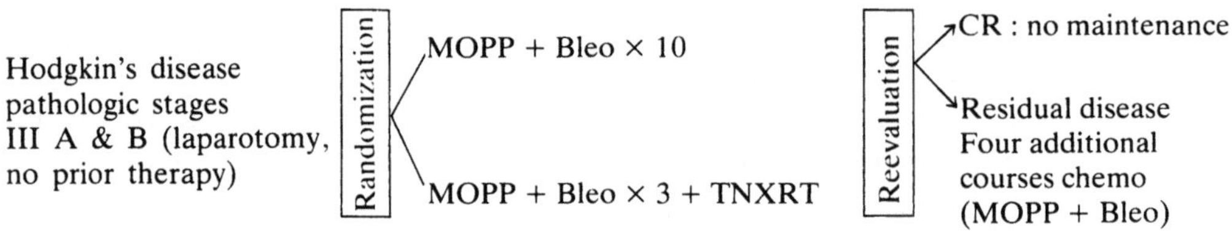

Fig. 1. SWOG 7518: Study schema

Table 1. MOPP–BLEO drug schema

	Day			
	1	2 3 4 5 6 7	8	9 10 11 12
Nitrogen mustard	6 mg/m^2		6 mg/m^2	
Vincristine (i.v.)	1.4 mg/m^2	(not to exceed 2 mg/injection)	1.4 mg/m^2	
Procarbazine (orally)		●—100 mg/m^2→		●—100 mg/m^2→
Prednisone (orally)[a, b]		●— 40 mg/m^2→		●— 40 mg/m^2→
Bleomycin (i.v.) (30 min after Vincristine)	2 mg/m^2		2 mg/m^2	

[a] Cycles 1, 4, 7, 10 [13] of chemotherapy only program
[b] Cycles 1 [4, 7] of combination chemotherapy + radiation therapy program

radiotherapy (XRT). There was no age limit. All cases were staged according to the Ann Arbor Symposium recommendations [10]. Patients had all pertinent pathologic material reviewed by the Lymphoma Pathology Panel and Central Repository. This study also featured a systematic restaging at the end of the induction phases to define the completeness of response [10]. TNI consisted of an upper mantle and inverted "Y" starting 4 weeks after completing chemotherapy (maximum "rest interval" was 10 weeks). The XRT requirements included (1) super voltage irradiation equipment of minimum energy 2.0 MeV, (2) central axis and off-axis tumor measurements, (3) beam verification films, (4) tumor dosage of 150–200 rad/day and a total of 4,000–4,500 rad during 4–6 weeks [NSD (nominal standard dose of Ellis) = 1,350–1,320 rets], and (5) monitoring of each institution for individual dose measurements and calculations by the Radiological Physics Center. Ordinarily the major or dominant involvement prior to chemotherapy was the first area to be treated by XRT. The usual sequence was upper mantle, then inverted "Y" designed as a single field or fractionated into an upper paraaortic, splenic pedicle, and a lower pelvic, inguinal-femoral area if there had been poor tolerance to chemotherapy with slow hematologic recovery. XRT was interrupted for grade 3 toxicity, i.e., white blood cell count (WBC) less than 2,000, or platelet count less than 50,000. Upon completion of the treatment, patients on both limbs of the study were followed in unmaintained remission at 3-month intervals to 2 years, then 6-month intervals to 5 years until relapse or death. No specific treatment was prescribed by the protocol for relapse. Relapse-free survival (RFS) and survival curves were calculated by the method of Kaplan and Meier [12] and survival curves were compared by the Gehan technique [5].

Results

As of February, 1980, 136 patients were registered (Table 2) and 112 of these were fully or partially evaluable. It was too early to consider the remaining cases statistically, or they were not evaluable. There were 61 patients evaluable on chemotherapy alone and 51 on combined treatment. This included patients in which a preliminary or a final evaluation could be made. Considering these fully or partially evaluable patients (Table 3) the CR rate of chemotherapy was 82%, and combined treatment 82% with a 26- and 23-week median time to completion, respectively. No significant differences in CR rates between the two limbs of the study have been detected thus far. With the given number of patients on each treatment, there was an

Table 2. Patient accession data

	10 MOPP + LDB[a]		3 MOPP + LDB + XRT[b]		Total	
Registered		68		68		136
Too early for statistical consideration		2		7		9
Fully evaluable	61	43	51	39	112	82
Partially evaluable		18		12		30

[a] Low-dose bleomycin
[b] Radiotherapy

Table 3. Response rate and time to complete remission (CR)

	MOPP + LDB	MOPP + LDB + XRT
Response rate (CR), fully and partially evaluable	82% (50 of 61)	82% (42 of 51)
Median time to CR	23 weeks	26 weeks

Table 4. Toxicity. BLEO indicates low-dose bleomycin, XRT indicates radiotherapy. Type and degree of toxicity: Total number evaluated = 125

	Code MOPP + BLEO						Code MOPP + BLEO + XRT					
	0	1	2	3	4	5	0	1	2	3	4	5
Leukopenia	26	7	18	8	7	0	21	6	18	14	1	0
Thrombocytopenia	45	2	7	7	5	0	39	3	4	7	7	0
Anemia	63	0	3	0	0	0	56	1	2	0	0	0
Nausea	36	7	16	7	0	0	36	5	10	8	0	0
Vomiting	27	9	22	8	0	0	35	6	10	8	0	0
Neurotoxicity	39	9	17	1	0	0	51	4	4	0	0	0
Pulmonary	66	0	0	0	0	0	56	0	1	2	0	0
Infection:												
H. zoster[a]	54			9	1		41	0	0	15	1	1[b]
Other	65	0	0	1	0	0	59	0	0	0	0	0

0 = None, 1 = mild, 2 = moderate, 3 = severe, 4 = life threatening, 5 = fatal

[a] The figures refer only to patients completing the program of treatment

[b] Died of systemic H. zoster; NED at autopsy

80% probability of detecting a 23% improvement in CR rate (or survival) for the combined-treatment patients. Hence, it is still possible that there is a difference between treatment regimens, but it may now be concluded that the difference will be less than 23%. The response rates were analyzed by treatment and various patient characteristics, such as sex, age, or race, initial hemoglobin (Hb) and WBC values, A or B symptomatology, clinical stage, and mediastinal disease. There were no significant differences found in these groups except, the suggestion that a Hb value below 10 or a WBC above 10,000 or below 5,000 was associated with a lower response. Also, for the averages of the clinical stages I and II compared to the averages of the clinical stages III and IV, there was a statistical difference approaching significance ($P = 0.064$). There were no differences within treatment arms.

The incidence of serious side effects were similar in the two programs, although they were to some extent of slightly different types (Table 4). There were comparable degrees of leukopenia and thrombocytopenia when considering the grades 3 and 4. There was more neurotoxicity on chemotherapy alone and there were two cases of pulmonary toxicity of a severe degree (grade 3) on combined treatment. Herpes zoster has been detected for combined treatment patients in 17 instances, including one fatality, and in ten cases on chemotherapy alone ($P = 0.15$) (three of these cases were systemic and two, on combined treatment). One case of second malignancy (AML) was recorded on combined treatment [14].

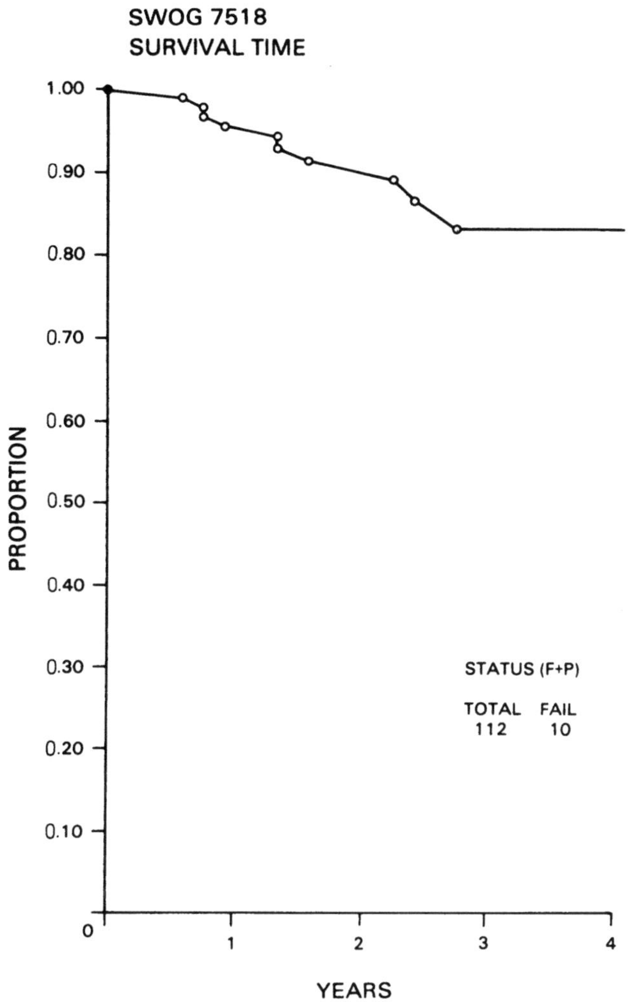

Fig. 2. Overall survival curve

Protocol compliance data show that of 54 patients on chemotherapy alone who had completed therapy and are fully or partially evaluable, 41% completed the minimum required ten cycles of MOPP plus LDB. These patients represent the group considered to be fully evaluable. Sixty-four percent completed eight, and 86% completed six cycles or more. The percent of drugs given throughout the entire program on the chemotherapy-alone limb was Mustargen (63%), Oncovin (59%), procarbazine (63%), prednisone (94%), and bleomycin (72%). For patients on combined treatment, all of the 41 partially or fully evaluable patients finished the XRT to the upper mantle except one (moderate hematologic toxicity). However, only 73% completed the program of XRT to the inverted "Y" when considering 3,000 rad as minimum therapy (61% of patients completed 3,500 rad and 39% completed 4,000 rad). In all cases except one (a pulmonary *Pneumocystis carinii* infection), the XRT dosage was low due to myelosuppression. This completion rate is comparable to the 22% of patients who were given low doses in the pelvis (median 2,000 rad) in the previous CAR 1 study [2]. No cases in CAR 1 or the present trial (CAR 2) has shown

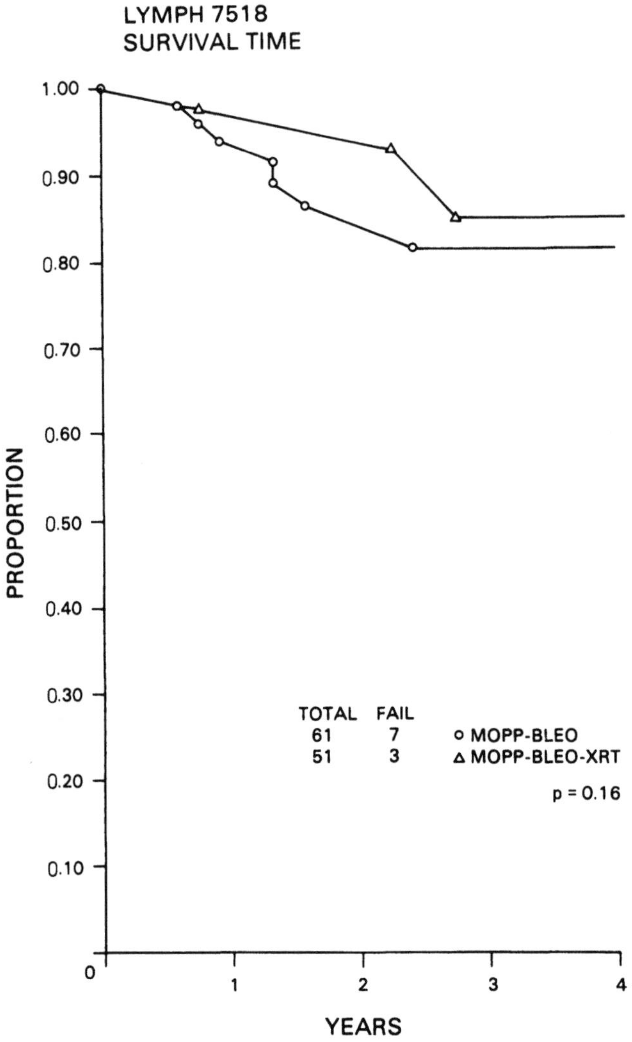

Fig. 3. Chemotherapy alone versus combined treatment

evidence of patients who received low doses in the pelvis relapsing at a higher rate than patients who received 4,000 rad.

Fig. 2 shows the overall survival curve. With a maximum follow-up time now at a little over 4.5 years and a median time on study of 2 years, there are only ten deaths from 112 patients, with an overall survival rate of 89% obtained in 2 years and 82% at 3 years. Fig. 3 shows the survival curves for chemotherapy alone versus combined treatment with no significant differences; seven deaths on chemotherapy alone and three on combined treatment.

The RFS curves, defined as the time interval from start of treatment to disease progression or relapse, are shown in Fig. 4.

Preliminary evaluation of the relapse rates show they have occurred as follows: Six relapses have been recorded on chemotherapy alone and all of these have been histologic nodular sclerosis; three relapses have occurred on combined treatment; and two had mixed cellularity, one lymphocyte predominance and one nodular sclerosis.

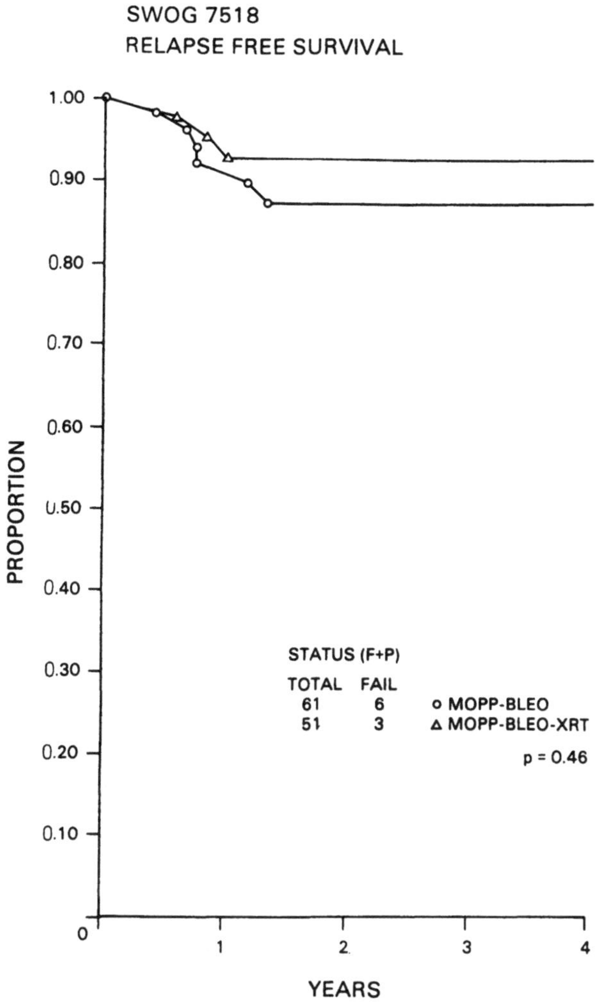

Fig. 4. Relapse-free survival: chemotherapy alone versus combined treatment

The comparison of relapses with histologic nodular sclerosis between the two limbs of the study yields a *P* value of 0.076. Three of the relapses on chemotherapy alone and none on combined treatment have died of Hodgkin's disease. There was no pattern to the relapses when they are grouped by substage $IIIA_1$ versus $IIIA_2$ [13] or when they are related to presence of absence of mediastinal involvement. Generally the relapses occurred in or contiguous to the original sites of involvement.

Discussion

The median time of data accrual in this clinical trial is only 2 years, thus the study will have to progress further before allowing comparison to results obtained by other programs.

The patients on this protocol were all entered through a multiinstitutional cooperative study group and we feel that this would yield results that are more in keeping with those that might be obtained in a community cancer center setting.

As of the February, 1980, statistical analysis of SWOG 7518, (CAR 2) a large number of the patients have completed the chemotherapy regimen. The majority have finished the course of XRT without any relapses in those patients with low doses in the pelvis. This is further evidence of the ability of this chemotherapy combination (MOPP plus LDB) to control microscopic deposits of disease.

The preliminary observation that more patients with nodular sclerosis histology have relapsed on chemotherapy alone than on combination therapy is important. Should this trend continue with time, it would indicate a combined modality treatment for this pathologic type.

The cases of Herpes zoster are following a known trend of increased incidence during combined treatment.

The overall results suggest that chemotherapy alone (MOPP plus LDB) may be as effective as combined therapy (MOPP plus LDB plus XRT) in the initial management of stages IIIA and IIIB Hodgkin's disease. However, further follow-up will be necessary to detect differences in long-term toxicities, relapse patterns, and to discern other small differences between the two treatment groups.

References

1. Coltman CA Jr (1980) Chemotherapy of advanced Hodgkin's disease. Semin Oncol 7: 155–173
2. Coltman CA Jr, Montague E, Moon TE (1977) Chemotherapy and total nodal radiotherapy in pathological stage IIB, IIIA, and IIIB Hodgkin's disease. In: Salmon SE, Jones SE (eds) Adjuvant therapy of cancer. Proceedings of the International Conference on the Adjuvant Therapy of Cancer held in Tucson, AZ, USA, March 2–5, 1977. North-Holland, Amsterdam Oxford New York, pp 529–536
3. De Persio EJ, Grozea PN, Fischer R, Jones SE, Coltman CA Jr (1979) Chemotherapy versus chemotherapy plus radiotherapy for stage IIIA, IIIB Hodgkin's disease. A Southwest Oncology Group Study. Int J Radiat Oncol Biol Phys [Suppl 2] 5: 138
4. DeVita VT Jr, Simon RM, Hubbard SM et al. (1980) Curability of advanced Hodgkin's disease with chemotherapy. Long-term follow-up of MOPP-treated patients at the National Cancer Institute. Ann Intern Med 92: 587–595
5. Gehan EA (1965) A generalized Wilcoxon test for comparing arbitrarily singly-censored samples. Biometrika 52: 203–223
6. Grozea PN, de Persio EJ, Fisher RJ, Coltman CA Jr, Jones SE (1979) Chemotherapy versus chemotherapy plus radiotherapy for stage III Hodgkin's disease. A Southwest Oncology Group (SWOG) study. Proc Am Assoc Cancer Res 20: 119
7. Hoogstraten B, Glidewell O, Holland JF et al. (1979) Long-term follow-up of combination chemotherapy-radiotherapy of stage III Hodgkin's disease: A cancer and acute leukemia group B study. Cancer 43: 1234–1243
8. Hoppe RT (1980) Radiation therapy in the treatment of Hodgkin's disease. Semin Oncol 7: 144–154
9. Johnson RE, Thomas LB, Schneiderman M, Glenn DW, Faw F, Hafermann M (1970) Preliminary experience with total nodal irradiation in Hodgkin's disease. Radiology 96: 603–608
10. Jones SE (1980) Importance of staging in Hodgkin's disease. Semin Oncol 7: 126–135
11. Kaplan HS (1980) Hodgkin's disease: Unfolding concepts concerning its nature, management and prognosis. (The General Motors Research Foundation prizes for research in cancer). Cancer 45: 2439–2474

12. Kaplan ES, Meier P (1959) Non-parametric estimations of incomplete observations. J Am Stat Assoc 53: 457–481
13. Stein RD, Golomb HM, Diggs CH et al. (1980) Anatomic substages of stage IIIA. Ann Intern Med 92: 159–165
14. Toland DM, Coltman CA Jr, Moon TE (1979) Second malignancies complicating Hodgkin's disease: The Southwest Oncology Group experience. Cancer Clin Trials 1: 27–33

15. *Maintenance Immunotherapy with BCG in Non-Hodgkin's Malignant Lymphomas: A Progress Report of a Randomized Trial*

B. Hœrni, M. Durand, H. Eghbali, G. Hœrni-Simon, P. Richaud, and A. de Mascarel

Fondation Bergonié, 180 rue de Saint-Genès, F-33076 Bordeaux Cedex, France

Summary

Ninety-eight patients with non-Hodgkin's malignant lymphoma were first put into complete remission by a combination of chemotherapy and radiotherapy, and then received one course of chemotherapy as reinforcement. They were then randomized to receive either maintenance BCG therapy or no other treatment. Ninety-three patients were available for this analysis. There was a significant difference ($P = 0.021$) in relapse-free survival times between the two groups of patients. This difference is particularly significant in male patients, in patients ages 50–65 years, in all histologic classes, in patients treated after an initial relapse, and in clinical stages I and II. There was also a difference in crude survival, but the difference was not significant.

Introduction

In a previous paper we presented our current results of a randomized trial on maintenance BCG therapy in non-Hodgkin's malignant lymphomas [3]. These results were significant in patients showing clinical stages I and II. The trial was then discontinued for these patients, but was pursued for clinical stages III and IV and was also extended to include patients over 65 years of age who were initially excluded from the study. We present here the overall results of this trial.

Patients and Methods

All patients included in the trial presented a histologic diagnosis of non-Hodgkin's lymphoma assessed after review in our institute and classified according to Kiel's classification [4, 5]. During a first period (January, 1973, to December, 1977), only patients less than 65 years old were included in the trial. As of January 1, 1978, patients with clinical stages I and II were excluded and were systematically treated with BCG because of the favorable results with this maintenance treatment [3]. Thus, from January, 1978, to April, 1980, the trial was continued for patients under 65 with stages III and IV and was extended to include patients over 65 years of age.

Recent Results in Cancer Research, Vol. 80

Besides data dealing with histologic diagnosis, age of the patients, and clinical stage of the disease, the design of the trial was first to obtain a complete remission with a treatment combining chemotherapy and radiotherapy in all involved areas and, secondly, to reinforce the complete remission with a further course of chemotherapy. The patients were then randomized into two groups to receive either BCG therapy or no further treatment. Chemotherapy consisted of a triple or quadruple association, according to previously published schedules [1, 2], with the same distribution in the two groups of patients: Each patient received one course of 15 days before radiotherapy and then one similar course immediately after radiotherapy. Radiotherapy was usually given in all areas primarily involved with clinically or radiographically apparent disease. Eighteen patients with low grade malignancy received only total body irradiation according to a previously published design [7]. Ninety-eight patients were randomized. Five were excluded for the following reasons: Two patients randomized in the control group died from another disease within the month following randomization; three patients (two in the control group, one in the BCG group) were inaccurately irradiated and all three relapsed in a primarily involved and erroneously nonirradiated area.

The distribution of the main prognostic criteria and treatments in the two groups of patients is shown in Table 1. There was no significant difference between the two groups, except for sex: There were significantly more females in the BCG-treated

Table 1. Prognostic criteria

		BCG	Control	*P* value
Total		49	44	
Patients	Male	25	32	0.03
	Female	24	12	
Age (years)	< 50	19	14	
	50–65	13	16	0.58
	> 65	17	14	
Histology	Low grade	33	30	0.93
	High grade	16	14	
Initial evolution		37	30	0.43
Relapse		12	14	
Clinical stage	I	14	13	
	II	10	11	0.71
	III	10	11	
	IV	15	9	
Treatment				
First chemotherapy	triple	13	15	0.42
	quadruple	36	29	
Radiotherapy	localized	23	22	
	segmental	17	13	0.86
	total body	9	9	
Second chemotherapy	triple	26	22	0.76
	quadruple	23	22	

group, though the results were not influenced significantly by the sex of the patient.
BCG was given by skin scarifications on a 5 × 5 cm area. We used BCG produced by the Institut Pasteur (BCG-S until December, 1975, and thereafter Immun BCG-F). These scarifications were done weekly and were discontinued in case of relapse or after 3 years.
All patients were followed-up until their death or June, 1980. No patients were lost from follow-up. Survival was calculated according to the actuarial method and the log rank test was used for statistical comparison between survival curves [6]. The direct Fisher's test was used for other comparisons.

Results

Remission

Thirty-six patients relapsed (12 of 49 BCG-treated patients and 24 of 44 control patients). Fig. 1 shows the actuarial curves of disease-free survival for each group of patients; there is a significant difference ($P = 0.021$) of about 30 percent between the plateaus of the two curves in favor of BCG-treated patients. As shown in Table 2, the difference is significant in male patients, in patients 30–65 years of age, in both classes of histology, and in patients already suffering relapse and in clinical stage I. These results seem to be particularly valuable concerning patients treated after a first or additional relapse ($P = 0.005$) (10 of 14 control patients relapsed again and only 2 of 12 BCG-treated patients relapsed). In male patients the difference was highly significant, whereas no difference was observed in females.
No relapse was observed after 28 months in BCG-treated patients and 14 patients have exceeded this date. None of the nine patients in whom BCG was discontinued at 36 months and who have exceeded this date have suffered relapse.

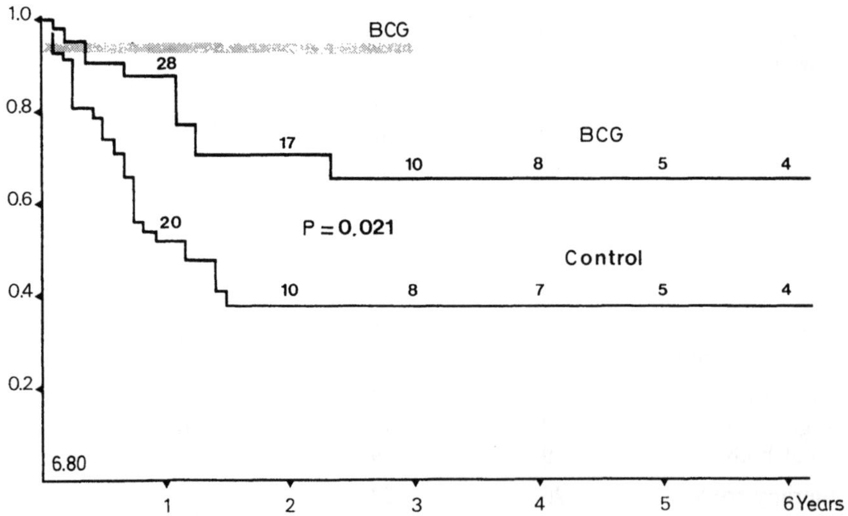

Fig. 1. Actuarial disease-free survival for all patients

Table 2. Rate of relapse according to main prognostic criteria (relapses/total)

		BCG	Control	*P* value
Total		12/49	24/44	0.003
Patients	Male	4/25	19/32	0.0009
	Female	8/24	5/12	0.62
Age (years)	< 50	6/19	9/14	0.06
	50–65	1/13	8/16	0.014
	> 65	5/17	7/14	0.24
Histology	Low grade	6/33	14/30	0.015
	High grade	5/16	10/14	0.028
Initial evolution		10/37	13/30	0.16
Relapse		2/12	10/14	0.005
Clinical stage	I	2/14	7/13	0.029
	II	4/10	7/11	0.27
	III	3/10	7/11	0.12
	IV	4/15	3/9	0.72

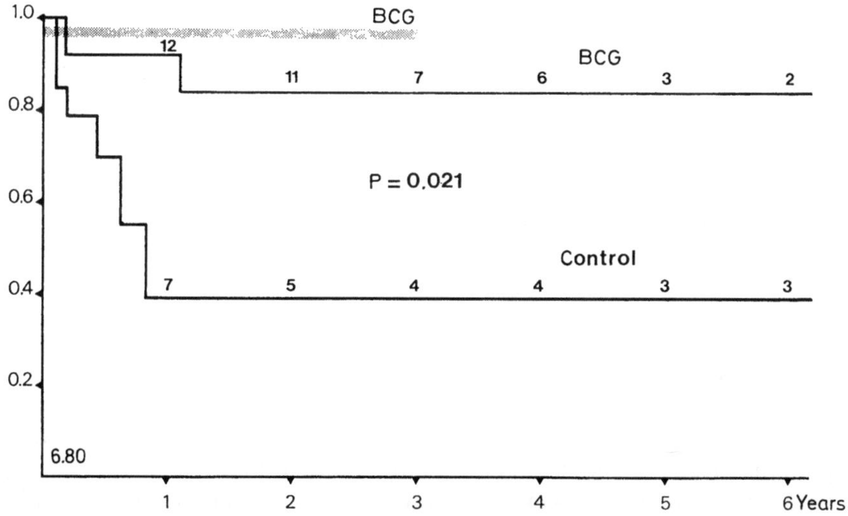

Fig. 2. Actuarial disease-free survival for patients < 65 years, clinical stage I and II

If we consider only stage I and II patients less than 65 years of age who were no longer included in the trial after January 1, 1978, the difference in disease-free survival remains significant (Fig. 2) with a difference of more than 40 percent between the two plateaus. Thus, for these latter patients, BCG seems useful in preventing relapses, at least in four of ten patients.

Except for BCG, no other prognostic criteria influenced the rate of relapse. There is no difference concerning the site of relapses between the two groups.

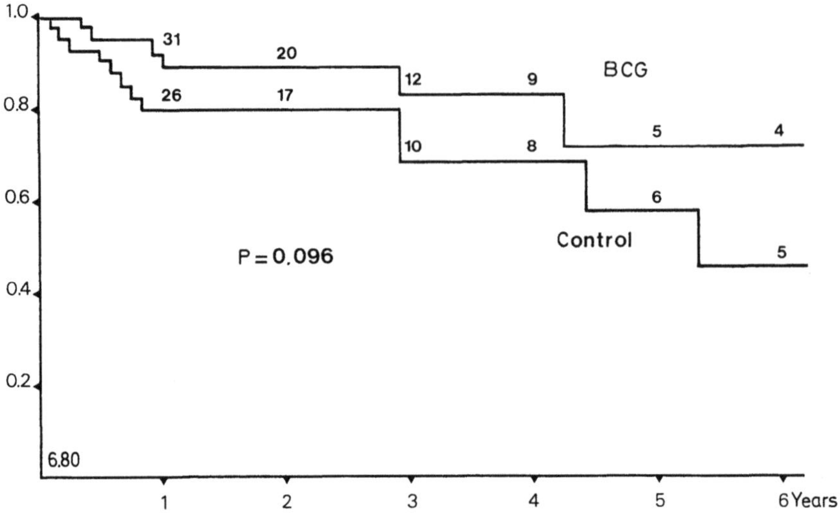

Fig. 3. Overall survival for all patients

Survival

Eighteen deaths occurred, all but three being due to malignant lymphoma: One BCG-treated patient succumbed to an autoimmune hemolytic anemia 51 months after the beginning of BCG, i.e., 15 months after its discontinuation; one ethylic control patient died while in complete remission from liver cirrhosis; and one control patient died from a stroke while his lymphoma was uncontrolled. From an overall point of view, there were six deaths among 49 BCG-treated patients and 12 deaths among 44 controls. If we consider the crude survival curves, the difference is not significant (Fig. 3).

Discussion

Our previous results [3] are confirmed by this analysis, which includes twice as many patients. BCG seems useful as maintenance treatment in preventing relapse in all varieties of non-Hodgkin's lymphomas. The difference is particularly striking in patients with clinical stages I and II in whom the trial was discontinued 2 years ago so that systematic BCG treatment could be instituted. However, until now the only difference in the rate of relapses seems very slight in female patients, in patients over 65 years of age, and in clinical stage IV.

Published elsewhere here is evidence that BCG may be useful in maintaining complete remission in patients with non-Hodgkin's lymphoma. Therefore, it seems necessary to see whether this is valid in all patients and in all tumors; thus, we are continuing our trial. At this point in our study the usefulness of BCG in clinical stages I and II seems no longer questionable. Clinical staging is particularly valuable in estimating the tumor volume, which is probably much more important than the topographic extension from the immunotherapeutic point of view. On the contrary, the role of BCG in females, in elderly patients, and in clinical stage IV remains doubtful and requires further study.

References

1. Chauvergne J, Hœrni B, Durand M, Hœrni-Simon G, Lagarde C (1973) Chimiothérapie des réticulosarcomes. Résultats d'un essai contrôlé portant sur 60 malades. Nouv Press Méd 2: 2039–2042
2. Durand M, Chauvergne J, Hœrni-Simon G et al. (1978) Chimiothérapie d'induction des lymphomes malins non hodgkiniens. Résultats d'un essai contrôlé comparant deux quadruples associations. Acta Haematol (Basel) 59: 80–87
3. Hœrni B, Durand M, Richaud P, de Mascarel A, Hœrni-Simon G, Chauvergne J, Lagarde C (1979) Successful maintenance immunotherapy by BCG of non-Hodgkin's malignant lymphomas: Results of a controlled trial. Br J Haematol 42: 507–514
4. Lagarde C, Hœrni B, de Mascarel A et al. (1980) Lymphomes malins non hodgkiniens. Caractères anatomocliniques et évolutifs dans une série de 370 malades. Bull Cancer (Paris) 657: 139–148
5. Meugé C, Hœrni B, de Mascarel A et al. (1978) Non-Hodgkin's malignant lymphomas. Clinico-pathologic correlations with the Kiel classification. Retrospective analysis of a series of 274 cases. Eur J Cancer 14: 587–592
6. Peto R, Pike MC, Armitage P et al. (1977) Design and analysis of randomized clinical trials requiring prolonged observation of each patient. II. Analysis and examples. Br J Cancer 35: 1–39
7. Richaud P, Hœrni-Simon G, Denépoux R, Durand M, Hœrni B, Lagarde C (1979) Total body irradiation (T.B.I.). Preliminary results of a new technique used in 30 patients with hematologic malignancy. Strahlentherapie 155: 736–739

III. Bone Tumors

16. *Role of Lung Irradiation in the Adjuvant Treatment of Osteosarcoma*

E. van der Schueren and K. Breur*

Academisch Ziekenhuis St. Rafaël, Division of Oncology, Department of Radiotherapy, Capucienenvoer 35, B-3000 Leuven, Belgium

Introduction

The vast majority of osteogenic sarcoma originates in bones of the limbs, and radical surgery can nearly always control the primary tumor. The prognosis of these patients is thus determined by the appearance of distant metastases, mainly in the lungs. The results of treatment of overt metastases are very limited, though the last decade has seen a great effort to improve therapeutic results by eliminating tumor deposits when they are not yet detectable, thus containing smaller numbers of tumor cells.

For such adjuvant therapies, treatment modalities are selected on the basis of their proven effectiveness in inducing regressions in visible tumor locations. Therefore, it is obvious that every form of such adjuvant treatment will result in tumor-growth delay in at least some of the treated patients, thus a higher percentages of patients will remain disease-free during and immediately after such therapies. When an adjuvant treatment, such as chemotherapy, is given up to and over 1 year, disease-free survival curves can be expected to change drastically in shape. However, the fundamental question in adjuvant therapy is not whether the tumor-free interval is lengthened, but whether the fraction of patients ultimately remaining disease-free increases by treating all the patients at an earlier stage.

All too often this principle has been overlooked and great successes have been claimed for adjuvant therapies based on data showing only tumor-growth delay. The critical factor has usually been an insufficient patient follow-up after discontinuation of treatment at the time of a premature publication. To assess whether a larger fraction of patients remains disease free is very difficult as it necessitates a dependable reference value which has to be selected.

The use of historical controls is a dangerous exercise as it requires a balance in composition of the compared patient groups, as well as balanced prognostic factors, such as diagnostic procedures before treatment. Also, comparison of the overall survival curve can be complicated by developments of the second line treatment which can lengthen survival after recurrence or even rescue patients definitively. Using historical controls can, thus, only give clear-cut answers in cases where a very large gain is obtained by the application of a new treatment policy.

* For the Cooperative Radiotherapy-Chemotherapy Group of the EORTC

Recent Results in Cancer Research, Vol. 80

It seems that in osteosarcoma, all problems have been compounded. In evaluating treatment results, the patients have been considered to be a homogeneous group with a very stable, dismal prognosis of 15–20% for metastses-free survival. As no effective treatment was available against metastases, the absolute survival for patients with this very rapidly growing tumor followed this prognosis very closely.

While this most likely still holds true when large groups of patients are considered [6, 8], it has been demonstrated several times that in smaller groups (around 50 patients or less), results have been widely divergent. The study from the Mayo Clinic has been particularly illustrative [14]. Evaluating the metastases-free fraction of patient groups treated over different periods of 3 years, they found a percentage of around 20% for three periods, but during 1969–1971 the percentage of patients remaining metastases-free was as high as 38%. The change in overall survival curves as a function of the time of diagnosis was even more pronounced: Although the patients diagnosed during 1972–1974 developed clearly more metastases than the patients initially treated during 1969–1971, they still had a higher survival percentage after 3 years. This reflects a more effective and aggressive treatment at the time of recurrence rather than a change in biologic behavior of the tumor. This initial divergence between the disease-free percentages and the surviving fractions is also reflected in the study of the National Cancer Institute (NCI) where aggressive surgical management was directed at the lung metastases [13]. Also the possible influence of other prognostic factors, such as histologic type and differentiation, sex, and site of the primary tumor, are mentioned in the study from the Mayo Clinics [14]. In view of all these facts, it seems extremely difficult to assess the value of adjuvant therapies in patients with osteosarcomas based on comparisons with historical controls.

A prospective randomized clinical trial of the value of lung irradiation, carried out by the Cooperative Group Radiotherapy/Chemotherapy of the EORTC during 1969–1972 had to be discontinued under the pressure of premature publication of overoptimistic chemotherapy results. From that point, nearly all studies have accepted the efficiency of adjuvant chemotherapy in osteosarcoma and all studies have only centered on the type of drugs to be used. However, although interesting results were obtained in some series, the majority of cases have shown results only marginally different from those expected without adjuvant treatment and, a few years ago, several centers felt compelled to return to the initial questions of the intrinsic value of the adjuvant therapies in osteosarcoma. The Mayo Clinic and the NCI carry out prospective randomized studies comparing groups of patients with adjuvant chemotherapy or without any form of treatment after the radical surgery for the primary tumor. The Cooperative Group Radiotherapy/Chemotherapy of the EORTC, in collaboration with the Société Internationale d'Oncologie Pédiatrique (SIOP) initiated a study comparing a simple lung irradiation to chemotherapy and to a combination treatment of chemotherapy and lung irradiation.

O2 Trial on Lung Irradiation

In 1969 the Cooperative Group Radiotherapy/Chemotherapy of the EORTC decided to investigate the values of lung irradiation in patients with osteosarcoma. The basis for this study came from earlier clinical data. It was found that a dose of 20 Gy (2,000 rad) given in ten sessions over 2 weeks could safely be given to the lungs. These data were later published with even longer follow-ups [1]. The radiation dose to reduce the number of viable tumor cells with a factor 10 (D 10) calculated to be 4 Gy (400 rad) from regression curves of irradiated lung metastases of osteosarcomal. Thus a dose of 20 Gy could be expected to sterilize tumor deposits of up to 10^5 cells.

From the time of appearance of metastases and their growth rate it was calculated that, at the time of treatment of the primary tumor, about 20% of the patients who would develop lung metastases have tumor localizations of 10^5 cells or less [2, 4, 7]. This gives a reasonable estimate of the possibilities and limitations of such a treatment in these patients.

The trial commenced in 1970 with the participation of five French and two Dutch centers. Patients up to 60 years of age were included and the treatment of the primary tumor consisted of surgery or radiotherapy, with or without delayed surgery.

After the initial treatment, patients were randomized to receive either no further treatment or whole lung irradiation of 20 Gy. The complete results are published and discussed [2, 3] and will therefore only be briefly reviewed here.

In 4 years, 86 patients were entered in the study (42 with lung irradiation and 44 without). At 5 years the disease-free survival was 43% for the patients who had received the lung irradiation and 28% for the patients without any adjuvant therapy. Due to the limited number of patients in the two groups, this difference is only significant at the 6% level ($P = 0.059$). In the pediatric age group (less than 17 years of age), this difference was larger, with an increase of disease-free survival from 28–48% ($P = 0.028$). Remarkable in this study were the differences in results obtained at the Institut Gustave-Roussy (Villejuif) and the other participating centers. In the group from Villejuif the metastases-free survival was 27% and 33%, respectively, without and with lung irradiation for a group of 38 patients. The other 48 patients had disease-free percentages of 30% and 50%, respectively. In the other centers, the disease-free fraction of pediatric patients ($N = 19$) was even as high as 61%. These large difference underline again the great danger of evaluating treatment results in small patient groups and reconfirm the need to carry out multicenter trials.

Several conclusions can be drawn from this study. The metastases-free survival of patients without adjuvant treatment is definitely higher than what is usually used as reference in most recent studies. Whether this is due to a better selection initially due to more careful staging, to a real change in the biologic behavior of the tumor, or to statistical deviation due to sample size is really irrelevant, as the size of most recent studies is similar. This fact should, however, be kept in mind while evaluating the results of therapies which are investigated without a control group of patients.

The percentage of patients remaining disease-free (42%) is higher than the untreated patients. This difference is only marginally significant, but becomes clearly significant when only the pediatric patients are considered. Still, the fact that in one center (Villejuif) with 38 patients, no difference was found after lung irradiation should indicate some caution in evaluating these results.

In addition, a parallel study carried out in the Mayo Clinic, in which lung irradiation was tested in combination with a single-agent alkylating chemotherapy, found no improvement in the disease-free fraction of patients [10]. However, the radiation dose in that study was only 15 Gy (1,500 rad) and, based on the previous calculations, an improvement of only slightly over 10% could be expected from such a dose. With about 20 patients in each group this would have been nearly impossible to detect. While the effect of the lung irradiation suggested by this study can thus not yet be considered as confirmed, the percentage of 48% disease-free patients is in the same range as that obtained in most studies on adjuvant chemotherapy.

It is apparent that to confirm these possible advantages, further studies are necessary and it seems unavoidable, in view of the small improvements which can be expected, that prospective randomized trials will have to be used in which several centers participate to increase the number of evaluable patients. It also seems that potentially more effective treatment policies have to be investigated. In view of all these data, a new trial was initiated by the Cooperative Group Radiotherapy/Chemotherapy of the EORTC in conjunction with the SIOP.

The first question asked in this study is whether heavy chemotherapy for about 1 year is better than simple lung irradiation. The second question is whether the potential gains, suggested to be present after both these treatment policies, can be combined by adding lung irradiation to the initial induction chemotherapy.

The radiotherapy uses the same modalities as those which were used in the first trial, namely, 20 Gy in ten sessions during 2 weeks. The chemotherapy starts with an induction phase of 9 weeks in which three doses of methotrexate (6 g/m^2) (with leukovorin rescue) in combination with vincristine (1.5 g/m^2) are alternated every 2 weeks with adriamycin (70 mg/m^2). After that a maintenance chemotherapy is given with the same drugs every 4 weeks, with cyclophosphamide (1.2 g/m^2) between cycles for up to 42 weeks. For the combination therapy only the induction chemotherapy is given during 9 weeks, followed by lung irradiation. The full treatment schedules have been published earlier [15].

The study started in 1978 and on June 1, 1980, already 117 patients were included. It was decided by the group of centers conducting the trial that no preliminary results of the study would be communicated until enough follow-up has been assembled on a group of patients large enough to make the results significant.

Conclusion

For the moment there is some confusion concerning the effect of adjuvant therapy in the treatment of patients with osteosarcoma. Irradiation of the lungs has been suggested to be able to eliminate the metastases in about 20% of the patients treated. If confirmed, this would also mean that for further progress other agents would have to be combined with the lung irradiation as it is not possible to raise the radiation dose.

The results of chemotherapy have been divergent. However, nearly all series with a follow-up which is long enough after the discontinuation of chemotherapy have reported disease-free fractions around 50% at best and many of them well below that number. So, in spite of some very impressive recent results [11, 12], it was concluded in a recent review paper that the role of chemotherapy in adjuvant treatment of osteosarcoma still needs evaluation [9]. The study from the Mayo Clinic, which has accrued about 40 patients up to now, detected no advantage of adjuvant chemotherapy in its first assessment [5]. All these data confirm the pressing need for the continuation of prospective randomized trials on this subject.

References

1. Abbatucci JS, Boulier A, Fabre J, Lozier JC (1979) Functional evaluation of pulmonary irradiation effects. Eur J Cancer 14: 781–785
2. Breur K, van der Schueren E (1979) Adjuvant therapy in the management of osteosarcoma: Need for critical reassessment. Recent Results Cancer Res 68: 5–15
3. Breur K, Cohen P, Schweisguth O, Hart AMM (1978) Irradiation of the lungs as an adjuvant therapy in the treatment of osteosarcoma of the limbs. Eur J Cancer 14: 461–471
4. Cohen P (1979) Osteosarcoma of the long bones. Eur J Cancer 14: 995–1004
5. Edmonson JH, Green SJ, Ivins JC, Gilchrist GS, Creagan ET, Burgert EO, Pritchard DJ, Hahn RG, Dahlin DC, Taylor WF (1980) Post-surgical treatment of primary osteosarcoma of bone-comparison of high dose methotrexate vs. observation: Preliminary report. Proc Am Soc Clin Oncol 620: 476
6. Gehan EA, Sutow WW, Uribe-Botero G, Romsdahl M, Smith TL (1978) Osteosarcoma: The M.D. Anderson experience, 1950–1974. In: Terry WD, Windhorst D (eds) Immunotherapy of cancer: Present status of trials in man. Raven Press, New York, pp 271–282
7. Jeffree GM, Price DHG, Sissons HA (1975) The metastatic patterns of osteosarcoma. Br J Cancer 32: 87–107
8. Marcove RC, Miké V, Hajek JV, Levin AC, Hutter RVP (1970) Osteogenic sarcoma under the age of 21. J Bone Joint Surg [Am] 52: 411–423
9. Pratt CB (1980) Chemotherapy of osteosarcoma: An overview. In: Van Oosterom AT, Muggia FM, Cleton FJ (eds) Therapeutic progress in ovarian cancer, testicular cancer and the sarcomas, vol 16. Leiden University Press, Leiden (Boerhaave Series, pp 329–348)
10. Rab GT, Ivins JC, Childs DS Jr, Cupps RE, Pritchard DJ (1976) Elective whole lung irradiation in the treatment of osteogenic sarcoma. Cancer 38: 939–942
11. Rosen G, Marcove RC, Caparros B, Nirenberg A, Kosloff C, Huvos AG (1979) Primary osteogenic sarcoma. The rationale for preoperative chemotherapy and delayed surgery. Cancer 43: 2163–2177
12. Rosen G, Caparros B, Nirenberg A, Juergens H, Huvos AG (1980) The successful management of metastatic osteogenic sarcoma: A model for the treatment of primary osteogenic sarcoma. In: Van Oosterom AT, Muggia FM, Cleton FJ (eds) Therapeutic progress in ovarian cancer, testicular cancer and the sarcomas, vol 16. Leiden University Press, Leiden (Boerhaave Series, pp 349–366)
13. Rosenberg SA, Sindelar WF (1980) Surgery and adjuvant chemo-immunotherapy in osteosarcoma: Review on treatment at the National Cancer Institute. In: Van Oosterom AT, Muggia FM, Cleton FJ (eds) Therapeutic progress in ovarian cancer, testicular cancer and the sarcomas, vol 16. Leiden University Press, Leiden (Boerhaave Series, pp 301–316)
14. Taylor WF, Inis JC, Dahlin DC, Pritchard DJ (1978) Osteogenic sarcoma experience at the Mayo Clinic, 1963–1974. In: Terry WD, Windhorst D (eds) Immunotherapy of cancer: Present status of trials in man. Raven Press, New York, pp 257–269
15. Van der Schueren E, Breur K, Schweisguth O, Voute PA, Cohen P, Machin D (1979) Assessment of the role of chemotherapy and radiotherapy as adjuvant in the treatment of osteosarcomas of the limbs. A trial of the EORTC (Clinical Group Radiotherapy/Chemotherapy) and of the SIOP. Eur J Cancer 15: 1001–1003

17. *Adjuvant Interferon Treatment of Human Osteosarcoma**

H. Strander, T. Aparisi, H. Blomgren, L. Å. Broström, K. Cantell, S. Einhorn, S. Ingimarsson, U. Nilsonne, and G. Söderberg

Karolinska Hospital, S-104 01 Stockholm, Sweden

Summary

This paper updates the results of the clinical trial to examine the efficacy of exogenous leukocyte interferon therapy as adjuvant treatment for osteosarcoma. So far the incidence of metastases is lower and the survival rate is better for the interferon-treated group than for the concurrent control group. The number of treated patients is too small at present to allow proper statistical calculations to be made.

Introduction

A clinical trial was initiated at the Karolinska Hospital in December, 1971, where exogenous leukocyte interferon (IF) therapy was given as adjuvant treatment to a consecutive series of osteosarcoma patients. Preliminary results have been given previously [1–4, 14–19]. The present communication is an update of the results obtained thus far in this ongoing trial.

Case Series

Only patients without signs of metastases on admission are included in both groups. Only patients with classical type of osteosarcoma are included in the different groups. The interferon group comprises all patients given IF therapy to date (at present, 46 patients). The concurrent control group comprises the rest of all the osteosarcoma patients in Sweden up to January 1, 1976, and treated during the same time period as the IF-treated group. Of these patients, 30 received no adjuvant therapy. Six patients received high-dose chemotherapy and are discussed separately. The control group will be enlarged by checking the patients treated in Sweden after January 1, 1976, and not receiving IF adjuvant therapy. All the patients in this group were treated elsewhere than at the Karolinska Hospital, i.e., at other university clinics in Sweden.

---

* This study was supported by the Cancer Society of Stockholm, the Swedish Cancer Society, and Dagmar Hasselgren's Fund

The age of the patients in the IF-treated group was 22 ± 20 years and in the concurrent control group 16 ± 8 years. There were 17 females (37%) in the IF-treated group and 12 females (40%) in the concurrent group.

Treatment Delay

The time period from the first symptom to biopsy was, for the IF group, 3.5 ± 5 months and, for the concurrent control group, 2.5 ± 2 months. The time period from the first symptom to treatment was, for the IF group, 4 ± 5 months and, for the control group, 3 ± 3 months.

Symptoms and Pathology

In the IF group 91% of the patients experienced pain and 63% had noticed a tumor; for the control group were 87% and 47%, respectively. The largest diameter of the tumors on the radiograms were, for the IF group, 10 ± 4 cm and, for controls, 9 ± 3 cm.

Pathology of most of the patients were checked by an American group of investigators [2]. All patients had classical osteosarcomas according to the criteria established by the American group. In the interferon group 61% of the patients had osteoblastic tumors, 17% chondroblastic, and 22% fibroblastic. The respective figures for the control group were 53%, 16%, and 30%. In the IF group 54% and, in the control group, 56% of the patients had grade IV tumors.

In the IF group, 59% of the tumors were localized at proximal sites, while the control group showed 60%. The IF group showed 71% and the controls showed 77% of the tumors to be localized in the knee region.

Irradiation

Thirteen percent of the IF group received more than 45 Gy cobalt irradiation to the primary site, 9% 10–45 Gy, and 78% received no irradiation. Corresponding figures for the control group were 40%, 3%, and 57%.

Surgery or Treatment of Pulmonary Metastases

In the IF group 13% were exarticulated, 48% amputated, 35% resected, and 2% received no surgery due to the development of pulmonary metastases after or during preoperative irradiation. In the control group the corresponding figures were 23%, 60%, 7% and 10%.

In the IF group 12 patients were operated for pulmonary metastases, 5 patients received 10–45 Gy irradiation, and 15 received chemotherapy upon development of pulmonary metastases. Corresponding figures for the control group were nine, two, and ten patients. Two patients in the control group received more than 45 Gy irradiation for pulmonary metastases.

Other Factors

The time between the last negative and the first positive X-ray were, for the IF group, 2 ± 2 months and, for the control group, 6 ± 6 months. It is therefore likely that some of the lung metastases would have been detected earlier in the control group if the pulmonary radiograms had been done more frequently.

Interferon

Two types of preparations were used, one being more pure (P-IF) than the other (C-IF) [5, 6, 13]. Properties of these preparations have been described in detail previously. All the IF which was used was prepared by exposing human leukocytes to Sendai virus in tissue culture.

The IF was administered according to a schedule described previously [1, 2]. During the first months after diagnostic open biopsy 3×10^6 standard IF units were given i.m. Thereafter, the preparation was given on an ambulatory basis, 3×10^6 IF units three times weekly for a further IF months.

Side Effects

The most prominent side effects experienced during C-IF administration were fever (62%), local pain (38%), shivering (38%), scalp hair loss (28%), and itching erythema (17%). As P-IF became routinely used in clinical experimental medicine, it was shown that this preparation was better tolerated by the patients [2]. Fever reactions and headache became the more prominent symptoms remaining. These symptoms were noticed mostly during the early course of P-IF treatment and all patients tolerated the IF treatment well.

The effect of long-term administration of IF on various blood parameters was studied. The erythrocyte sedimentation rate (ESR) decreased significantly and the hemoglobin concentration rose significantly after cessation of IF therapy.

Sera were saved regularly for testing anti-IF activity and in no sera was this demonstrated. On the other hand, all patients showed antibody responses to heterologous antigens present in the IF preparations.

Infections

The patients receiving IF had significantly fewer incidences of symptoms indicating acute infections than their family members [11, 18]. Viral serology done on the patients and patient groups developing and not developing metastases were compared. It could be shown that some clinical and subclinical viral infections took place in the group later developing metastases while, in the group not developing metastases, no subclinical infections were detectable by serology during IF therapy. These findings suggest a common denominator for the susceptibility to certain infectious agents and progression of osteosarcoma during the course of interferon therapy.

Immunologic Findings

IF has been shown to affect the immune system in vitro. Studies were therefore initiated to investigate whether treatment by human leukocyte IF affects the immune system also in vivo. Prolonged treatment with exogenous IF did not significantly change the mitogen responsiveness of lymphocytes in vitro [8]. Nor did the sensitivity of lymphocytes to IF-induced inhibition of mitogen responsiveness in vitro change during therapy. The natural killer cell activity of peripheral lymphocytes increased following the first injection of IF [7] and was maintained an increased level during prolonged IF therapy [9]. The proportion of lymphocytes showing sheep redblood cell (SRBC) receptors increased after the first IF injection, whereas the proportion of lymphocytes showing Fc and C3 receptors did not change to any major extent [10].

Metastases and Survival Rate

In the IF group, 17 of 35 patients who had been followed-up for 2 years were free of metastases and, after 3, 4, and 5 years of follow-up, were 13 of 27, 12 of 26, and 8 of 16, respectively. The corresponding figures for the concurrent control group were 10 of 30, 9 of 29, 9 of 29, and 7 of 26.
The survival rate for the IF group was, at 2 years, 25 of 35, at 3 years 17 of 27, at 4 years 12 of 20, and at 5 years 8 of 16. Corresponding figures for the concurrent control group were 18 of 30, 10 of 29, 10 of 29, and 8 of 26. In the concurrent control group there were six additional patients who received adjuvant high-dose chemotherapy. Of these six patients, four died of tumor disease while two are alive and free of metastases.

References

1. Adamson U, Aparisi T, Broström LÅ et al. (1979) Interferon treatment of human osteosarcoma. Study week of the Pontifical Academy of Sciences, Vatican city, Oct. 17–21, 1977. The role of non-specific immunity in the prevention and treatment of cancer. Pontif Accad Sci Scripta Varia 43: 383–406
2. Adamson U, Aparisi T, Broström LÅ et al. (1979) Adjuvant interferon treatment of human osteosarcoma. EORTC Annual Meeting June 21–24, 1978, Paris. Recent Results Cancer Res 68: 40–44
3. Broström LÅ (1979) On the natural history of osteosarcoma. Acta Orthop Scand [Suppl] 183: 1–38
4. Broström LÅ, Ingimarsson S, Strander H, Söderberg G (to be published) Adjuvant interferon treatment and late development of cerebral metastases in a patient with osteosarcoma. Acta Orthop Scand
5. Cantell K, Hirvonen S (1978) Large scale production of human leukocyte interferon containing 10^8 units per ml. J Gen Virol 39: 541–543
6. Cantell K, Strander H (1977) Human leucocyte interferon for clinical use. In: Högman CF, Lindahl-Kiessling K, Wigzell H (eds) Blood leucocytes, function and use in therapy. Almqvist & Wicksell, Stockholm, pp 73–75
7. Einhorn S, Blomgren H, Strander H (1978) Interferon and spontaneous cytotoxicity in man. II. Studies in patients receiving exogenous leukocyte interferon. Acta Med Scand 204: 477–483

8. Einhorn S, Blomgren H, Cantell K, Strander H (1979) Effect of prolonged in vivo administration of leukocyte interferon on the mitogen responsiveness of human lymphocytes. Acta Med Scand 206: 345–350
9. Einhorn S, Blomgren H, Strander H (to be published) Interferon and spontaneous cytotoxicity in man. V. Enhancement of spontaneous cytotoxicity in patients receiving human leukocyte interferon. Int J Cancer
10. Einhorn S, Blomgren H, Strander H (to be published) Effect of one intramuscular injection of human leukocyte interferon on blood leukocyte counts and proportion of lymphocytes forming E-, EA-, and EAC-rosettes. Int Arch Allergy Appl Immunol
11. Ingimarsson S, Strander H (1980) The frequency of acute infections in patients receiving interferon. In: Khan A, Hill NO, Dorn GL (eds) Interferon: Properties and clinical uses. Leland Fikes, Dallas, pp 633–644
12. Ingimarsson S, Cantell K, Strander H (1979) Symptomatic side-effects in patients receiving long-term therapy with human leukocyte interferon. J Infect Dis 140: 560–563
13. Mogensen KE, Cantell K (1977) Production and preparation of human leukocyte interferon. Pharmacol Ther [C] 1: 369–381
14. Nilsonne U, Strander H (to be published) Clinical experience of interferon treatment in osteosarcoma. 12th International Immunobiological Symposium. Yugoslav Academy of Sciences and Arts. Symposium on interferon, 1979
15. Strander H, Cantell K, Jakobsson PÅ, Nilsonne U, Söderberg G (1974) Exogenous interferon therapy of osteogenic sarcoma. Acta Orthop Scand 45: 958
16. Strander H, Cantell K, Ingimarsson S, Jakobsson PÅ, Nilsonne U, Söderberg G (1975) Interferon treatment of osteogenic sarcoma. 3rd International Congress for Virology. Madrid, Sept. 10–17
17. Strander H, Cantell K, Ingimarsson I, Jakobsson PÅ, Nilsonne U, Söderberg G (1975) Interferon treatment of osteogenic sarcoma. 7th Meeting of the International Society of Pediatric Oncology. Stockholm, Sept. 17–20
18. Strander H, Cantell K, Carlström G, Ingimarsson S, Jakobsson P, Nilsonne U (1976) Acute infections in interferon-treated patients with osteosarcoma: Preliminary report of a comparative study. J Infect Dis 133: A245–A248
19. Strander H, Cantell K, Ingimarsson S, Jakobsson PÅ, Nilsonne U, Söderberg G (1977) Interferon treatment of osteogenic sarcoma: A clinical trial. Conference on "Modulation of host immune resistance in the prevention or treatment of induced neoplasias", Dec. 9–11, 1974. Fogarty Int Center Proc 28: 377–381

18. A Strategic Adjuvant Therapy of Osteosarcoma*

C. Jasmin**

Hôpital Paul Brousse, Institute of Cancerology and Immunogenetics, Department of Virology, 14–16 Avenue Paul Vaillant Couturier, F-94800 Villejuif, France

Summary

Twenty-one patients with osteogenic sarcoma of the limbs were treated with an early combination of 1,750 rad whole lung irradiation, alternate cyclic chemotherapy with high-dose methotrexate, vincristine, mitomycin C, adriamycin, immidazol carboxamide (DTIC), cyclophosphamide, and intercalated immuno-BCG. The primary lesion was treated either by amputation or an 8,000 rad irradiation. Patients have been followed up for 6–29 months. Three patients relapsed, respectively, after 8, 11, and 22 months. All three patients had a long delay in completing the first part of treatment (first cycles A and B and lung irradiation). The 18 other patients are disease-free. Local relapses have not been observed. The toxicity of this protocol appears to be acceptable, but a longer follow-up is necessary to more precisely discern the efficacy and tolerance of the lung to this combined treatment.

Introduction

The failure of radical surgery to prevent the development of lung metastases in the vast majority of patients bearing osteosarcomas of the limbs has led most investigators to propose an adjuvant therapy associated with the treatment of the primary tumor. Many types of treatment have been tried during the last 10 years.

Prophylactic lung irradiation of 1,750 rad (equivalent to 2,000 rad with correction for air absorption) has increased the percentage of disease-free patients, by 15–20% in an EORTC randomized study. The difference observed between control and treated patients was significant [1]. Apparently this dose, which corresponds to the maximum tolerated dose for the lung, is critical. Indeed, a randomized trial performed at the Mayo Clinic (Rochester) with a 1,500 rad prophylactic lung irradiation was not effective [6]. It has been estimated that a 1,750 rad lung irradiation cannot kill more than approximately 10^5 tumor cells.

* French-American Cooperation on Cancer

** For the GETO-EORTC Working Party. Participating members: P. Cappelaere, P. Fumoleau, B. Le Mevel, D. Guerin, R. Hansen, D. Liegey-Bagarry, X. Meyer, G. Mathé, A. Mazabraud, R. Metz, J. Stines, G. Meynard, B. Serrou, A. Trifaud, M. Verhaeghe, and R. Wallaert

Recent Results in Cancer Research, Vol. 80

During the last 10 years many studies have demonstrated that chemotherapy is active against osteosarcoma on the primary tumor and lung metastases [4]. Although there is still some controversy as to its efficacy as adjuvant treatment, chemotherapy is widely used. Adriamycin and high-dose methotrexate are currently used most in the various published chemotherapeutic regimens [5].

The possible role of immunotherapy in osteosarcoma has not yet been adequately evaluated. However, it has been suggested that BCG may induce a better hematologic tolerance to the hematotoxic effects of chemotherapy. In 1978, our group started a strategic protocol of adjuvant therapy in patients with osteosarcoma of the limbs according to the following principles: (1) early combination of prophylactic lung irradiation and intensive chemotherapy; (2) alternating cycles of chemotherapy, combining drugs which have shown activity in metastatic osteosarcoma, to decrease the possibility of selecting subpopulations of resistant tumor cells; and (3) interspersed immunotherapy with immuno-BCG to increase the hematologic tolerance of patients to chemotherapy.

We report here the results of the 21 patients treated with this protocol since 1978.

Patients and Methods

The criteria for entry were (1) histologically proven osteosarcoma characterized by osteoid substance or bone apposed to tumor cells (none of the patients had parosteal osteosarcoma, radiation-induced sarcoma, or osteosarcoma after Paget's disease); and (2) no evidence of metastases (by standard lung tomography) at the start of therapy.

Table 1. Adjuvant therapy SO478: Characteristics of patients

Male/female		14/7
Age median (years)		15 (9–27)
Mean delay between first symptoms and diagnosis (months)		2.47 (1–6)
Localization of the primary tumor		
Proximal femur		2
Distal femur		5
Proximal tibia		8
Proximal fibula		3
Proximal humerus		3
Size of the primary tumor (product of two diameters in cm^2)		
	10	2
	10–19	2
	20–29	3
	30–49	4
	50–79	4
	100	2
	Not determined	4

Treatment of primary tumor consisted of either radical surgery for large tumors (when the function of the limb was definitively compromised by large soft-tissue invasion, by articular dysfunction, or by a bone fracture) or 80 Gy in 8 weeks on the tumor zone and 60 Gy over a 10 cm zone above and below the limits of the tumor in the case of small tumors or tumors on the superior limb.
The scheme for the adjuvant therapy is summarized in Table 1. The adjuvant therapy was given for 1 year. Thereafter, clinical observation was continued without any further drug administration. If metastases became evident during the course of the chemotherapy or after the patient was considered to be a treatment failure and other therapy was administered. Regular examination, blood counts, blood urea nitrogen (BUN), liver function test, blood levels of alkaline phosphatase, chest roentgenograms, EKG before each course of adriamycin, and respiratory function tests were performed.

Results

From January, 1978, to January, 1980, 21 patients were entered in the study. The age, sex, site of primary tumor, mean size of the tumor, interval between first symptoms

Table 2. Treatment of primary tumor

1. Histologic diagnosis
2. If possible, immuno-BCG 1 AMP/GRID (3 GRIDS at each time, one per limb), 3× week for 2 weeks, then pyocycanic vaccine (3 AMP. IM/day) on 3 consecutive days
3. Radical treatment (surgery or radiotherapy) of the primary tumor
4. Alteration for 11 months of immunochemotherapy A and B

Cycle A:	Day 1 mitomycin C (6 mg/m^2)
	Day 2 vincristine (1.4 mg/m^2) ($\leq$ 2 mg) methotrexate (10–25 mg/kg) with citrovorum factor rescue
	Days 13 and 15 immune-BCG (2 AMP/2 GRIDS)
Cycle B:	Day 1 adriamycin (60 mg/m^2)
	Day 2 vincristine (1.4 mg/m^2) ($\leqslant$ 2 mg)
	Days 3 and 6 DTIC (200 mg/m^2), cyclophosphamide (300 mg/m^2)
	Days 16 and 18 immuno-BCG AMP/2 GRIDS

5. Between the first cycle A and B, intercalate 2,000 rad lung irradiation

Table 3. Osteosarcoma adjuvant therapy SO478: Treatment of the primary tumor

Radiotherapy	9
Radical surgery	10
Radiotherapy followed by radical surgery	1 (Progression of tumor during radiotherapy)
Resection followed by radiotherapy	1 (Fibula)
Duration of observation	100% 6 months Median 12 months Range 6–30 months

Table 4. Characteristics of the three patients with metastases after adjuvant treatment SO478

Patient	Sex	Age (years)	Site of the primary tumor	Site of recurrence	Disease-free interval (months)	Remarks
S. I.	M	11	Proximal femur	Distant bone then lung metastases	11	Chemotherapy started more than 2 months after diagnosis. Doses of ADM and other drugs unduly decreased by 30%
B. O.	M	26	Proximal tibia	Lung	8	Chemotherapy was started 2 months after diagnosis: Reduction of doses of chemotherapy due to an hematologic toxicity 2-month interval between the first cycles A and B
A. L.	F	16	Proximal tibia	Lung	23	Primary tumor progressed during irradiation. Amputation was done secondarily. A second distal site of tumor was found in the inferior tibia by anatopathologic examination of the amputated limb. There was a 2-month interval between the first and the second course of chemotherapy

and diagnosis, and the treatments of the primary tumor are shown in Tables 2 and 3. At the time of this analysis, the follow-up time was 6–29 months.
Of the 21 patients, three have developed metastases. Table 4 summarizes the history of these three patients. Two patients relapsed after 8 and 11 months of adjuvant chemotherapy respectively, and one patient relapsed 10 months after the end of treatment. In two patients, metastases developed initially in the lungs. In one patient, a bone metastasis was detected in the absence of any sign of lung metastases and remained isolated for several months. Two patients died after 10 and 28 months, respectively. One metastatic patient is alive. Figure 1 represents the curve for the disease-free state and the survival curve is represented in Fig. 2. The estimated

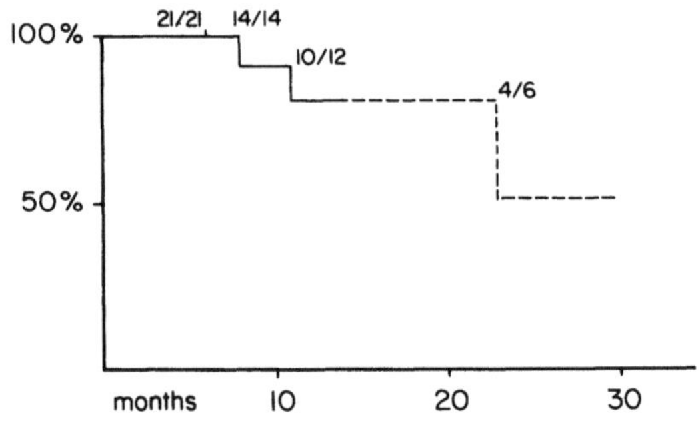

Fig. 1. Disease-free survival of osteosarcoma patients treated with protocol SO478. The Kaplan-Meier method was used to draw the curve

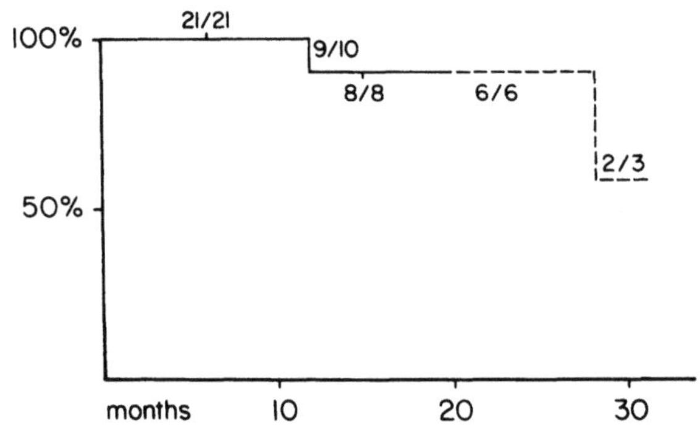

Fig. 2. Survival of osteosarcoma patients treated with protocol SO478. The Kaplan-Meier method was used to draw the curve

Table 5. Toxicity of protocol SO478

Hematologic toxicity	Twelve percent of chemotherapeutic courses with grade 2 toxicity (delay of the following cycle)
Nausea, vomiting	100% of patients
Alopecia	100% of patients
Infection	Two infectious episodes (grade 2)
Fever	Four episodes (3%) (grade 1)
Lung toxicity	Restriction of lung capacity without dyspnea in four patients, two patients with dyspnea (one heavy smoker)
Cardiac toxicity	One patient (grade 2)
Hepatic toxicity	Two patients (grade 1)

percentage of disease free patients at 16 months is 80% and the survival is 90%, using the Kaplan-Meier method of estimation.
The toxicity of the treatment is summarized in Table 5. Alopecia was consistently present. Digestive troubles were very frequent. Hematologic toxicity occurred after approximately 20% of the chemotherapeutic cycles. For the moment, the observed lung toxicity of combined lung radiotherapy and chemotherapy consisted of restrictive ventilatory effects. Allergy to BCG was seen in one case and immunotherapy was suspended for this patient.

Discussion

This trial is a phase II strategic protocol of adjuvant therapy characterized by the triple association of chemotherapy, prophylactic lung irradiation, and nonspecific active immunotherapy with BCG.
To our knowledge, there are only two published reports in which prophylactic lung irradiation was combined with chemotherapy. In the trial of Rab et al. [6] 15 Gy of whole lung irradiation combined with actinomycin D did not show any value as adjuvant therapy. More recently, Caceres et al. [2] treated 18 patients with 20 Gy whole lung irradiation over 21–28 days immediately after primary surgical resection of the primary tumor. Additionally, 11 of these patients received adriamycin at a dose of 20 mg/m^2 i.v. × 3 days repeated every 6 weeks (total dose 550 mg/m^2): In this small nonrandomized study no difference was found between the two groups, leading the authors to conclude that whole lung irradiation had no efficacy. The EORTC clinical cooperative group on radiotherapy and the SIOP (International Society of Pediatric Oncology) are presently conducting a trial in which they are comparing prophylactic whole lung irradiation versus intensive chemotherapy followed by whole lung irradiation. The results are not yet known and this trial is still in progress. Differing with the previous EORTC trial, we have chosen to combine, as early as possible, chemotherapy and whole lung irradiation. We were afraid that the lung toxicity of radiation might increase with chemotherapy, but at the present time there are no clinical signs of lung function impairment. We have only seen frequent restrictive ventilatory effects without alteration of the diffusing capacity of the lung. A longer follow-up is necessary for a better evaluation of the feasibility of this combined treatment.
Although cycle A was expected to have low hematotoxicity, the hematologic tolerance of the patients was often limited and in 20% the cycles were delayed to allow hematologic recovery. It is possible that the lung irradiation, which includes a large zone of active bone marrow, decreased the hematologic tolerance of the patient. The intercalation of BCG was not apparently sufficient to obtain a complete hematopoietic restoration between cycles in all patients. In summary, it can be said that this protocol has an acceptable toxicity and no toxic death has occurred. It is too early to fully evaluate the antitumor activity of this protocol. Only three patients of 21 have relapsed, and this figure differs from our previous experience with high-dose adriamycin or a protocol combining a sequential administration of high-dose methotrexate-citrovorum factor, high-dose adriamycin, and high-dose cyclophosphamide [3].
The three patients who have relapsed have had a long delay in completing the first period of treatment (first cycles A and B and lung irradiation). We think that this may

be a critical factor and that a great deal of attention should be given to this early period. It should be noticed that many primary tumors were treated by irradiation. It will be interesting to know whether these irradiated patients will present more local recurrences and/or more lung metastases than amputation patients.
In conclusion, we hope that this study will provide useful information as to the feasibility and the possible clinical interest of an early combination of lung irradiation and intensive cyclic chemotherapy, which may represent one way to improve the results of adjuvant therapy of osteogenic sarcoma.

References

1. Breur K, Cohen P, Schweisguth O, Hart AMM (1978) Irradiation of the lung as an adjuvant therapy in primary treatment of osteogenic sarcoma. Eur J Cancer 14: 461–471
2. Caceres F, Zaharia M, Moran M, Fejada F (1978) Adjuvant whole lung irradiation with or without adriamycin treatment in osteogenic sarcoma. Cancer Treat Rep 2: 297–300
3. European Group for Bone Tumors (GETO) (1978) The use of high and low doses of methotrexate on the treatment of osteogenic osteosarcomas. Chemother Oncol 2: 201–204
4. Jaffe N, Frei E III, Treggis D, Watts H (1977) Weekly high-dose methotrexate-citrovorum factor in osteogenic sarcoma: Pre-surgical treatment of primary tumor and of overt pulmonary metastases. Cancer 39: 45–50
5. Muggia F, Catam R, Lee YJ, Rozencweig M (1979) Factors responsible for therapeutic success in osteosarcoma: A critical analysis of adjuvant triam results. In: Jones SE, Sydney E (eds) Proceeding of the Second International Conference on the Adjuvant Therapy Cancer II. Salmon, Arizona, 28–31, 1979. Grune & Stratton, New York, pp 383–390
6. Rab GT, Ivins JC, Childs DS, Cupps RE, Pritchard DJ (1976) Elective whole lung irradiation in the treatment of osteogenic sarcoma. Cancer 38: 939–942

19. *Ewing's Sarcoma: Treatment with High-Dose Radiation and Adjuvant Chemotherapy*

A. Goldman*,**

Royal Marsden Hospital, Fulham Road, London SW3, United Kingdom

Summary

Twenty-nine patients with pathologically proven Ewing's sarcoma without overt metastases at diagnosis were treated with a protocol designed by The Royal Marsden and St. Bartholomew's Hospital Children's Solid Tumour Group. They received megavoltage radiotherapy to the involved bone and adjuvant chemotherapy with a combination of four cytotoxic drugs. Comparison with a historical control group of 19 patients treated with local surgery or radiotherapy but no initial chemotherapy shows a significant improvement in survival for the study group ($P = 0.022$). Thirteen patients have failed on the protocol: eight at the original site, four in other bones and only one in the lungs. Sixteen patients remain alive and disease free, 11 of these for over 33 months. The treatment regimen was moderately toxic but there were no treatment-related deaths. These results confirm that an improved survival time and, hopefully, cure rate can be expected by treating Ewing's tumour with high-dose megavoltage radiation and combination chemotherapy. Future goals must be better control of primary lesions and eradication of micrometastases in other bones.

Introduction

Ewing's sarcoma is a rare malignant bone tumour affecting children and young adults. In the past, 90% of patients with this disease died within 5 years in spite of local radiotherapy (RT) or surgery [1]. Today there is evidence that early treatment with megavoltage irradiation and chemotherapy is lowering this mortality [2, 4, 7].

---

* For the Children's Solid Tumour Group. Participating members: A. Barrett, H. J. G. Bloom, J. Graham-Pole, D. N. Lawson, T. J. McElwain, J. S. Malpas, D. Phil, J. Pritchard, and R. Sandland

** I would like to thank Professor Malpas for his helpful advice, Miss Mary Jones for her assistance with the statistical analysis and Prof. M. Peckman (Royal Marsden Hospital), Dr. S. Cartwright (Cookridge Hospital Leeds) and Dr. J. Darmady (Basingstoke District Hospital) who referred patients to this study

Patients and Methods

In 1974 the members of the Children's Solid Tumour Group designed a protocol for the treatment of stage I and II Ewing's sarcoma. The aims were to test the effectiveness of high-dose megavoltage irradiation in controlling the primary tumour and adjuvant chemotherapy in eradicating micrometastases. The treatment regimen, as it is in use now, is shown in Fig. 1. Vincristine (VCR), adriamycin (ADM), and cyclophosphamide are used initially. Two courses of chemotherapy are given prior to RT to decrease the tumour bulk. During irradiation the ADM is omitted because of sensitising effects [2], but it is subsequently used to a total dose of 400 mg/m^2. Actinomycin D is then substituted into the three-drug maintenance programme because of the dose-related cardiotoxic effects of ADM [6]. The intention is to maintain therapy for 2 years, but this has not been tolerated by all the children. The RT was administered using a cobalt 60 machine or 4 or 6 megavolt linear acelerator. The whole tumour-bearing bone received a dose of 4,000–5,000 rad and an additional 1,500 rad were given to the tumour field.

The study patients consisted of 29 children with stage I or II disease. None had evidence of metastases at the time of diagnosis. There were 19 boys and ten girls with a median age of 13 years (range 1–19 years). Their primary sites were pelvis (nine), humerus (four), fibula (four), femur (three), scapula (three), ribs (two), facial bones (two), cervico-dorsal spine (one), and foot (one).

A control group of patients were taken from the records of the Royal Marsden and St. Bartholomew's Hospital and used for comparison. This contained 19 patients, 11 boys and eight girls with a median age of 12 years (range 6–37 years) at diagnosis. Their primary sites were femur (six), pelvis (four), tibia (two), humerus (two), ribs (two), clavicle (one), mandible (one), and foot (one). These patients received a variety of primary surgical or radiation procedures for their local tumours. None had combination chemotherapy from the time of diagnosis, although many did receive drugs following the development of overt metastases.

The actuarial survival and duration of remission of both groups were compared statistically using the method of Peto et al. [3].

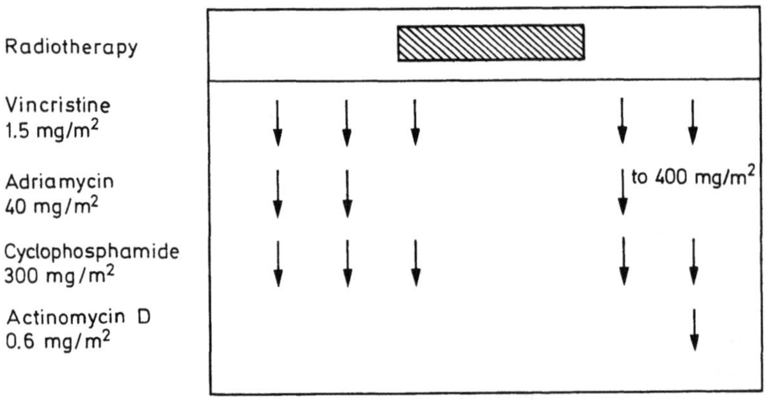

Fig. 1. Regime for treating Ewing's sarcoma. Drugs administered 3× weekly for up to 2 years

Results

The treatment regimen was moderately toxic but there were no treatment-related deaths. Common, expected complications of the chemotherapy were nausea, vomiting, alopecia and myelosuppression. In two cases vomiting was severe enough to result in curtailing the length of chemotherapy. One boy developed a pathological fracture through the site of his primary tumour 20 months after RT. This subsequently healed with conservative management. One boy, with a primary tumour of the fibula, has an unstable ankle. One patient, with a primary pelvic tumour, developed congestive cardiac failure which followed a cumulative dose of ADM (232.5 mg/m^2). He had received no thoracic radiation. In spite of the low ADM dose, this was felt to be the cause [4]. He responded to diuretics and, with the withdrawal of ADM from his treatment scheme, has had no further cardiac problems. A 15-year-old girl with a pelvic primary, developed severe cyclophosphamide cystitis, which was probably aggravated by infiltration of the bladder and pelvic irradiation.
Fig. 2 shows the actuarial survival of the study patients compared with the control group. The expectancy of survival is plotted against the time from diagnosis. The patterns of survival were compared using a χ^2 test which shows an increased expectancy of survival in the study group at the 5% significance level.
Fig. 3 shows the actuarial duration of remission. The probability of remaining in remission is plotted against the time from diagnosis. Recurrences occurred both during and after treatment up to 33 months from diagnosis. There are now 11 children in remission beyond this time.
There have been 13 patients who have failed on this protocol (Table 1). In two patients, local control was never achieved. Both of these had primary disease in the pelvis. One has since died but the other is only 6 months into treatment and may still achieve a remission. Recurrences occurred in 11 patients. In six of these, disease recurred locally before appearing in other sites. Four children developed their first evidence of metastases in another bone and only one girl had secondary deposits in her lungs. Those children whose disease recurred locally had several primary sites; two children with pelvic disease and rib primaries and one with tumours of the humerus and frontal bone. The sites of original disease in those who first had bone recurrence were one each in the femur, scapula, humerus and pelvis. The girl who developed lung metastases had a pelvic primary.

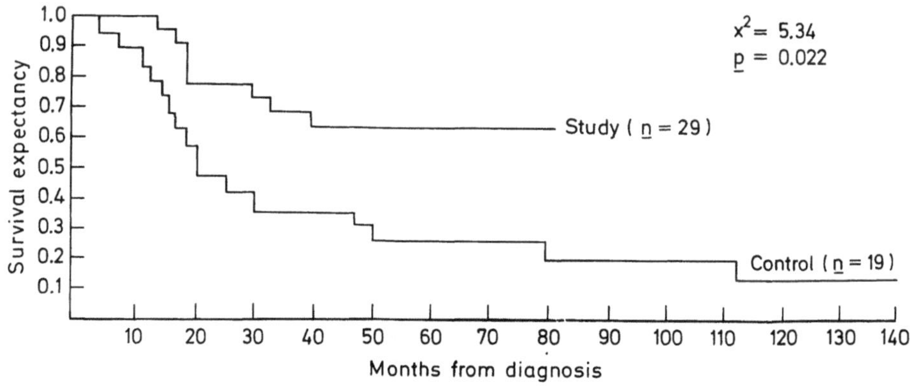

Fig. 2. Actuarial survival of study group and controls

Table 1. Treatment failures

Patient	Age at diagnosis	Sex	Site of primary tumour	Date of diagnosis	Time of recurrence (months)	Site of recurrence	Time to death (months)
V.B.	5	F	Rt. humerus	March 74	17	Rt. humerus	39
P.S.	14	M	R. femur	April 75	28	cervical spine	21
B.J.	13	F	R. scapula	April 75	33	R. femur	
M.Q.	10	M	R. humerus	Nov 75	13	L. femur	16
P.K.	16	F	Pelvis	June 76	24	Lung	
S.W.	15	F	Pelvis	July 76	No remission		13
R.G.	9	M	Pelvis	Sept 76	12	Pelvis	18
T.D.	19	M	Frontal bone	Nov 76	25	Frontal bone	29
L.S.	7	M	Pelvis	Jan 77	9	Pelvis	18
P.B.	16	M	Pelvis	July 77	17	Humerus	18
R.B.	11	F	Rib	May 78	20	Rib	
R.W.	6	M	Rib	Aug 78	17	Rib	
S.S.	1	F	Pelvis	Oct 79	No remission		

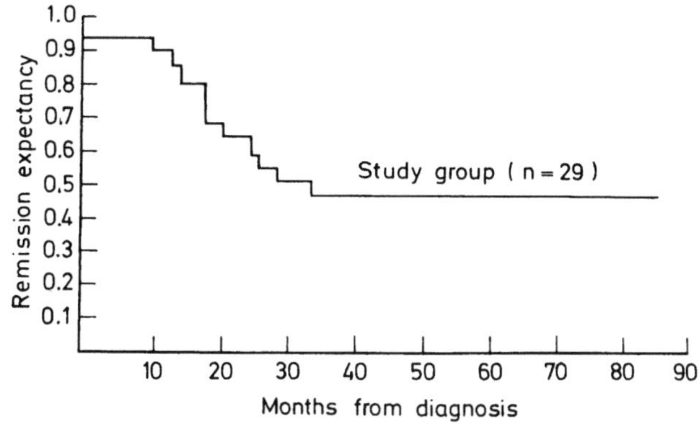

Fig. 3. Actuarial duration of remission

Discussion

There appears to be a statistically significant improvement in the pattern of survival of the patients who have been treated on this protocol, compared with the historical controls. There is improved control of the primary site, but initial disease in the pelvis and axial skeleton remains particularly difficult to eradicate. It may be of value to review the place of surgery in the treatment of the primary site and use RT either in the form of a split course or post-operatively to the tumour bed.

Chemotherapy has helped to control metastatic disease particularly to the lungs. The use of additional agents or more effective use of established drugs against micrometastases to the bony skeleton must be considered in the future.

Reference

1. Dahlin DC, Coventry MB, Scanlon PW (1961) J Bone Joint Surg 43: 185
2. Graham-Pole J (1979) Med Pediatr Oncol 7: 1–8
3. Lefrake EA, Pitha J, Rosenheim S, Gottlieb JA (1973) Cancer 32: 302–314
4. Perez CA, Razek A, Tefft M, Nesbit M, Burgert EO, Kissane J (1977) Cancer 40: 2864–2873
5. Peto R, Pike MC, Armitage P, et al. (1977) Br J Cancer 35: 1
6. Phillips TL, Fu KF (1976) Cancer 37: 1186–1200
7. Rosen G, Capparros B, Mosende C, McCormick B, Huvos AG, Marcove RC (1978) Cancer 4: 888–899

20. *Adjuvant Chemotherapy in Ewing's Sarcoma Patients*

M. Gasparini and F. Lombardi

Istituto Nazionale Tumori, Division of Clinical Oncology F, Via Venezian 1, Milano, Italy

Summary

At the Istituto Nazionale Tumori of Milan 60 patients with clinically localized Ewing's sarcoma were treated during 1965–1978 according to three different protocols. From 1965–1971, 18 patients received almost exclusively local therapy and 17 of 18 (94%) relapsed in a median time of 6 months. From 1971–1978 adjuvant chemotherapy according to two different drug schedules was employed after radiotherapy. Twenty-five of 42 (59%) are surviving and relapse-free at this time (follow-up 20–101 months).

Introduction

In the majority of patients with clinically localized Ewing's sarcoma, local treatment utilizing either radiotherapy (RT) or surgery does not appear to prevent distant relapse, mainly in lungs and bones. Median relapse-free survival (RFS) in about all series of patients who received only local treatment was less than 8 months [1–3]. In the early seventies, adjuvant chemotherapy was administered after local therapy to destroy the undetectable metastatic foci of malignant cells, which are believed to be present at the time of initial diagnosis. Results were promising and several papers reported a substantial increase in the RFS and, in some cases, an improvement of the cure rate was also claimed [3–5]. This paper reports the results obtained in our institute in the treatment of localized Ewing's sarcoma with and without adjuvant chemotherapy.

Patients and Methods

Patients with localized Ewing's sarcoma were treated in Milan with different modalities during various periods of time as shown in Table 1. From 1965–1971 treatment consisted mainly of RT delivered to the primary tumor site. Doses were from 40–70 Gy delivered only to the tumor area. Five of eighteen patients received adjuvant chemotherapy with cyclophosphamide (CTX) or vincristine (VCR) for a short period of time with different dose schedules. From 1971–1973, treatment

Recent Results in Cancer Research, Vol. 80

Table 1. Treatment modalities

Period of time	No. patients	Local therapy[a]			Adjuvant chemotherapy
		S	R	S + R	
1965–1971	18	3	13	2	5 (28%)
1972–1973	6	–	5	1	6 (100%)
1974–1978	36	2	28	6	36 (100%)

Types of adjuvant chemotherapy

Period of time	
1965–1971	Single-agent chemotherapy (CTX, VCR) for 1–2 months
1971–1973	ADM 20 mg/m^2/8 weeks. Every month VCR 1.4 mg/m^2/weekly, CTX 300 mg/m^2/weekly, and MTX 20 mg/m^2/weekly were alternated for 2 years
1974–1978	ADM 60 mg/m^2 day 1 + VCR 1.4 mg/m^2 day 1 and 8 monthly alternated with CTX 1 g/m^2 day 1 + VCR 1.4 mg/m^2 day 1 and 8 for 18 cycles

[a] S indicates surgery and R indicates radiotherapy

Table 2. Patient characteristics

	Period of study		
	1965–1971	1972–1973	1974–1978
No. of patients	18	6	36
Males/females	13/5	6/0	21/15
Age range (years)	5–29	8–21	2–37
Mean	15	13	13
Primary tumor site			
Extremities	7	3	24
Axial skeleton	11	3	10
Extraosseous	–	–	2

became more systematic and included an adjuvant chemotherapy program employing adriamycin (ADn), VCR, CTX, and methotrexate (MTX) once 50–70 Gy were delivered to the whole tumor-bearing bone. In 1974, the chemotherapy program was modified to administer higher pulse doses of ADM and CTX (Table 1).

Sixty consecutive patients were treated from 1965–1978. In all cases the diagnosis of Ewing's sarcoma was histologically proven and the extent of the disease was assessed with chest X-ray and skeletal survey. The systematic use of bone scans, bone marrow aspiration, and bipedal lymphangiogram was introduced only in 1974.

The patient characteristics are shown in Table 2. During the different periods of observation, patients' characteristics were not similar. In fact, the sex ratio of cases treated from 1965–1971 favored males. Furthermore, in this group there was a prevalence or primary tumor in the axial skeleton, which has a poor prognosis. In the two patients with tumor located in an extraosseous site, the histologic diagnosis was confirmed by electron microscopy.

Results

Table 3 summarizes the treatment results obtained in the three study periods. When treatment consisted mostly of local therapy, 50% of patients relapsed in a median time of 6 months (range 1–18 months). A total of 94% patients have relapsed. Starting from 1972, a total of 42 patients received adjuvant chemotherapy after local therapy. At the time of the present analysis, 25 patients (59%) are alive and relapse-free. Table 4 shows the primary sites of relapse according to the different types of treatment modalities employed. Lung metastases were more frequent in the group of patients treated without adjuvant chemotherapy. Local relapse as the first manifestation of treatment failure was observed only in patients given adjuvant chemotherapy. In fact, in the group treated only with local therapy, reactivation of the tumor at the level of the primary site was always associated with distant metastases.

Conclusions

In our series, adjuvant chemotherapy has improved RFS in patients with localized Ewing's sarcoma. However, it is difficult to compare present results with our historical

Table 3. Treatment results

	Period of study		
	1965–1971	1972–1973	1974–1978
Total treated	18	6	36
Relapsed	17 (94%)	2 (33%)	15 (41%)
Median time to relapse	6 months	Not reached	42 months (actuarial analysis)
Follow-up range	–	101 months	20–78 months (median 38 months)

Table 4. Sites of first relapse

Site of relapse	Period of study		
	1965–1971	1972–1973	1974–1978
Local	–	–	3
Local + distant	6	–	–
Distant	11	2	12
Lungs	8	1	2
Bones	3	1	9
Other	–	–	1
Total relapsed	17	2	15

controls. The poor outcome of patients who belong to this group could be due both from the more ominous sites of the primary tumor and from a less refined RT technique. Furthermore, diagnostic staging procedures were not as systematic as those utilized in more recent years. A fraction of patients treated from 1965–1971 were not studied with osseous scans, bone marrow aspiration, and lymphangiograms and they could have had undetected metastatic deposits at the time of the initial diagnosis. For these reasons, it is difficult to establish whether the improvement of RFS is only from the use of adjuvant chemotherapy. This impression should be demonstrated through randomized trials or in prospective studies carried out in a larger series of patients. However, it is worthy of note that the incidence of lung metastases was reduced in the group of patients given multimodality treatment.

References

1. Boyer CW Jr, Brickner TJ Jr, Perry RH (1967) Ewing's sarcoma. Case against surgery. Cancer 20: 1602–1606
2. Falk S, Alpert M (1967) Five-year survival of patients with Ewing's sarcoma. Surg Gynecol Obstet 24: 319–324
3. Gasparini M, Fossati Bellani F, Bonadonna G (1978) Current results with a combined treatment approach to localized Ewing's sarcoma. Recent Results Cancer Res 68: 45–51
4. Nesbit M, Vietti T, Burgert O et al. (1978) Intergroup Ewing's sarcoma study (IESS): Results of three different treatment regimens. Proc Am Assoc Cancer Res 323: 81
5. Rosen G (1978) Primary Ewing's sarcoma: The multidisciplinary lesion. Int J Radiat Oncol Biol Phys 4: 527–532

21. *Early Results of Combined Modality Therapy of Patients with Ewing's Sarcoma*

D. K. Hossfeld, S. Seeber, E. Siemers, C. G. Schmidt, and E. Scherer

Medizinische Universitätsklinik, Abteilung für Onkologie und Hämatologie, Martinistraße 52, D-2000 Hamburg 20, Germany

Summary

Fourteen patients with localized Ewing's sarcoma were treated with radiation therapy to the involved bone and systemic chemotherapy. Nine patients remained free of disease for a median follow-up period of 3 years. The actuarial 5-year disease-free survival rate is 60%.

Introduction

Ewing's sarcoma is a rare disease and it is even rarer in adults. Since only patients older than 14 years of age are admitted to our clinic, we thought it would be interesting to compare the results obtained in such patients with the usually much younger patient population reported in the literature.

Patients and Methods

Between December, 1973, and December, 1978, 14 untreated patients with localized Ewing's sarcoma entered our clinic. Eighty percent of the patients were 16–25 years of age. The diagnosis had been established by histologic examination of a representative biopsy. The stage of the disease had been evaluated by chest films, a bone scan with technecium pyrophosphate, and eventually a bone survey. The anatomic distribution of the primary lesions is given in Table 1.

Table 1. Anatomic distribution of primary lesions (n = 14)

Pelvis	3
Lower extremities	5
Upper extremities	1
Rib, scapula, clavicula	3
Maxilla	1
Spine	1

Recent Results in Cancer Research, Vol. 80

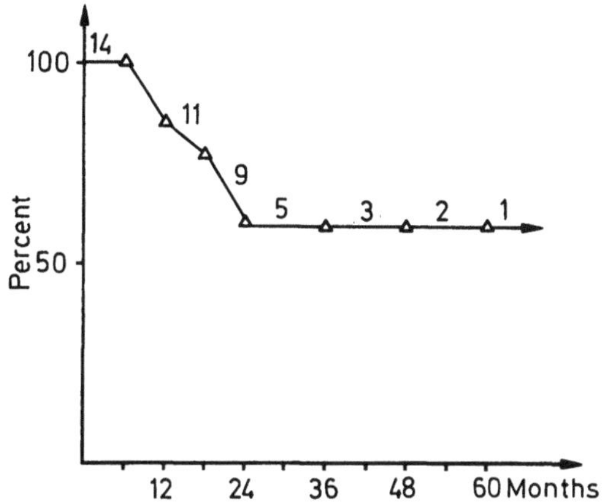

Fig. 1. Actuarial 5-year survival rate of 14 patients with localized Ewing's sarcoma is 60%

Table 2. Locations of relapse. Numbers in parentheses indicate time of recurrence in months after diagnosis

Primary lesion	Local treatment	Local recurrence	Distant metastases	Survival (months)
Tibia	Amputation Femoris	–	Epidural (12) Lung (18)	18
Scapula	Resection + 4,000 rad	(15)	Femur (12) Epidural (25)	49
Femur	5,600 rads	(16)	Pleura (18)	21
Sacrum	7,000 rads	(20)	Retro-orbital (22)	24
Rib	Partial resection + 5,000 rads	(40)	Epidural (42) Lung Ribs	50

Except for two patients who showed ablatio femoris before entering our clinic, all patients received megavoltage radiation therapy to the entire involved bone. Using the shrinking-field technique, the doses were 4,200–5,500 rad delivered in 4–6 weeks. One patient with a tumor located in the os sacrum got a tumor dose of 7,000 rad. Chemotherapy consisted of the combination adriamycin (ADM) (60 mg/m^2), vincristine (VCN) (1 mg/m^2), and cyclophosphamide (600 mg/m^2). This regimen was given every 3–4 weeks for six to eight courses. ADM was then substituted by methotrexate (MTX) (40 mg/m^2) and four to six such courses were added. During the early part of the study, dimethyl triazo imidazol carboxamid (DTIC) (250 mg/m^2/day) for 5 consecutive days was included. The duration of chemotherapy varied between 10–18 months depending on the size of the tumor and the degree of toxicity. In case of marked myelosuppression the intervals between chemotherapy courses were extended rather than reducing the drug doses.

Follow-up examinations were performed every 3–4 weeks during the first 18 months after diagnosis and every 3–6 months thereafter. They included films of the chest and of the involved bone. A bone scan was repeated if indicated, otherwise once a year.

Results

After a median follow-up period of 3 years, 9 of the 14 patients remained free of disease for 12 + to 59 + months. The actuarial 5-year disease-free survival rate is 60% (Fig. 1).

The relevant data of the five patients who relapsed are given in Table 2. Except for the patient who showing an ablatio femoris, all patients developed local recurrence which was followed shortly by distant metastases. In four patients the relapse became evident 3–22 months after discontinuation of chemotherapy. Spinal cord compression due to epidural tumor growth as the first sign of generalized disease was observed in three patients. Resumed chemoradiotherapy, using drugs such as actinomycin D, high-dose MTX, cisplatin, and ifosphamide, was unable to induce significant response, in contrast to our results obtained in patients with primary metastatic disease. Five of eight such patients went into complete remission; three of them are disease free 18–22 months after chemotherapy had been stopped.

Discussion

About 65% of all patients with Ewing's sarcoma are younger than 16 years [3]. Eighty percent of our patients, however, were 16–25 years of age. Because the results we obtained are comparable to those achieved in younger patients [2–5] we conclude that, in Ewing's sarcoma, age is not a significant prognostic factor.

The number of patients with local recurrences is disturbingly high. We do not believe that this is due to our treatment policy because Rosen et al. [5], with more aggressive chemotherapy and simultaneous radiochemotherapy reported a similar local recurrence rate. Also, it is known that radiation therapy exceeding 5,000 rad does not improve results [1, 3]. More importantly, local control is only a part of the problem, considering that our patients almost simultaneously developed distant metastases. The simultaneous local recurrence and distant metastases make it unlikely that an amputation or wide resection of the tumor-bearing limb or bone would have been able to solve the problem. Thus, we presently are reluctant to further maximize treatment modalities in patients with Ewing's sarcoma.

Epidural tumor growth with spinal cord compression occurs rather frequently in Ewing's sarcoma [2, 3, 5]. It may originate from vertebrae with metastatic involvement [2] or may be due to hematogenous spread of the disease. Epidural tumor growth is unrelated to meningeosis sarcomatosa, and, accordingly, cannot be prevented by prophylactic CNS treatment. Prophylactic irradiation of the spine is not indicated because it would limit chemotherapy with regard to bone marrow tolerance.

References

1. Fernandez CH, Lindberg RD, Sutow WW, Samuels ML (1974) Localized Ewing's sarcoma: Treatment and results. Cancer 34: 143–148

2. Le Mevel B, Mathé G, Jasmin C et al. (1980) Treatment of Ewing's sarcoma by radiotherapy and adjuvant chemotherapy: Results at 3 and 5 years. Nouv Presse Med 9: 359–362
3. Perez CA, Razek A, Tefft M et al. (1977) Analysis of local tumour control in Ewing's sarcoma. Cancer 40: 2864–2873
4. Pomeroy TC, Johnson RE (1975) Combined modality therapy of Ewing's sarcoma. Cancer 35: 36–47
5. Rosen G, Caparros B, Mosende C, McCormick B, Huvos AG, Marcove RC (1978) Curability of Ewing's sarcoma and considerations for future therapeutic trials. Cancer 41: 888–899

22. *Ewing's Sarcoma: 5-Year Survival Under Adjuvant Chemotherapy*

B. P. Le Mevel*,**

Centre René Gauducheau, Quai Moncousu, F-44035 Nantes Cedex, France

Summary

The results at 5 years of an adjuvant chemotherapy trial in primary Ewing's sarcoma, started in 1973, are presented. Twenty-three eligible patients were treated with radiotherapy (60 Gy) to the tumor site and given polychemotherapy either using the E_3 protocol (12 patients) or the E_{76} protocol (11 patients). Overall survival at 5 years was 37%, with 34% disease-free survival. There was no significant difference between the two chemotherapy groups. Only three local relapses and one major orthopedic failure were reported. Among the distal relapses, no metastases to the brain have been observed. These results are encouraging and show a clear improvement over the classical survival rate. However, further improvement is necessary and may be obtained by using new active drugs, as well as earlier and probably more aggressive cyclic chemotherapy. But primary surgical amputation and prophylactic CNS irradiation are not indicated for treatment of primary Ewing's sarcoma.

Introduction

The very poor prognosis of Ewing's sarcoma [1], the rapid appearance of distant metastasis [6], as well as the objective results obtained by chemotherapy [4, 6] led the EORTC Osteosarcoma Working Party and the Groupe d'Etude des Tumeurs Osseuses to start, in 1973, a therapeutic trial of adjuvant chemotherapy in primary Ewing's sarcoma.

Patients and Methods

The local treatment consisted of radiation therapy: 45 Gy to the entire involved bone, plus 15 Gy to the tumor in 6 weeks. In 1973, the adjuvant therapy was the E_3 protocol

* For the EORTC Osteosarcoma Working Party and Groupe d'Etude des Tumeurs Osseuses. Participating members: B. Le Mevel, P. Fumoleau, G. Mathé, C. Jasmin, M. Delgado, H. Sancho-Garnier, J. Durand, D. Guerin, C. Kenesi, R. Brossel, C. Chenal, P. Mazabraud, R. Metz, and J. Stines

** We thank Mrs. Brigitte Lapouyade and Mrs. Francoise Durand for their excellent assistance in the preparation of this manuscript

Recent Results in Cancer Research, Vol. 80

Vincristine (VCR)	1.5 mg/m^2	i.v., day 1, 10, and 20
Cyclophosphamide (CPM)	1 mg/m^2	i.v. or i.m., day 2, 11, and 21
Adriamycin (ADM)	60 mg/m^2	i.v., day 35 and 50
Procarbazine (PCB)	200 mg/m^2	orally, day 70 and 80

Chometherapy cycles: every 20 days for 18 months

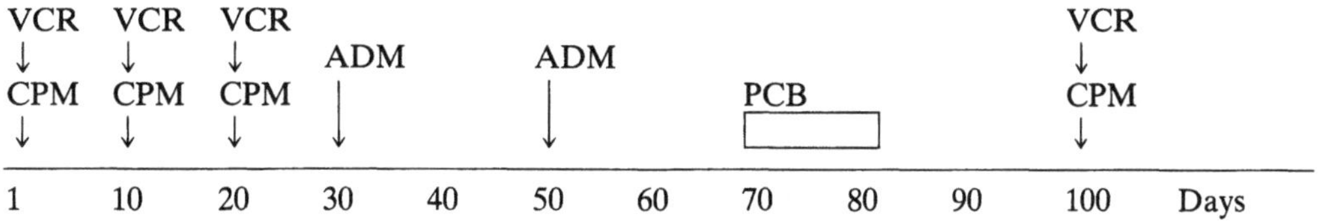

Fig. 1. E_3 protocol of adjuvant chemotherapy for primary Ewing's sarcoma

Starting with radiotherapy

Vincristine (VCR)	1.5 mg/m^2	i.v., day 1
Cyclophosphamide (CPM)	300 mg/m^2	i.v. or i.m., day 2, 3, 4, and 5

Disease-free interval, 3weeks

After radiotherapy

Adriamycin (ADM)	30 mg/m^2	i.v., day 1 and 2
Vincristine (VCR)	1.5 mg/m^2	i.v., day 3
Cyclophosphamide (CPM)	300 mg/m^2	i.v. day 4 and 5
Actinomycin D (act D)	0.3 mg/m^2	i.v., day 4 and 5

Chemotherapy cycles: every 3 weeks for 9 Cycles

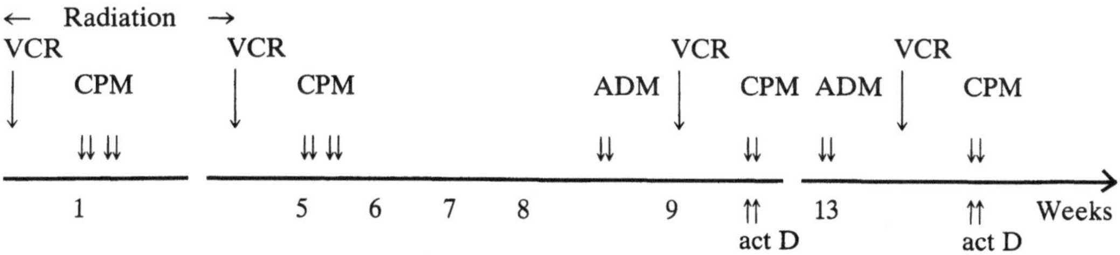

Fig. 2. $E_{76\text{-}5\text{-}170}$ protocol of adjuvant chemotherapy for primary Ewing's sarcoma

of the International Society of Paediatric Oncology (SIOP), a combination of vincristine (VCR), cyclophosphamide (CPM), adriamycin (ADM), and procarbazine (PBC) given for 18 months (Fig. 1).

In 1976, the appearance of early relapses with E_3 led us to follow another protocol ($E_{76\text{-}5\text{-}170}$). This protocol (Fig. 2) starts a combination of VCR, CPM, ADM, and

Maintenance chemotherapy

Methotrexate (MTX)	(20 mg/m^2 i.m. every weeks)
Cyclophosphamide (CPM)	(150 mg/m^2/day orally, 7 days, every 4 weeks)
Procarbazine (PCB)	(200 mg/m^2/day orally, 7 days, every 4 weeks alternately with CPM)

for 12 months

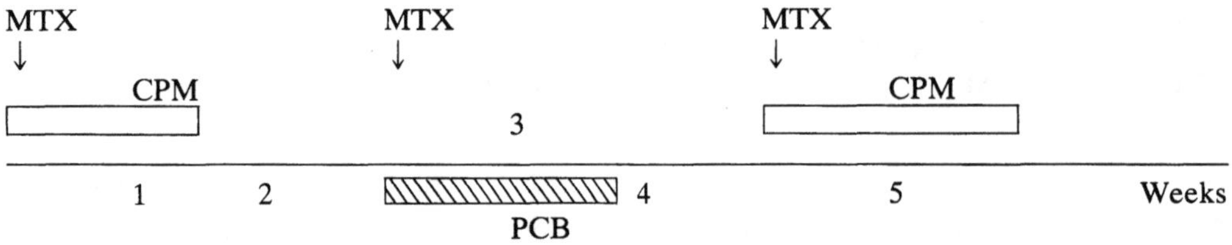

Fig. 3. $E_{76\text{-}5\text{-}170}$ protocol maintenance therapy

actinomycin D as early as possible, for 9 months; ADM and actinomycin D are used only after radiotherapy is completed. After nine cycles, a maintenance chemotherapy (Fig. 3) with methotrexate (MTX), CPM, and PCB is given for 12 months. Since 1973, 31 previously untreated nonmetastatic patients with primary Ewing's sarcoma entered our trial. Eight have been excluded for various reasons (incorrect diagnosis or staging and lost to follow-up). Twenty-three patients have been correctly followed-up, 12 under E_3 and 11 under E_{76} protocols. The distribution of these patients with respect to age, sex, and site of primary tumor is very similar in both groups. The median age is 17 years (range 7–37 years). There are more males (17) than females (six). The number of tumors of bad prognosis is very high (19 of 23); nine pelvis, one vertebrae, six femur, and three humerus. The other tumors are one rib, two tibia, and one calcaneum. This high number of poor-prognosis tumors has to be kept in mind in the evaluation of survival and for comparison with other trials.

Results

The 12 patients who entered the E_3 protocol were followed-up for a mean period of 59 months (range 33+ to 88+ months). We observed seven relapses (three skeletal of which one was local and four pulmonary) at 7, 8, 15, 18, 22, 22, and 24 months, respectively, after a mean period of 19 months. One patient in complete remission for 41 months developed an acute myeloid leukemia (AML) without evidence of recurrent Ewing's sarcoma. These eight patients died after rapid failure of medical treatment at 9, 11, 21, 26, 30, 38, 44, and 47 months, respectively. Four patients remained free of disease for a mean period of 67+ months (range 41+ to 88+ months). The mean follow-up of the 11 patients under E_{76} protocol is shorter (33+ months, range 25+ to 48+ months). We observed seven relapses (four skeletal of which one was local and three pulmonary) at 8, 9, 10, 18, 21, 22, and 29 months, after a mean period of 17 months. Five of these patients died within 2 years (18, 20, 22, 24, and 24 months). Four patients remained free of disease for a mean period of 36+ months (range 26+ to 48+ months).

Although the number of our patients is small, actuarial survival curves have been drawn using the method of Kaplan and Meier [7]. As shown in Fig. 4, a disease-free survival at 5 years is observed in 37% of the patients under E_3 protocol and in 34% under E_{76}. And as shown in Fig. 5, an overall survival at 5 years is obtained in 37% of the patients with E_3 protocol and in 54% of the patients with E_{76}, but the follow-up is shorter. There is no significant difference between the two groups. For the whole group of 23 patients under adjuvant chemotherapy we observed an overall survival at 5 years in 37% of the patients and a disease-free survival at 5 years in 34% of the patients (Fig. 6).

It is noticeable that the 14 relapses observed in these 23 patients occurred mainly within 2 years (after a mean period of 18 months) and usually led quickly to death.

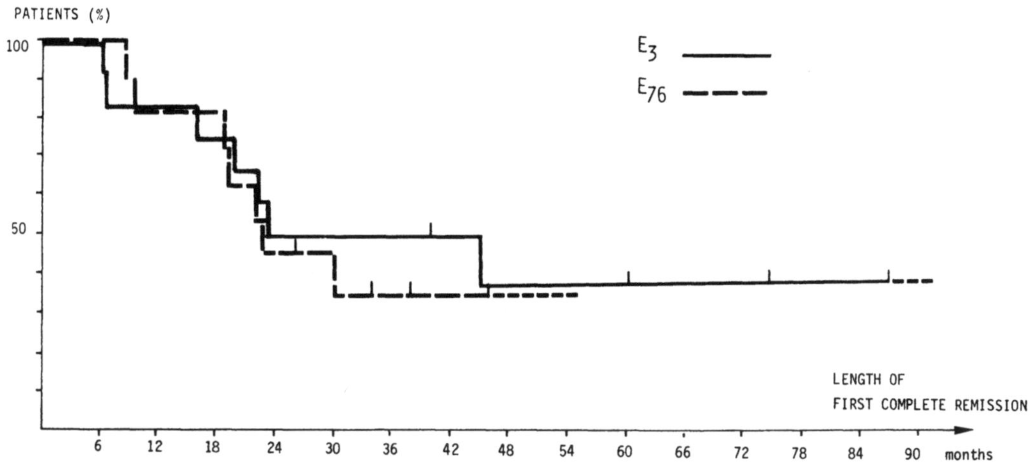

Fig. 4. Disease-free survival of primary Ewing's sarcoma patients on E_3 or E_{76} adjuvant protocols

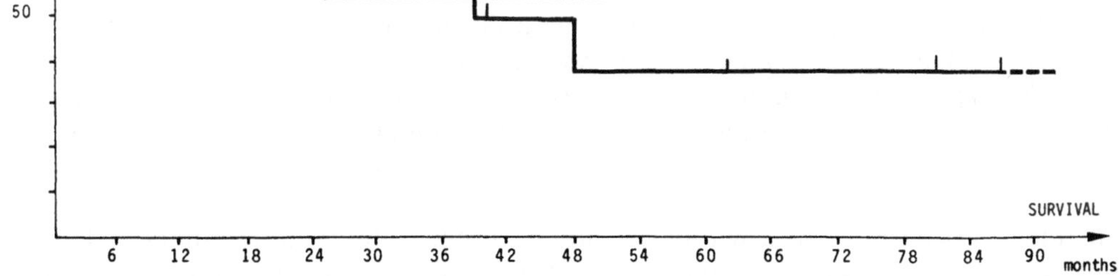

Fig. 5. Overall survival of primary Ewing's sarcoma patients on E_3 or E_{76} adjuvant protocols

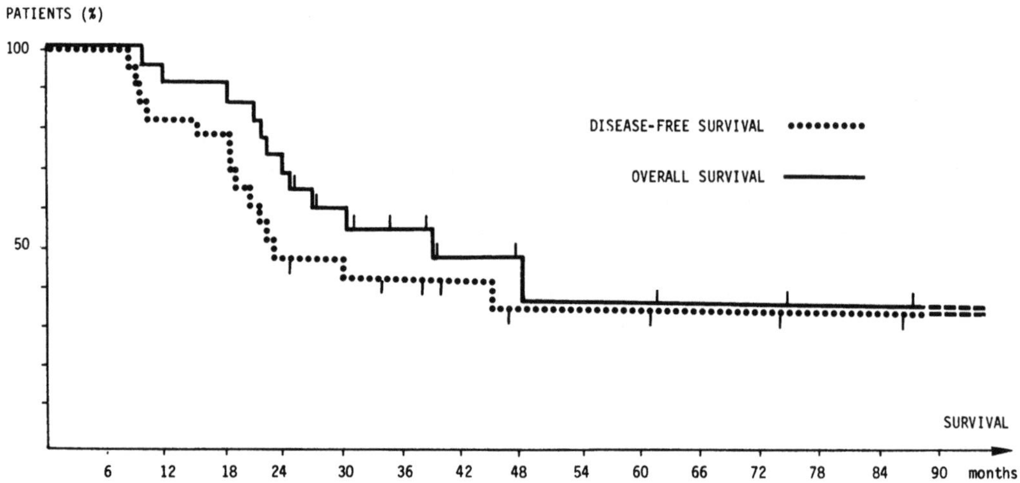

Fig. 6. Disease-free and overall survival of primary Ewing's sarcoma patients on adjuvant chemotherapy (E_3 and E_{76})

These relapses were skeletal (seven cases), pulmonary (five cases), or both (two cases). Most of the relapsing patients were male (12 of 14) with tumor of bad prognosis (six pelvis, four femur, three humerus). There were only two local relapses (one pelvis, one humerus). We observed no brain metastases. However, in three patients, metastasis to the vertebrae resulted in paraplegia.

Tolerance to both protocols was good. Reversible cardiomyopathy due to ADM occurred in one patient. Among the eight long-term survivors, we noticed one major orthopedic sequellae (hip).

Discussion

The results of our therapeutic trials are encouraging, although somewhat less than anticipated 2 years ago [8]. The 37% survival at 5 years is of no doubt a real progress over the classical 10–15% survival after local treatment alone [1], in the same range as the results obtained recently by Jaffe et al. [5], Pomeroy and Johnson [10], Rosen et al. [11], and Glaubiger et al. [2].

However, these results have to be improved by selection of new drugs in phase II trials with relapsing patients, as well as by making a distinction between patients of good prognosis with distal long-bone lesions (we observed only one relapse out of four patients) and patients of bad prognosis with central and proximal long-bone lesions (13 relapses out of 19 patients in these cases). A reinforcement of the treatment of these latter patients using, for example, alternate cycles of chemotherapy, may be necessary [2].

Our relapses occurred early, within 2 years, as already observed by others [11]. We think that prevention of these relapses might be possible by the use of an earlier and more aggressive combination therapy. However, we must emphasize that AML occurred in one patient after 41 months of complete remission. Although Ewing's tumor arises from immature blast cells,leukogenesis could be due to the combination of radiation and chemotherapy [3, 12].

In January 1980, our group started a new protocol for poor-prognosis patients based inclusion of new drugs like (dimethyl-3,3 triazéno-1)-5 imidazole-4 carboxamide (DTIC) and (chloro-2 ethyl)-1 cyclo hexyl-3 nitroso-1 urea (CCNU) and alternate cycles of polychemotherapy. We observed only two local relapses and one major dysfunction of the limb. This is consistent with previous results [9] obtained by a combination of local radiation at 6,000 rad and a polychemotherapy including ADM. It is obvious that surgical amputation is not the primary treatment of Ewing's sarcoma, in view of its clear radiosensitivity.

We did not observe any brain metastasis and see no indication for prophylactic CNS irradiation, with its uncertain future risks.

Ewing's sarcoma is rare and we would like to stress that only inclusion of such patients in therapeutic trials will allow us to improve its prognosis. However, it is possible to say that the treatment of Ewing's sarcoma should be a multidisciplinary approach and the best modality has yet to be defined.

References

1. Falk S, Alpert M (1967) Five years survival of patients with Ewing's sarcoma. Surg Gynecol Obstet 124: 319–324
2. Glaubiger DL, Makuch R, Scwarz J, Levine AS, Johnson RE (1980) Determination of prognostic factors and their influence on therapeutic results in patients with Ewing's sarcoma. Cancer 45: 2213–2219
3. Greene MH, Glaubiger DL, Mead GD, Graunneni JF (1979) Subsequent cancer in patients with Ewing's sarcoma. Cancer Treat Rep 63: 2043–2046
4. Hustu JD, Pinkel D, Pratt CB (1972) Treatment of clinically localized Ewing's sarcoma with radiotherapy and combination chemotherapy. Cancer 30: 1522–1527
5. Jaffe N, Paed D, Traggis D, Saliàn S, Cassady JR (1976) Improved outlook for Ewing's sarcoma with radiotherapy and combination chemotherapy. Cancer 38: 1925–1930
6. Johnson RE, Pomeroy TC (1972) Integrated therapy for Ewing's sarcoma. AJR 114: 532–535
7. Kaplan EL, Meier P (1958) Nonparametric estimation from incomplete observation. J Am Stat Assoc 53: 457–481
8. Le Mével B, Mathé G, Jasmin G, Durand M, Brassel R, Chenal C, Guerin D, Kenesi C, Tomeno B, Mazabrand A, Sancho H. (1979) Five-years survival of Ewing's sarcoma patients treated by radiotherapy and adjuvant chemotherapy. In: Jones SE, Salmon SE (eds) Adjuvant therapy of cancer II. Grune & Stratton, New York, pp 403–408
9. Perez CA, Razek A, Tefft M, Nesbet M, Burger EO, Kissane J, Vietti T, Gehan EA (1977) Analysis of local tumor control in Ewing's sarcoma: Preliminary results of a cooperative intergroup study. Cancer 40: 2864–2873
10. Pomeroy TC, Johnson RE (1975) Combined modality therapy of Ewing's sarcoma. Cancer 35: 36–37
11. Rosen G, Caparos B, Massende C, McCornik B, Huros AC, Marcove R (1978) Curability of Ewing's sarcoma and considerations for future therapeutic trials. Cancer 41: 888–899
12. Youness D, Rosik G, Benjamin R, Trujillo JM, et al. (1978) Acute myeloid leukemia following a chemotherapeutic regiment for metastatic sarcoma. Cancer Treat Rep 62: 1513–1516

IV. Breast Carcinoma

23. *Natural History of Breast Cancer*

S. Gore, A. Langlands, S. Pocock, and G. Kerr*

MRC Biostatics Unit, Medical Research Council Centre,
Hills Road, Cambridge CB2 2QH, United Kingdom

Summary

Retrospective analysis was made of 3,918 cases of breast cancer seen during 1954–1964. Median survival was 4.5 years and 30% of patients survived through a 10-year period. For stages I, II, and III patients, the mortality increased during 1–4 years after diagnosis and then slowly declined. Beyond 15 years, stage III patients assumed the same mortality (5%) as those with lesser disease; 58% excess of deaths from all causes after 15–20 years showed that breast cancer was not curable within 20 years but ultimately, taking account of clinical status, 51% of 5-year survivors with stages I–III disease are cured.

Introduction

Important observations on the natural duration of cancer were made by Greenwood [10]. He noted that the risk of dying (or hazard) increases during the first 3 years after onset, and was then constant or slowly declined. He wrote of breast cancer, "At no observed epoch from onset is the rate of mortality of the same order of magnitude as normal mortality." Early descriptions of the natural history of treated breast cancer, nevertheless, usually admitted a cured group [4, 5, 11] due to an overriding concern to counter fears which could delay referral. Theories about the aetiology of breast cancer were naive; insight was gained by identifying covariates (physical signs, histology, demographic data, etc.) associated with prognosis. Cancer registries were an important data source and case histories, then subject to review, were done more carefully. Communication of results between centres led to the staging of breast cancer and marked the inadequacy of current series for treatment comparison.
Three major consequences of these early researches have been, firstly, a recognition that conventional fixed-time survival at 5 or 10 years is not synonymous with cure. As a

* We are grateful to colleagues, past and present, and to the Department of Radiotherapy, Edinburgh, for access to case records, the high quality of which made this study possible. We wish to thank Mr. W. Lutz, Medical Computing and Statistics Unit, Edinburgh, for making our collaboration possible

result there has been increasing use of life-table analysis [15]. Secondly, the diversity of the disease has been incorporated as covariate data into descriptions of survival. Finally, the fact that relapse can occur many years after initial treatment has made it necessary not only to continue follow-up for 20 years or more, but also to allow for the normal mortality in the general population.

Several authors have analysed survival taking these considerations into account. Myers et al. [14] developed a systematic model relating survival to prognosis. They considered that survival was exponentially distributed when patients were classified by nuclear grade, nodal status, sinus histiocytosis and tumour size. By implication, they doubted the existence of a cured cohort. Their method was adopted by Cutler and Myers [8], who made some progress towards staging breast cancer by grouping patients with similar survival rates. Berg and Robbins [3] showed that the exponential model failed to predict survival in the second decade, when observed deaths were fewer than expected.

Easson and Russell [9] could not identify a cured cohort by year 15 after treatment, though the observed mortality in their main study group of 1,812 operable cases was only 1% per annum in excess of expected mortality during the 10–15 year period. They emphasised the need for a follow-up of more than 15 years. Brinkley and Haybittle [6], in a 25-year study of 704 women, suggested that, after 21 years, observed and expected mortalities were the same and interpreted this to mean that 18% of all patients and 30% of women with stages I and II disease were cured. Haybittle [12] also showed that the mortality from cancer in the Birmingham series was not constant (which would suggest incurability) but decreased with time: He calculated that more than a quarter of those patients could be considered cured.

In spite of these estimates of curability, careful analysis of the deaths that occur more than 20 years after treatment has shown that breast cancer remains significantly more common as a cause of death than in the general population [10]. Of all women who die after developing cancer of the breast, 80–85% do so from their disease. Definition of cure in terms of general population mortality may have serious limitations.

Langlands et al. [13] reported the effect of three prognostic variables singly (stage, tumor size and menstrual status) on the curability of breast cancer. Further results are presented in this paper.

Patients and Methods

All 3,922 patients referred to the Department of Radiotherapy, Edinburgh, for a primary decision on the treatment of breast cancer from January, 1954, to March, 1964, were followed-up. Four who had bilateral disease were excluded. Patients were reviewed on every anniversary of first treatment and were dismissed from follow-up after 20 years. The standard treatment was simple mastectomy plus radiotherapy. Seventy-three percent of all patients in the series, and over 90% of those with stages I or II disease, were treated in this way.

Life-table analyses are based on 6-month intervals during the first 5 years of follow-up and yearly intervals thereafter. In the analysis of curability, 40 patients are excluded who were over 85 years of age at presentation, and others are removed from follow-up on reaching age 85; since national age-specific death rates are not accurately known for people 85 years of age or more and to prevent analytical effects of undue concentration on elderly deaths. The main results concern deaths from all causes. Allowance is made for the expected mortality from causes other than breast cancer by reference to age-specific death rates in the Scottish national population. The bases for statistical comparison are the ratio of observed to expected deaths and the excess death rate. By modifying the extrapolated actuarial model [11] we assess simultaneously the effect of several prognostic factors on curability.

Results

Overall Survival

Figure 1 shows the life-table for 3,918 patients with unilateral carcinoma of the breast. Median survival was 4.5 years and 30% of patients survived for at least 10 years. Survival was also analysed by considering the percentage who died of those alive at the start of each year of follow-up. The rate of dying decreases steadily from a peak mortality of 16.6% in year 1 to an average mortality of 4.9% over the 14–16 years of follow-up. In the later period there is slight upturn in hazard, probably due to elderly deaths, while the form of the hazard is changed dramatically when allowance is made for prognostic factors.

Staging

International staging separates patients into four groups with progressively poorer survival. Sixty-nine percent of stage I and 57% of stage II patients survive for at least 5 years compared with 35% and 7% respectively of stages III and IV patients. Hazard decreases for stage IV patients (473): More than 60% of such patients die within 1 year of diagnosis. For patients with stages I–III breast cancer (1,301, 641, 1,417, respectively) Fig. 2 shows that rate of death increases during the first few years after treatment and then slowly declines. Peak hazard is apparently earlier for more advanced breast cancer: For stage III patients hazard is maximum (23% mortality)

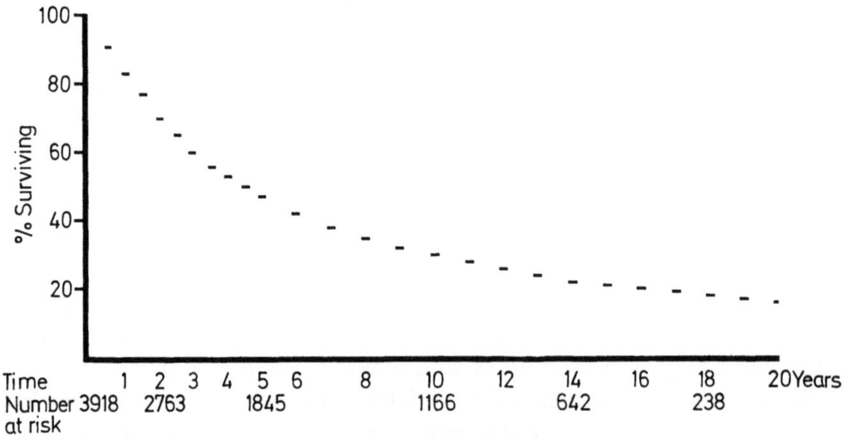

Fig. 1. Life-table: All patients (3918), unilateral breast carcinoma

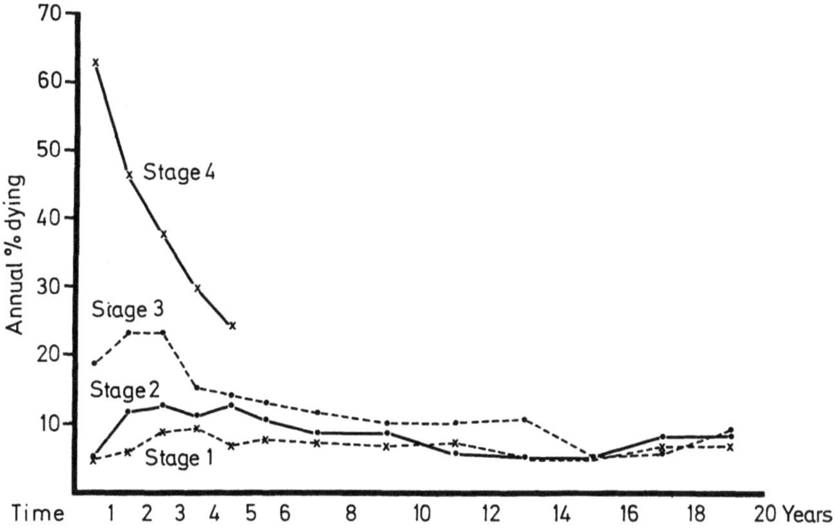

Fig. 2. Mortality by year, according to International stage

2–3 years after diagnosis, while, for women with stage I breast cancer, peak hazard (9%) is 3–4 years after diagnosis. Hazards corresponding to stages I–III are distinct during the first 10 years of follow-up, but thereafter the mortality converges. Beyond 15 years, stage III patients assume the same mortality (about 5%) as those with stages I or II. Only eight patients with stage IV breast cancer survived for more than 8 years.

Menstruation

Survival rates at 5 and 10 years are summarised in Table 1. Survival is most favourable for women diagnosed as premenopausal. These women, of course, are the group least depleted by deaths from other causes. From year 6 of follow-up, the distributions for menopausal and postmenopausal survival diverge so that only 14% of postmenopausal patients survive for more than 15 years, compared with 24% who, at diagnosis, were menopausal. Mortality for the three menstrual classes are shown in Fig. 3. During the first 4–5 years, mortality is as high for menopausal patients as it is for the postmenopausal group but, thereafter, postmenopausal patients have the worst overall prognosis. By year 10 of follow-up the outlook is as good for menopausal patients as it is for the premenopausal group, despite significantly older mean age (cf. 10-year survivors at 61.2 and 52.9 years respectively).

Aetiology

An index was constructed from clinical variables to identify tumours diagnosed as premenopausal [1]. The aggressive features of such tumours were size ($\leqslant 2$ or $\geqslant 5$ cm) and moderate clinical involvement of the axillary nodes. Nevertheless discrimination was poor: 94% of patients who were menopausal or postmenopausal were identified,

Table 1. Menstruation. Menstrual status was not recorded for 199 patients

Time (years)	Survivors after ± (years)		
	Premenopausal	Menopausal	Postmenopausal
0	1,064	450	2,205
5	596 (56%)	196 (44%)	952 (43%)
10	437 (41%)	134 (30%)	522 (24%)

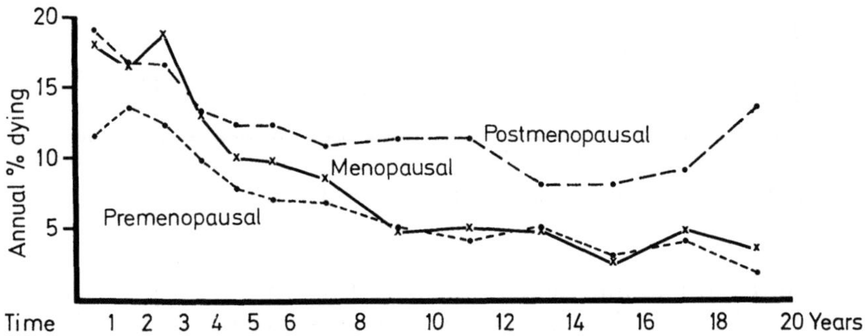

Fig. 3. Mortality by year, according to menstrual status

compared to only 17% of premenopausal patients. Menstrual status does not determine clinical profile at presentation.

Terminal Survival

Defined as time from relapse (local or distant) to death, terminal survival is significantly longer for patients whose disease-free interval was long. Median terminal survival is 8 months for the 1,019 patients who relapsed within 2 years of initial treatment; 17 months if disease-free interval was 2–4 years (421 patients) and 28 months for patients (534) who were disease-free for at least 4 years. For 1,944 patients, neither local nor distant recurrence was noted.

Comparison with Expected Mortality

Langlands et al. [13] showed that the ratio of observed to expected deaths ($O : E$) for the series as a whole (3,878 patients) fell from 8.3 in year 1 to 2.6 in year 10 of follow-up. Thereafter the ratio varied from year to year but remained greater than 1 throughout. Table 2, from their data, shows an excess mortality among patients up to 15 years after initial treatment. From 15–20 years there was still a 58% excess mortality which was very highly significant ($P < 0.001$). The 95% confidence limits indicated that the real excess for all breast cancer patients at this stage was somewhere between 25–98%.

Table 2. Comparative mortality in 3,878 cases of breast cancer

Follow-up (years)	Observed deaths	Expected[a] deaths	Ratio[b] $O:E$	95% Confidence limits for ratio	Excess death[c] rate/1,000 woman-years
0– 5	2,013	298.5	6.74	6.45–7.05	130.8
5–10	638	186.0	3.43	3.17–3.71	63.1
10–15	268	123.9	2.16	1.91–2.44	33.4
15–20	77	48.7	1.58	1.25–1.98	18.8

[a] Based on Scottish age-specific death rates
[b] $O:E$ indicates observed-expected death ratio ($P < 0.001$ comparing observed ratio with 1)
[c] Defined as (observed-expected deaths) × 1,000/woman-years at risk

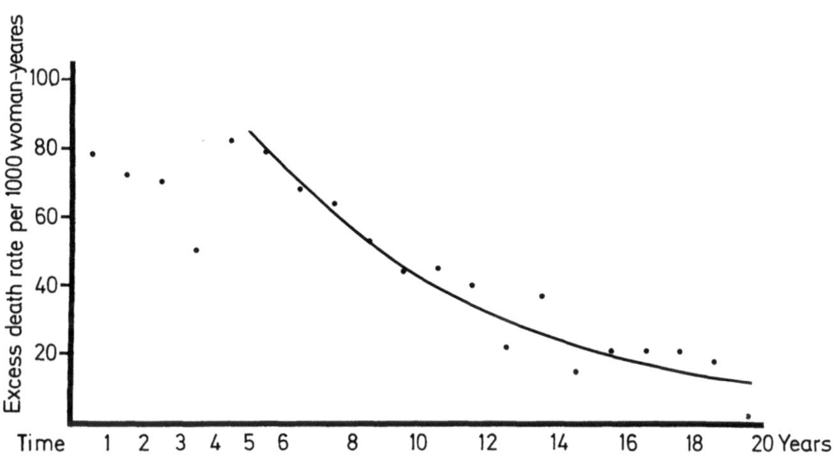

Fig. 4. Excess death rate: Exponential decay

The lethality of breast cancer is most extreme, in relative terms, at younger ages (compare $O:E$ during 0–5 years for respectively pre-, menopausal and postmenopausal women; 25.13, 17.26, and 3.70), but that is not evidence for the hypothesis that the disease is more aggressive in younger women. An alternative method of expressing the mortality of breast cancer patients is an excess death rate [13]. At 15–20 years follow-up the excess death rate was 18.8 per 1,000 woman-years, or just under 2% a year. Fig. 4 shows that excess death rate declines exponentially after 5 years after diagnosis. Perhaps we could describe the hazard for a breast cancer patient as the sum of the underlying force of mortality (Scotland) and an exponentially decaying excess hazard which depends on the patient's clinical status at presentation. Haybittle [11] applied this extrapolated actuarial model from time of diagnosis, but found it necessary to choose the early time intervals carefully to mask the initial rise in hazard.

Sixteen-hundred and ten patients with known tumour size and menstrual status who had stages I, II, or III disease were alive after 5 years. Taking account of clinical status

Table 3. Exponential fit of stage and menstruation

Covariate	Weight	SE	t-Value
β_1 Constant (all patients)	−8.0123	0.1100	
Stage I	−0.6108	0.1168	−5.23[a]
Stage II	−0.3095	0.1360	−2.28[b]
Premenopausal I	−0.0965	0.1122	−0.86
Menopausal	−0.0017	0.1584	−0.01
β_2 Decay per annum (all patients)	0.1263	0.0188	6.73[a]

[a] Highly significant
[b] Significant at $P < 0.03$

we fitted the model

hazard at time (t) for years of age (x) with clinical status (z) = hazard for woman aged $x + t$ years in Scottish population (approximation) + exp $[\beta_1(z)\text{-}\beta_2(z)t]$

to the survival from 5 years of these 1,610 women, where $\beta_1(z)$, $\beta_2(z)$ are weighted sums of covariates (estimation by maximum likelihood). Table 3 shows the result of fitting stage and menstruation. Log excess hazard decays at the rate of 0.1263 per annum so that at 20 years after diagnosis the excess hazard is estimated to be

$$\exp[-8.0123 - 0.0965 - 0.3095 - 0.1263 \times 15] = 3.321 \times 10^{-5}$$

for a patient who was referred as premenopausal with stage II disease and who had survived for 5 years after initial treatment. The time-specific risk of death for a woman 60 years of age in the Scottish population is 3.314×10^{-5}.

A better description is given by fitting several clinical covariates together with menstruation, but the terms for menstruation can be dropped so that the virulence of breast cancer is seen to depend only on clinical signs at diagnosis and does not change with age. Remarkably the penalty associated with skin fixation was higher than for involvement of axillary nodes. Mortality rate increased with tumour size. Following Haybittle [11] we estimated that 826.3 (51%) of the 1,610 5-year survivors constituted a cured cohort. There have been 867 deaths up to December, 1976, of which 219 were recorded as deaths from other causes. A further 208 patients are expected to die from breast cancer. The ratio 826.3 : 3068 is a conservative estimate of the cure rate (27%) in this series (3,068 is the number of stages I, II or III patients younger than 85 years at diagnosis on whom data were complete).

Discussion

Patients in the menopausal group are conventionally regarded as carrying the poorest prognosis. In the Western General series, this was so for the first 5 years, but the difference disappeared with longer follow-up. The clinical profile at presentation did not differ between patients who were diagnosed before and after menopause, although mobile axillary nodes were a pointer to premenopausal status.

Stage-separated patients into four groups with progressively poorer survival. The hazard associated with dire covariates decreased sharply, but for patients with a more favourable prognosis the rate of dying increases during the first 1–4 years after diagnosis, and then slowly declines. This could have implications for breast cancer as a systemic disease [2]. The hazards associated with different disease profiles converge with time (an exception is skin fixation). By implication, the exponential (constant hazard) and Cox (proportional hazard) models [7] are not appropriate for describing survival in breast cancer patients.

The Western General series (3,878 cases) is considerably larger than that reported by Brinkley and Haybittle [6]. The 58% excess of deaths from all causes at 15–20-year follow-up provides strong evidence that breast cancer patients as a whole cannot be considered cured within 20 years, particularly since the excess includes a 20-fold increase in deaths from breast cancer [13].

This prolonged increase in mortality should not be interpreted too pessimistically since the excess mortality rate beyond 15 years is less than 2% per annum and, taking account of clinical status, we estimate that 51% of 5-year survivors with stages I, II, or III disease are ultimately cured.

References

1. Armitage P, Geham EA (1974) Statistical methods for the identification and use of prognostic factors. Int J Cancer 13: 16–36
2. Baum M (1976) The curability of breast cancer. Br Med J I: 439–442
3. Berg JW, Robbins GF (1967) Failure of a model to predict cancer survival. J Chronic Dis 20: 809–814
4. Berkson J, Gage RP (1952) Survival curve for cancer patients following treatment. J Am Stat Assoc 47: 501–515
5. Boag JW (1949) Maximum likelihood estimates of the proportion of patients cured by cancer therapy. J R Stat Soc [B] 11: 15–44
6. Brinkley D, Haybittle JL (1977) The curability of breast cancer. World J Surg 1: 287–289
7. Cox DR (1972) Regression models and life-tables. J R Stat Soc [B] 34: 178–202
8. Cutler SJ, Myers MH (1967) Clinical classification of extent of disease in cancer of the breast. J Natl Cancer Inst 39: 193–207
9. Easson EC, Russell MH (1968) The curability of cancer at various sites. Pitman, London
10. Greenwood M (1926) Natural duration of cancer. Her Majesty's Stationary Office, London (Report on Public Health and Medical Subjects No 33)
11. Haybittle JL (1965) A two-parameter model for the survival curve of treated cancer patients. J Am Stat Assoc 60: 16–26
12. Haybittle JL (1968) Letter to the editor. Br J Radiol 41: 639
13. Langlands AO, Pocock SJ, Kerr GR, Gore SM (1979) Long-term survival of patients with breast cancer: A study of the curability of the disease. Br Med J 2: 1247–1251
14. Myers MH, Axtell LM, Zelen M (1966) The use of prognostic factors in predicting survival for breast cancer patients. J Chronic Dis 19: 923–933
15. Peto R, Pike MC, Armitage P, Breslow NE, Cox DR, Howard SV, Mantel N, McPherson K, Peto J, Smith PG (1977) Design and analysis of randomised clinical trials requiring prolonged observation of each patient. Br J Cancer 35: 1–39

24. *Adjuvant Chemotherapy in Breast Cancer*

R. Nissen-Meyer, K. Kjellgren, and B. Mansson*

Tyribakken 10, Oslo 2, Norway

Summary

One single course of i.v. cyclophosphamide (30 mg/kg) was given over a 6-day period to 559 mastectomized patients. During a follow-up period of up to 15 years, 241 recurrences and 234 deaths are registered in this group, and 294 recurrences and 283 deaths in the randomized control group of 577 patients. Analysis of the life-table curves shows an increased cure rate of about 10%.

Introduction

When we add a systemic treatment to the surgical removal of the primary tumor, we may theoretically obtain two principally different types of effect: We may increase the definite cure rate, or we may reduce the speed of the subclinical tumor tissue growth in the patients not cured, resulting in an increased disease-free interval and increased survival time. There may of course also be a combination of these two effects.

Often necessary for increasing the cure rate is killing of the last remaining tumor cell. This may only be achieved when the tumor burden at the time of treatment is very small. Since such cases need a long time to develop clinically detectable metastases, a long follow-up is also needed. In a clinical trial, such an effect may be demonstrated by the curve A in Fig. 1.

Necessary for obtaining a delay in tumor growth is long-lasting influence of the delaying factor. We can assume that every systemic treatment which reduces disease progression in advanced cases will also do so in the subclinical phase, and prolong the disease-free interval. In a clinical trial, such an effect may be demonstrated by the curve B in Fig. 1.

There are two experimental animal models relevant to the study of cure by adjuvant chemotherapy. In the first, tumor cell suspensions are injected i.v. In the second, a

* For the Scandinavian Adjuvant Chemotherapy Study Group. Participating members: L. Kolsaker, M. Tangen, C.-A. Ekman, B. Mansson, G. Hellström, T. Norin, G. Odén, A. Järvinen, K. Malmio, L. Iacobaeus, B. Martensson, I. Hareide, S. K. Hjort, J. Sääf, D. Turesson, K. Kjellgren, R. Peterhoff, G. Blanco, T. Larmi, P.-O. Grönblom, and R. Nissen-Meyer

Recent Results in Cancer Research, Vol. 80

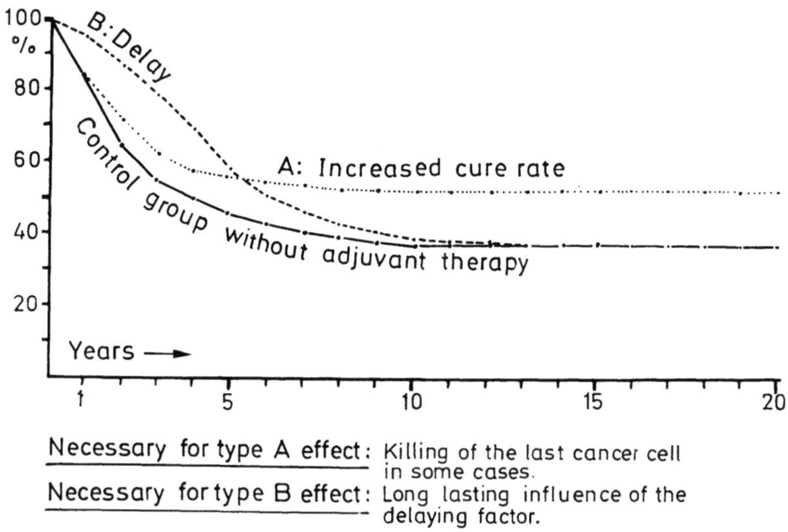

Fig. 1. Theoretically possible effects of adjuvant therapy

small piece of a solid tumor is transplanted under the skin of the animal and allowed to grow for a few days. Then this primary tumor is removed surgically, only the micrometastases which have disseminated during these days are left in the animal. In both these models a definite cure may be obtained by a single, short chemotherapy course.

For obtaining this effect, however, two factors are essential. The chemotherapy course must be given immediately after dissemination of the cancer cells, since a delay of a few days may spoil the effect, and near the maximum tolerated dose must be given, since a 30% reduction of this dose will reduce the effect considerably.

If, in a patient, the first dissemination of distant metastases takes place during mastectomy or shortly before, she will be in the same situation as the animals in the experimental models, and a cure by chemotherapy seems theoretically possible. The Scandinavian Adjuvant Chemotherapy Study Group decided in 1964 to study if this could be a practical reality.

Patients and Methods

In January, 1965, we started a cooperative, randomized clinical trial with one single, short chemotherapy course. We decided, in this series, not to give repeated courses, since that would have introduced a factor of delay and made evaluation of the possible effect on the cure rate difficult.

The chemotherapy group received one single 6-day course with i.v. cyclophosphamide (5 mg/kg body weight per day, to a total of 30 mg/kg). This drug and dose was our choice in 1964, today we would probably have chosen a short multidrug course. An extensive review of the case material and our methods has recently been published [1].

Results

Our total material was 559 patients in the chemotherapy group, with 241 recurrences and 234 deaths. In the control group we had 577 patients, with 294 recurrences and 283 deaths. The difference of 53 recurrences is significant ($P < 0.01$), and the difference of 49 deaths is also significant ($P < 0.02$). Regardless of how we stratified this total material (if the groups were of 50 patients or more), the results were invariably in favor of the chemotherapy group, with one important exception.
Figure 2 illustrates the results from the five participating hospitals which contributed more than 100 cases each. The four to the left belong to what we have called the

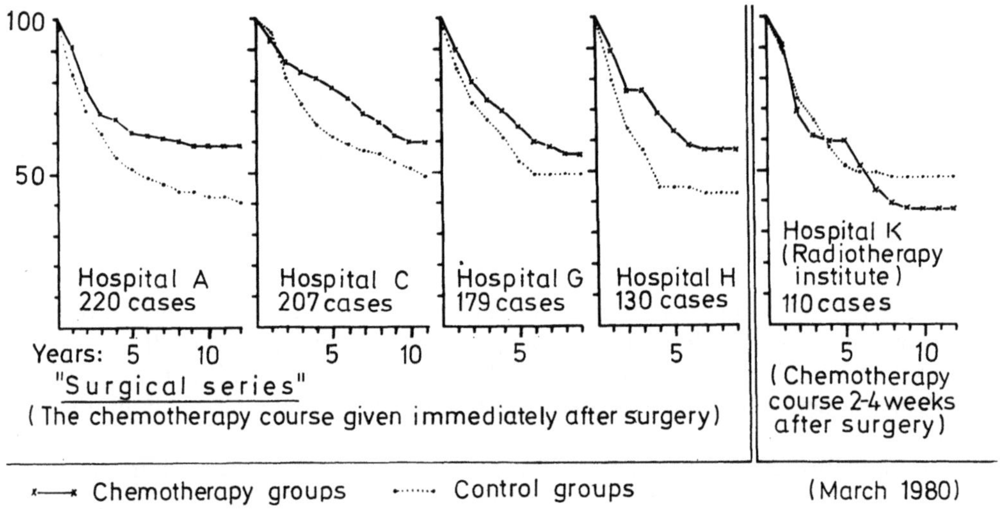

Fig. 2. Results in the five hospitals contributing with more than 100 cases each

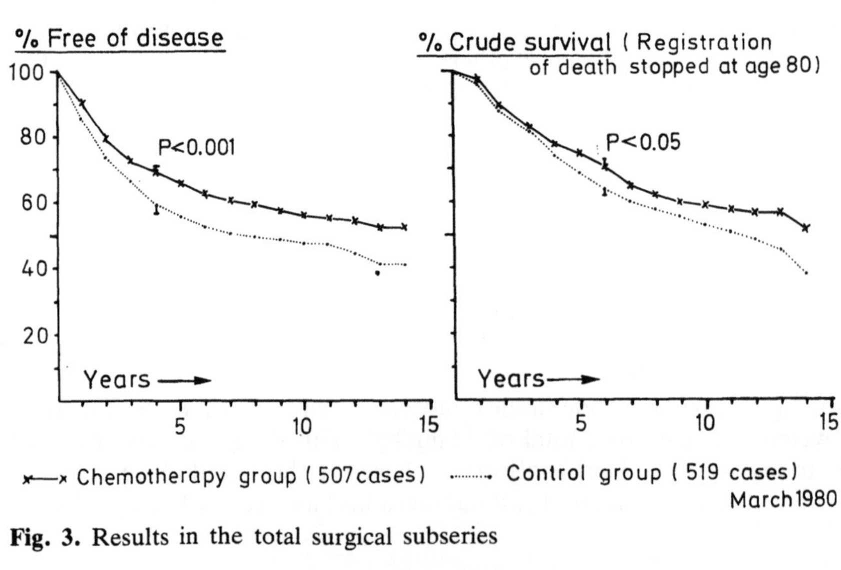

Fig. 3. Results in the total surgical subseries

surgical subseries. The randomization here was made by telephone from the operating theatre, and the first injection was given immediately after mastectomy. In all four hospitals the curves follow a pattern typical for a type A effect, an increased cure rate.

The hospital K is a radiotherapy institute and, in one respect, different from all the other participating hospitals. Here, the patients came for treatment 2–4 weeks after surgery, and, after randomization, chemotherapy started an average of 3 weeks after mastectomy. The patients from this institute were called the radiologic subseries. But, to avoid mistakes, we must stress that the patients of the surgical subseries also received postoperative radiotherapy. The only difference between the two subseries is the delay between mastectomy and chemotherapy in the radiologic subseries.

Hospital K was the only exception to the general rule, namely, showing no trend of effect on recurrence rates. This indicates that 3 weeks after mastectomy is beyond the optimal time for obtaining an increased cure rate. This corresponds closely with the experience gained from the animal experiments.

Figure 3 shows the results from the total surgical subseries (1,026 cases from ten hospitals). The difference in recurrence-free rates increased gradually during the first 4 years after mastectomy, and was then highly significant ($P < 0.001$). The difference then maintained a plateau at about 10% and, after 14 years, it was 11%.

It would be unreasonable to suggest that this result could be due to a simple delay of clinical manifestation of recurrences caused by the single 6-day chemotherapy course. It must be an increased cure rate which has been obtained.

Logically enough, the effect on survival rates shows later than the effect on recurrence rates. The difference in survival rates did not exceed 10% before 13 years after surgery and, after 14 years, it was 13.2%. This difference is also statistically significant. We used crude survival rates, but as soon as a patient reached the age of 80 years, she was withdrawn from the calculation of survival to avoid dilution of relevant data by too many noncancer deaths in the highest age groups.

In Fig. 4, the cases are stratified according to involvement of axillary nodes and tumor size. The best results of adjuvant chemotherapy seem to be obtained in the cases without involvement of the axillary nodes and with a tumor of less than 2 cm. This is also logical, and in accordance with the experience gained from animal experiments.

Considering the minimal side effects from this type of adjuvant chemotherapy, there is no point in restricting it to high-risk groups!

In Fig. 5, the cases are stratified according to premenopausal and postmenopausal patients. Whether the menopause was spontaneous or induced by oophorectomy or ovarian irradiation was disregarded. The effect of this short-term immediate chemotherapy seemed as good in the postmenopausal patients as in the younger patients with functioning ovaries. This demonstrates that a possible chemotherapy-induced ovarian suppression could have no influence on the results, as has been suspected for long-term chemotherapy treatment.

What does the effect cost in terms of side effects, inconvenience, and risk for the patient? The immediate side effects of one short cyclophosphamide course are very moderate, of short duration, and easy to palliate since the patient is still in the hospital [1].

During the later years, there has been much concern about possibly delayed, serious side effects of chemotherapy. Certainly long-term intensive chemotherapy carries the risk of late-developing secondary malignant disease, especially acute myelogenic

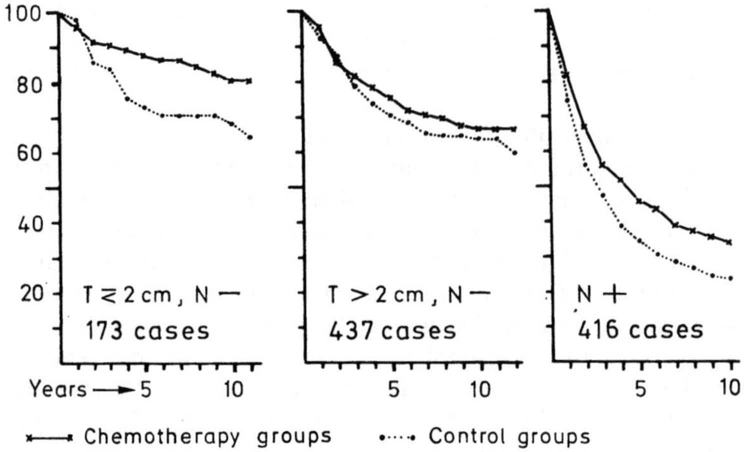

Fig. 4. Results by extent of primary disease

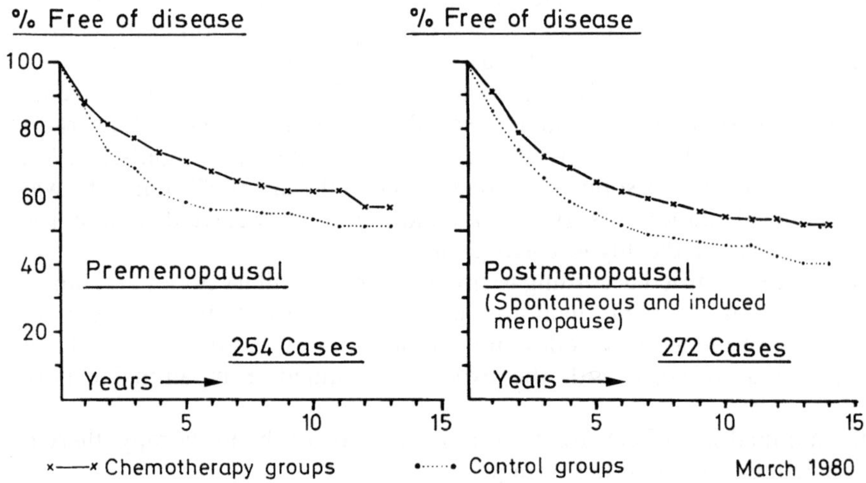

Fig. 5. Results by ovarian function

Table 1. Secondary malignant disease observed (excluding ca. mammae and ca. basocellulare)

	Treatment group	Control group
Gastrointestinal cancer	5	6
Gynecologic cancer	2	6
Malignant lymphomas	1	1
Other cancers	2	2
	10	15

leukemia. We cannot expect to see these complications before more than 5 years of observation in a large group of patients, but then they will probably increase in number. We have been looking for indications that such secondary malignancies could also be induced by the short-term chemotherapy employed in our series, but have not found the slightest trend of this. Among the 1,136 patients, observed an average of more than 10 years, we have found ten secondary cancers in the treatment group and 15 in the control group, with no remarkable distribution (Table 1).

Discussion

With 14 years of follow-up after the 6-day treatment we may conclude that there are, after mastectomy, patients with residual cancer cells who can definitely be cured by one short chemotherapy course, as it has been established in experimental animal models. To have proven that this is also the case under clinical conditions in a human carcinoma is probably the most important result of our study. One short cyclophosphamide course (30 mg/kg) immediately after mastectomy increased the cure rate about 10%, without significant side effects or inconvenience to the patients. This simple adjuvant treatment schedule may now safely be recommended for routine use in stages I and II, in premenopausal as well as in postmenopausal women.

However, the question arises whether our 10% gain in cure rate can be increased. There are two possibilities: (1) increase of the intensity of the immediate chemotherapy course; and (2) prolongation of the treatment.

An increase in dose, or use of a multiple drug course, may increase the effect, but may at the same time give more side effects. It might seem desirable to compare different doses and combinations in a new randomized trial, but this would be too time- and resource-consuming. Extremely large series and about a 10-year follow-up would be necessary to verify statistically a possible small improvement in the cure rate. It seems justified to take advantage of studies on the effectiveness of different doses and schedules in advanced breast cancer cases, and apply the best schedules as adjuvant courses.

Extension of adjuvant chemotherapy to intense treatment for 1–2 years may perhaps increase the definite cure rate more than a single short course does, and it would certainly introduce a factor of delay. It will, however, also certainly cause side effects and considerable distress for the patient during the entire treatment period, and it may perhaps also cause late serious complications, such as acute myelogenic leukemia, in some patients.

During recent years, several clinical trials have started comparing a group with long-term adjuvant chemotherapy with an untreated control group. Some of them will be reported later in this session. From such trials, however, it will be difficult to figure out how much of the observed effect is a result of the primary, real adjuvant chemotherapy, and how much is due to the continued treatment. Unfortunately, in most series the first chemotherapy course has been given after a delay of several weeks postmastectomy.

The Scandinavian Adjuvant Chemotherapy Study Group started in March, 1977, a new randomized series to compare directly the two principles of adjuvant chemotherapy. In this new series all patients receive one short multidrug chemotherapy course immediately after mastectomy, and one-half of the node-positive patients continue with CMF courses for 1 year. We have up to now about 600 patients randomized, but cannot hope to have conclusive results before another 10 years.

References

1. Nissen-Meyer R, Kjellgren K, Malmio K, Månsson B, Norin T (1978) Surgical adjuvant chemotherapy. Results with one short course with cyclophosphamide after mastectomy for breast cancer. Cancer 41: 2088–2098

25. *Multimodal Therapy with CMF in Resectable Breast Cancer with Positive Axillary Nodes: The Milan Institute Experience*

G. Bonadonna, P. Valagussa, A. Rossi, G. Tancini, C. Brambilla, S. Marchini, and U. Veronesi

Istituto Nazionale Tumori, Division Medical Oncology,
Via Venezian 1, I-20133 Milan, Italy

During the past few years, we have systematically published the short-term and the intermediate analysis of prospective randomized studies [4, 6, 15] with adjuvant combination chemotherapy in operable breast cancer having histologically positive axillary lymph nodes (N+). More recently, the 5-year results of the first trial were reported [11] as well as a retrospective analysis on the dose-response effect of adjuvant chemotherapy [2].
This paper will summarize the most important updated findings which emerged from our studies. Through comparative analyses we will attempt to draw some practical, though not yet definitive, conclusions on the efficacy of multimodal therapy in high risk groups with resectable breast cancer. For the characteristics of study patients as well as for the types of surgical and medical treatments, the readers are referred to our previous publications [1, 2, 4, 11, 15].

CMF vs Control: 6-Year Results

The essential findings of this study started in June 1973 and comparing radical mastectomy (RM or control group) vs RM followed by 12 cycles of CMF (cyclophosphamide, methotrexate and fluorouracil) are summarized in Table 1 and

Table 1. CMF vs control: 6-year results (data are in percentages)

	Control (179)	CMF 12 (207)	*P* Value
RFS, total	43.8	55.7	0.001
Nodes 1–3	45.6	65.1	< 0.001
Nodes > 3	31.8	35.7	0.27
Premenopause	42.7	59.8	< 0.001
Postmenopause	44.9	50.5	0.35
Survival, total	64.5	73.9	0.12

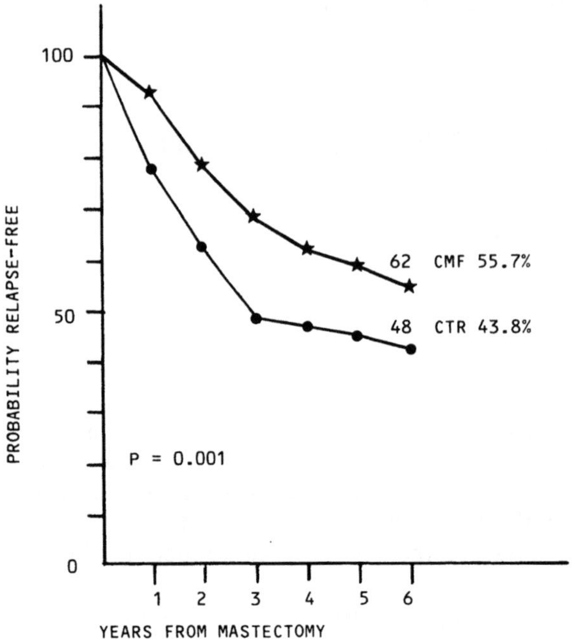

Fig. 1. First CMF Program: probability of relapse-free survival: all patients

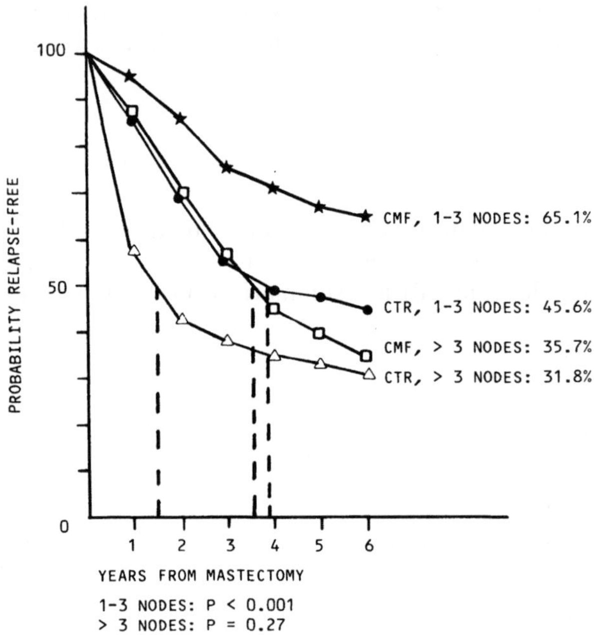

Fig. 2. First CMF Program: probability of relapse-free survival related to degree of nodal involvement

illustrated in Figs. 1 and 2. The results also confirm that at 6 years from RM the relapse-free survival (RFS) remains statistically superior in patients treated with multimodal therapy compared to those treated with the conventional local-regional therapy. The analysis of subgroups forming the stratification parameters also confirms that the *P* value remains significant in women with minimal tumour burden in the axilla (one to three nodes) and with premenopausal status. In this analysis, total survival for controls was 64.5% and 73.9% for CMF-treated patients with a P value of 0.12 (premenopausal: $P = 0.02$, postmenopausel: $P = 0.57$).

CMF 12 vs 6 Cycles

This trial initiated in September 1975 is now available for the 4-year analysis. It is important to recall that the accrual for postmenopausal women was discontinued in March 1977 because the 3-year analysis of the previous study (CMF vs control) had indicated that CMF was apparently ineffective in postmenopausal patients [1, 4]. Table 2 presents the comparative results. Since the 4-year analysis has indicated that in patients treated with 12 CMF cycles the results between the first and the second study were almost superimposable (RFS: first study 62.5%, second study 62.7%; survival: first study 81.9%, second study 76.8%); all women randomized to received 12 cycles were grouped together (total 450 patients). The control group remains that of the previous study (see Table 1). The essential findings can be described as follows (1) the RFS of groups given either 12 or 6 cycles is significantly superior to control for the total group of patients, those with 1–3 nodes and all premenopausal women as well as women given six cycles and having more than three nodes, (2) there are no significant differences in both RFS and survival rates between the groups treated with 12 or 6 cycles and (3) in women with more than three nodes and with postmenopausal status there is a trend in the RFS in favour of patients given six cycles compared to those given 12 cycles (more than three nodes: $P = 0.13$, postmenopause: $P = 0.22$). The trend in the survival is also present for patients with more than three nodes (CMF 6: 76.2% vs CMF 12: 65.2%, $P = 0.09$) but not for postmenopausal women (CMF 6: 80.4% vs CMF 12: 78.9%, $P = 0.81$).

Sequential Combinations

With the aim of testing a more aggressive form of drug therapy in postmenopausal women, a trial utilizing two non-cross-resistant regimens (six cycles of CMF-P followed by four cycles of adriamycin plus vincristine or AV) was started in May 1977

Table 2. CMF 12 vs 6 cycles: 4-year results (data are in percentages)

	Control (179)	CMF 12 (450)	CMF 6 (216)
RFS, total	48.4	62.7	69.4
Nodes 1–3	53.2	76.8	77.5
Nodes > 3	36.5[a]	43.6[a]	56.9
Premenopause	44.2	66.5	69.4
Postmenopause	52.4[a]	57.4[a]	68.8[a]
Survival, total	75.2[a]	79.4[a]	82.1[a]

[a] Difference not significant. CMF 12 vs 6: not significant

Table 3. Comparative percent age of 2-year RFS CMF vs CMFP → AV in postmenopausal women older than 65 years

	Total patients	Axillary nodes	
		1–3	> 3
Control	64.6	69.4	54.8
12 CMF[a]	79.3	85.0	69.8
6 CMF	76.5	82.7	66.7
CMFP → AV int.	78.6	90.8	66.9
no int.	83.0	96.1	67.0

[a] First and second study

[4, 6]. No dose reduction regimen was planned; rather, in the presence of myelosuppression, treatment was delayed until full marrow recovery occurred. In the attempt to evaluate in humans the Norton and Simon hypothesis [10], patients were randomly allocated to receive sequential adjuvant treatment either with no dose intensification (i.e., full dose from the first cycle) or with progressive intensification (i.e., cyclophosphamide, methotrexate, fluorouracil and adriamycin given during the first two cycles at low dose followed by progressive dose escalation). A total of 115 postmenopausal women aged 65 years or less are presently evaluable. Table 3 reports the 2-year actuarial analysis. The comparison also takes into account the results of previous CMF studies. With the limits of this type of retrospective comparison, there seems to be no clear evidence in favour of sequential chemotherapy except in the subgroup with one to three nodes and treated with initial full dose (96.1% vs CMF 12: 85% vs CMF 6: 82.7%). However, it should be stressed that the 2-year analysis is too premature to allow for the detection of meaningful comparative results. The initial observation indicating that patients started on a full dose regimen fared significantly better than those started on a low dose regimen [6] could not be confirmed at this point in the analysis.

CMF plus Tamoxifen

This prospective non-randomized trial utilizing low-dose CMF for 12 cycles with the concomitant administration of tamoxifen (20 mg/day for 12 months) was started in May 1977 and limited to women older than 65 years or with medical contraindication to treatment with adriamycin. The results in this study are also premature; however, it can be mentioned that the 2-year RFS in patients older than 65 years is 90.6% (one to three nodes: 95.6%, more than three nodes: 85.0%). Whether present findings indicate that low dose chemotherapy plus hormone therapy is really useful in this specific age group remains to be demonstrated.

Estrogen Receptors and CMF

The predictive value of estrogen receptors (ER) could be analysed in a large fraction of women who belonged to the second adjuvant study (CMF 12 vs 6 cycles). The

Table 4. Comparative percentage of 4-year RFS and survival after adjuvant CMF related to ER status

	ER+	ER−	*P*
RFS			
Premenopause	69.8	59.4	0.18
Nodes 1–3	84.0	70.1	0.20
> 3	53.4	52.0	0.61
Postmenopause	61.7	59.3	0.41
Nodes 1–3	67.2	65.8	0.84
> 3	49.3	50.0	0.87
Survival			
Premenopause	80.3	70.9	< 0.04
Postmenopause	84.4	76.5	0.48

comparative 4-year results (Table 4) essentially confirm our previous findings [5]. In fact, the analysis of RFS failed to detect a significant difference between ER-positive and ER-negative tumours both in pre- and postmenopausal patients. The survival of premenopausal women with ER-positive tumours was significantly superior to that of women with ER-negative tumors ($P < 0.04$), and this observation supports the evidence against an initial report [9] suggesting that ER-negative tumours could be more responsive to combination chemotherapy. Our updated findings further minimize the possible therapeutic role of drug-induced adjuvant castration [3].

Role of Dose Level

This important aspect has been extensively evaluated in a recent publication [2]. Table 5 presents the updated results on all patients treated with 12 CMF cycles. The findings confirm that also at 6 years after RM there is evidence in favour of a dose response effect. In fact, the RFS was dependent on the percentage of dose received (Level I: > 85%; Level II: 84–65%; Level III: < 65%) and the relation held true both in premenopausal and postmenopausal women. Furthermore, within each dose level, the results were related to the number of axillary lymph nodes, and within each patient subgroup with a certain number of nodes, the 6-year RFS was dose related. It is important to point out that in the total series of patients the first two levels of CMF were significantly superior vs controls (Level I: $P = 0.0002$; Level II: $P = 0.01$). The *P* value for Level I vs control was higher in pre- vs postmenopausal women and in patients with one to three vs more than three lymph nodes. Comparative results similar to those recently published [2] are confirmed in the analysis of total survival related to dose levels. Table 6 indicates that there are no significant differences within each dose level between patients treated with 12 or 6 CMF cycles. In women who received full or near full drug dose there remains the same trend in favour of 12 CMF cycles as has been recently reported [2]. Also in the group treated with six cycles of CMF both Level I ($P < 0.001$) and Level II ($P < 0.01$) were significantly superior compared to control.

Table 5. Six-year RFS related to dose levels after 12 CMF cycles[a]

	Total %	Axillary nodes		Menopause	
		1–3 %	> 3 %	Pre %	Post %
I	68.1	77.2	50.4	70.6	64.1
II	54.6	68.3	32.6	55.6	52.0
III	49.1	56.8	30.2	45.9	49.5
Total CFM	56.2	66.1	34.0	59.8	51.2
Control	43.8	45.6	31.8	42,7	44.9
P values					
I vs CTR	0.0002	< 0.0005	0.05	< 0.001	0.03
I vs II	0.03	0.07	0.25	0.23	0.09
I vs III	< 0.02	0.07	0.22	< 0.04	0.07
II vs CTR	0.01	0.02	0.35	< 0.01	0.33
II vs III	0.67	0.90	0.93	0.23	0.89
III vs CTR	0.10	0.09	0.45	0.07	0.33

[a] First and second study

Table 6. Four-year RFS related to dose levels: 12[a] vs 6 CMF cycles

Level	CMF 12 %	CMF 6 %	*P*
I	76.9	70.3	0.28
II	60.0	68.2	0.09
III	53.7	59.5	0.97
Total CFM	62.7	69.4	0.33
Control	48.4	48.4	

[a] First and second study

Comments

The results of our first adjuvant trials in operable breast cancer with N+ have become mature enough to allow for some conclusions which could form the basis to design new multimodal studies.

1. The observation that the therapeutic effect of CMF remains evident up to the 6th year from surgery confirms that the scientific and biological hypotheses forming the basis of multimodal therapy were correct. Although it is still premature to draw firm conclusions about total survival, which remains the endpoint of the multimodal strategy, the trend is for improved survival in patients treated with surgery plus chemotherapy. The 5-year analysis has indicated that second-line treatment at first relapse yielded comparable results between patients initially treated with surgery and surgery plus CMF [11]; thus salvage therapy in relapsing breast cancer was ineffective.

2. The therapeutic effect appears related to the percent of drug administered. Therefore, efforts should be made to improve current drug schedules to allow for constant administration of full doses. For this reason, all drugs should be given intravenously and treatment delayed for 1–2 weeks rather than reduced in the presence of moderate suppression. At present, all new studies being performed in Milan for early as well as for advanced breast cancer utilize a new CMF regimen (cyclophosphamide 600 mg/m^2 i.v., methotrexate 40 mg/m^2 i.v., and fluorouracil 600 mg/m^2 i.v.), where all drugs are administered intravenously on day 1 and courses repeated at 3-week intervals.

3. The most interesting new finding which emerged from the present update consists in the observation that also at 4 years both RFS and survival were not significantly different between the groups who received six cycles and those who were treated with 12 cycles. The important practical problem of the duration of CMF effectiveness was critically reviewed by Skipper [12]. By analysing our results on the rate, degree and duration of response with CMF in advanced breast cancer, he concluded that in clinically metastatic disease the nadir in surviving tumour cells is probably reached in the majority of patients in less than six cycles. Thus, subsequent cycles (i.e., from 6–12 cycles) do not reduce the surviving tumour cells by the same fraction as initial cycles, e.g., cycles one to three. Although there will probably be a correlation between the total amount of CMF given and the peak levels, our data would indicate that the main important pharmacological factor is the peak level of the drugs and not their total amount [2, 13]. Our clinical observation would substantiate the above-mentioned statement, i.e., cycles 7–12 provide little or no substantial therapeutic benefit in the majority of patients, even when comparative dose levels were considered. Also the M.D. Anderson group [8] noticed that the duration of complete remission in advanced breast cancer was not clearly related to the duration of further treatment once complete response was achieved. Therefore, both in the presence of advanced disease as well as in an adjuvant situation, the real therapeutic usefulness of prolonged treatments with the same cytotoxic drugs, even in the presence of continued response or absence of relapse, should be critically re-evaluated. Since the peak levels of CMF during the first cycles are probably of utmost importance, switching to some other effective agents after about four to five full-dose cycles of the first drug regimen (e.g., CMF) has the potential of increasing remission durations over those observed on continuation with repetitive cycles of the same drug regimen.

4. The observation that in an adjuvant situation utilizing effective chemotherapy the ER status does not predict the RFS and that in advanced disease it does not predict objective response to a variety of cytotoxic regimens [5, 14] should not discourage the design of randomized trials where the simultaneous administration of full-dose chemotherapy plus hormones is tested in patients with ER-positive tumours against either chemotherapy alone or hormones alone.

5. Although in Sprague-Dawley rats given three different doses of CMF a strong dose-related carcinogenic response was recently reported by Habs and Schmähl [7], we failed to detect also in the 5-year analysis an increased incidence of second neoplasms compared to controls [11].

References

1. Bonadonna G, Rossi A, Valagussa P, Banfi A, Veronesi U (1977) The CMF program for operable breast cancer with positive axillary nodes. Updated analysis on the disease-free interval, site of relapse and drug tolerance. Cancer 39: 2904–2915
2. Bonadonna G, Valagussa P (1981) Dose-response effect of adjuvant chemotherapy in breast cancer. N Engl J Med 304: 10–15
3. Bonadonna G, Valagussa P, De Palo G (1981) The results of adjuvant chemotherapy in breast cancer are predominantly due to the hormonal change such therapy induces: The view against. In: Van Scoy-Mosher MB (ed) Controversies in medical oncology. G. K. Hall & Co., Boston (in press)
4. Bonadonna G, Valagussa P, Rossi A et al. (1978) Are surgical adjuvant trial altering the course of breast cancer? Semin Oncol 5: 450–464
5. Bonadonna G, Valagussa P, Tancini G, Di Fronzo G (1980) Estrogen-receptor status and response to chemotherapy in early and advanced breast cancer. Cancer Chemother Pharmacol 4: 37–41
6. Brambilla C, Valagussa P, Bonadonna G, Veronesi U (1980) Sequential adjuvant chemotherapy in postmenopausal (≤ 65 year) breast cancer. Proc Am Assoc Cancer Res 21: 189
7. Habs M, Schmähl D (1981) Carcinogenic activity of cyclophosphamide, methotrexate, 5-fluorouracil treatment in rats. Int J Cancer (in press)
8. Legha SS, Buzdar AU, Smith TL et al. (1979) Complete remissions in metastatic breast cancer treated with combination drug therapy. Ann Intern Med 91: 847–852
9. Lippman ME, Allegra JC, Thompson EB et al. (1978) The relation between estrogen receptors and response rate to cytotoxic chemotherapy in metastatic breast cancer. N Engl J Med 298: 1223–1228
10. Norton L, Simon R (1977) Tumor size, sensitivity to therapy and design of treatment schedules. Cancer Treat Rep 61: 1307–1317
11. Rossi A, Bonadonna G, Valagussa P, Veronesi U (1981) Multimodal treatment in operable breast cancer: 5-year results of the CMF program. Br Med J (in press)
12. Skipper HE (1980) Response of advanced breast cancer to CMF (cyclophosphamide, methotrexate, 5-fluorouracil). Birmingham, Ala., Southern Research Institute (Booklet 2)
13. Skipper HE (1980) Breast cancer treated by means of mastectomy and mastectomy followed by 12 or 6 cycles of CMF. Birmingham, Ala., Southern Research Institute (Booklet 4)
14. Steroid Receptors in Breast Cancer. An NIH Consensus Development Conference (1980) Bethesda, Maryland, June 27–29, 1979. Cancer 46: 2759–2963
15. Tancini G, Bajetta E, Marchini S, Valagussa P, Bonadonna G, Veronesi U (1979) Preliminary 3-year results of 12 versus 6 cycles of surgical adjuvant CMF in premenopausal breast cancer. Cancer Clin Trials 2: 285–292

26. *Follow-Up Results from a Randomized Trial for T_3 and T_4 Breast Cancer Patients: Previous BCG Immunotherapy Improves Response to Chemotherapy in the Relapse Patient*

B. Serrou, H. Sancho-Garnier, P. Cappelaere, R. Plagne, R. Metz, M. Schneider, P. Chollet, N. Namer, H. Pujol, J. Gary-Bobo, G. Meyer, and G. Mathé*

Hôpital Saint-Eloi, Centre Paul Lamarque, Department of Immuno-Chemotherapy, F-34033 Montpellier Cedex, France

Summary

Following locoregional treatment, patients were randomized into three groups: The first group received no complementary treatment; the second group received adjuvant chemotherapy (vincristine, cyclophosphamide, and 5-fluorouracil once a month for 12 months); and the third group was treated by immunotherapy (150 mg BCG once a week for 1 year). Sixty-two of the 82 patients studied were menopausal. No significant difference was observed between the three groups. All patients were followed-up for at least 18 months. The disease-free interval difference between the chemotherapy group and the control and immunotherapy groups is not significant. But it should be noted that only 21.8% of the control group did not relapse compared to 57% in the chemotherapy group. BCG immunotherapy in such patients must be considered ineffective. However, our results suggest that patients first treated with BCG respond better to chemotherapy than patients not receiving any previous therapy.

Introduction

A number of randomized clinical trials suggest that adjuvant chemotherapy of predetermined duration can significantly prolong remission and survival of premenopausal breast cancer patients [1, 2, 8, 9]. We have previously reported [17, 18] encouraging preliminary findings with chemotherapy based on a clinical trial involving mostly menopausal (natural or artificial) patients with local advanced tumors (T_3 and T_4).

We here report our latest findings in this population. We show that adjuvant chemotherapy is associated with a nonsignificant prolongation of remission and survival time for the overall patient population considered. BCG immunotherapy did not improve results compared to controls. However, the overall survival of the group treated by chemotherapy and that treated with immunotherapy is similar. These results suggest that patients treated first with immunotherapy respond better to chemotherapy that the control group which did not receive any previous therapy prior to relapse.

* For the EORTC Cancer Immunology and Immunotherapy Group (GI2C)

Recent Results in Cancer Research, Vol. 80

Patients and Methods

Choice of Patients

Five anticancer centers participated in this trial: Clermont-Ferrand (12 patients); Lille (30 patients); Montpellier (19 patients); Nancy (ten patients); and Nice (nine patients).
The following criteria were employed: the number of relapses; the number of metastases; length of disease-free interval; toxicity; and survival time.
The patients chosen were T_3 and T_4 (TNM, UICC classification) breast tumor-bearing women irrespective of lymph node involvement. They were less than 70 years of age and had not received any previous treatment. Fifty-nine patients were classified as having adenocarcinoma, five as having undifferentiated tumors, two atypical cases, seven with positive cytology, and two with adenocarcinoma of unspecified origin. No significant difference in tumor type could be shown in the three randomized groups. Tumors in 47 patients were grade T_3 and in 32 were grade T_4 (no significant difference was observed in the three randomized groups).
Twenty of the 80 patients were premenopausal, with no significant difference in the three groups, and 60 patients were in a natural or artificial postmenopausal state. No significant difference was noted among the three groups.

Primary Lesion Treatment

All patients in this trial received radiotherapy according to a protocol prepared by each center. Surgery, when performed, was as follows: in the first group, without complementary treatment (22 patients), two axillary lymph node excisions and two mastectomies associated with lymph node dissection; in the group receiving chemotherapy (29 patients), one axillary lymph node dissection and ten mastectomies associated with lymph node dissection; and in the immunotherapy group (29 patients), eight mastectomies associated with lymph node dissection. No statistically significant difference in primary treatment could be shown among these groups.

Adjuvant Therapy and Randomization

Following locoregional treatment, the patients were randomized into three groups. The first group received no complementary treatment. The second group received adjuvant chemotherapy, i.e., vincristine (1 mg/m^2 i.v.) on days 1 and 2 and cyclophosphamide (300 mg/m^2 i.v.) and 5-fluorouracil (400 mg/m^2 i.v.) on days 3, 4, 5, and 6. This cyclic chemotherapy was repeated once a month over a 12-month period. The third group received immunotherapy (150 mg fresh BCG from the Institut Pasteur) administered once a week either by scarification or by the Sterneedle (Heaf gun) technique. In addition, 150 mg BCG was given orally. Immunotherapy was given for 1 year. In all cases, the complementary treatment was initiated 4 weeks after the end of radiotherapy.
All patients were followed-up for at least 18 months.

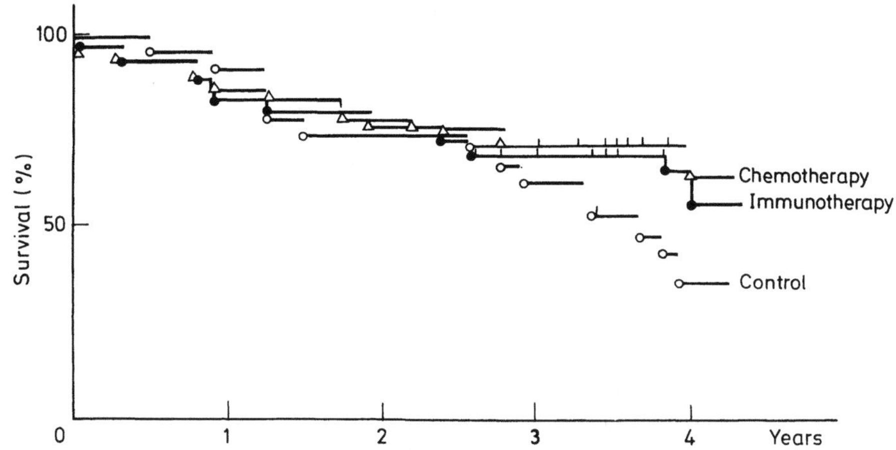

Fig. 1

Results

The results show no significant difference for disease-free survival between the three groups, i.e., chemotherapy, immunotherapy, and no therapy. A disease-free survival of 30 months was noted for 54% of the chemotherapy group and 40% of the no treatment and immunotherapy groups. No difference was observed between the 60 menopausal patients and the 20 nonmenopausal patients. Regarding age, the results are less encouraging as the patient becomes older (over 70 years of age) and conversely the results are more promising in the younger age groups (less than 50 years of age). Between 50–70 years of age, the results are less conclusive. There is no significant difference for those patients under 50 years of age treated with chemotherapy. Furthermore some patients had been treated either by radiotherapy alone, or with radiotherapy followed by complementary surgery, or by surgery followed by radiotherapy. At 30 months, the results show an increased disease-free survival time for patients treated first with surgery followed by radiotherapy then by chemotherapy, but this difference is not significant.

In no way can any differences be demonstrated in favor of the BCG immunotherapy group. It is interesting to note that we observed a difference (not yet significant) for overall survival (Fig. 1) between the chemotherapy and immunotherapy groups on one hand and the control group on the other. No difference was noted between the chemotherapy-treated group and the immunotherapy-treated group.

Discussion

Three significant points arose from our study. Firstly, BCG immunotherapy does not improve the results in the control group. However, since no significant difference with the control group was observed, this suggested that BCG had no adverse effects. To some extent, these clinical results do not confirm previous experimental data which showed that BCG given after local irradiation of a tumor could significantly decrease local tumor growth, the number of lung metastasis, and animal survival [6, 17, 18]. However, it has to be remembered that such results were in part at least dependent on the timing and on the dose administered. Beneficial effects were only noted in animals receiving BCG on the first 4 days following cessation of irradiation and one injection was as effective as repeated injections. Another important consideration could be the residual tumor volume at the end of the local treatment, to explain less effective BCG treatment effects. On the whole, these results are quite similar to those presented by Buzdar [3] who also used BCG but whose results did not confirm those recently presented by Rojas [15] and Klefstrom [12] using levamisole after radiotherapeutic treatment of identical tumor masses. However, BCG and levamisole are believed to have different effects on the immune response, which could explain these discrepancies.

Secondly, it clearly demonstrates that efficacy decreases as patient age increases. This aspect requires an in-depth study designed to determine whether the decreased sensitivity of tumor cells to chemotherapy is due to a decrease or loss of estrogen receptors, and whether a close relationship can be established between this chemotherapeutic response and an immune deficiency [4, 5, 11, 13, 14, 22] related, for example, to age, especially for the patient over 70 years of age, or treatment, especially where radiotherapy is involved [6, 16]. These factors are not mutually exclusive. An additional variable is the amount of chemotherapy received by each group, but no significant difference was noted in our group.

Thirdly, an interesting point is that we did not find any difference for overall survival between the chemotherapy and the immuntherapy groups, although there was a difference for disease-free survival time between these two groups. It should be recalled that no difference for disease-free survival was noted between the control and BCG-treated groups. This suggests that patients first treated by BCG respond better to chemotherapy than patients not receiving any previous therapy. This point is quite important to consider in the light of recent results that immunorestored patients show improved response to chemotherapy compared to nonimmunorestored patients [4, 10, 11]. If confirmed, this finding may open the way to new original trials and restimulate interest in chemotherapy with immunomodulating drugs.

References

1. Bonadonna G, Brusamolino E, Valagussa P et al. (1976) Combination chemotherapy as an adjuvant treatment in operable breast cancer. N Engl J Med 294: 405–408
2. Bonadonna G, Rossi A, Valagussa P, Banfi A, Veronesi U (1977) The CMF program for operable breast cancer with positive axillary nodes. Cancer 39: 2904–2915
3. Buzdar A, Blumenschein G, Hortobagyi G, Campos L, Hersh E (to be published) Adjuvant therapy with 5-fluorouracil, adriamycin and cyclophosphamide with or without BCG in stage II or III breast cancer. In: Terry WD (ed) Immunotherapy of cancer: Present status of trials in man. Elsevier North-Holland, New York Oxford
4. Caraux J, Thierry C, Serrou B (1979) Human autologous rosettes. II. Prognostic significance of variations in autologous rosette-forming cells in the peripheral blood of cancer patients. J Natl Cancer Inst 63: 593–597
5. Cuttner J, Glidewell O, Holland J (to be published) A controlled trial of chemoimmunotherapy in acute myelocytic leukemia (AML). In: Terry WD (ed) Immunotherapy of cancer: Present status of trials in man. Elsevier North-Holland, New York Oxford

6. Dubois JB, Serrou B (1976) The treatment of the mouse Lewis tumor by the association of radiotherapy and BCG immunotherapy. Cancer Res 36: 1731–1734
7. Dubois JB, Serrou B, Pourquier H (1975) Influence des traitements par rayonnements ionisants sur la réponse immunitaire du cancereux. Bull Cancer 62: 1–20
8. Fisher B, Carbone P, Economou SG et al. (1975) L-Phenylalanine mustard in the management of primary breast cancer. N Engl J Med 292: 117–120
9. Fisher B, Glass A, Redmont C et al. (1977) L-PAM in the management of primary breast cancer. An update of earlier findings and comparison with those utilising L-PAM plus 5 FIU. Cancer 39: 2883–2903
10. Gallagher JG, Louie AC, Sihora K, Levy R, Rosenberg SA, Merigan TC (to be published) The evaluation of human leukocyte interferon in patients with non-Hodgkin's lymphoma and Hodgkin's disease: A phase II study. In: Terry WD (ed) Immunotherapy of cancer: Present status of trials in man. Elsevier North-Holland, New York Oxford
11. Jones S, Salmon S, Haskins C (to be published) Chemoimmunotherapy of non-Hodgkin's lymphoma. In: Terry WD (ed) Immunotherapy of cancer: Present status of trials in man. Elsevier North-Holland, New York Oxford
12. Klefstrom P, Holsti P, Grohn P, Heinonen E (to be published) Combination of levamisole immunotherapy with conventional treatments in breast cancer. In: Terry WD (ed) Immunotherapy of cancer: Present status of trials in man. Elsevier North-Holland, New York Oxford
13. Mathé G (1978) Systemic active immunotherapy is shifting from the middle ages to a renaissance period I. The multiplication of randomized trials showing significant effect of active immunotherapy on residual minimal disease. Cancer Immunol Immunother 5: 149–152
14. Mathé G, Serrou B (1979) Immunomodulateurs à visée cancérolytique et/ou cancérostatique. In: Giroux JP, Mathé G, Meyniel G (eds) Traité de pharmacologie clinique, vol 2. Expansion scientifique. Paris, pp 1797–1824
15. Rojas A, Seierstein J, Glait H, Olivari A (1977) Levamisole action in breast cancer stage III. In: Terry WD, Windhorst D (eds) Immunotherapy of cancer – Present status of trials in man. Raven Press, New York, pp 635–645
16. Serrou B (to be published) Detrimental and favorable effects of radiotherapy on immune response of cancer patients. Toward a rational approach to radio-immunotherapeutic associations. In: Dubois JB, Serrou B, Rosenfeld C (eds) Immunopharmacological effects of irradiation. Raven Press, New York
17. Serrou B, Dubois JB (1977) Combination of radiotherapy and immunotherapy in the treatment of Lewis's tumor. Eur J Cancer 13: 489–494
18. Serrou B, Dubois JB (1978) Efficacy of BCG treatment after local radiotherapy in Lewis and MBL_2 tumor-bearing mice. Cancer Immunol Immunother 4: 209–213
19. Serrou B, Sancho-Garnier H, Cappelaere P et al. (1979) Results of a randomized trial of prophylactic chemotherapy in T_3-T_4 breast cancer patients previously treated by radiotherapy. In: Bonadonna G, Mathé G, Salmon S (eds) Adjuvant therapies and markers of post-surgical minimal residual disease II. Springer, Berlin Heidelberg New York (Recent results in cancer research, vol 68, pp 105–108)
20. Serrou B, Sancho-Garnier H, Cappelaere et al. (1979) Improvement of disease-free interval by chemotherapy in T_3-T_4 breast cancer including majority of menopausal patients. 2nd International Conference on the Adjuvant Therapy of Cancer. Abstract p 27 – TUCSON
21. Serrou B, Goldstein AL, Thierry C, Caraux J (1979) Regulation of human suppressor cell function by thymosin. Biomedicine 31: 89
22. Serrou B, Gauci L, Caraux J, Cupissol D, Thierry C, Esteve C (to be published) Immune imbalance in cancer patients. In: Mathé G, Muggia F (eds) Recent results in cancer research. Springer, Berlin Heidelberg New York

27. *Adjuvant Treatment of Node-Positive Breast Cancer with Adriamycin-Cyclophosphamide with or Without Radiation Therapy: Interim Results of an Ongoing Clinical Trial**

S. E. Jones, S. E. Salmon, H. Allen, G. F. Giordano, S. Davis, E. Chase, T. E. Moon, and R. S. Heusinkveld

Arizona Health Sciences Center, Department of Internal Medicine, Section of Hematology/Oncology, Tucson, AZ 85724, USA

Summary

During 1974–1980, 138 women with node-positive stage II breast cancer were treated with either eight courses of adriamycin-cyclophosphamide (AC) chemotherapy (82 patients) or AC chemotherapy plus comprehensive regional radiotherapy (56 patients). The overall relapse-free survival of the treated patients was significantly superior ($P < 0.001$) to a comparable group of women who underwent surgery alone. This effect of adjuvant therapy was clearly manifest in all groups of patients irrespective of nodal involvement or menopausal status. To date, relapse-free survival for patients receiving AC compared to AC plus radiotherapy is not different ($P = 0.7$). In summary, we have demonstrated that a brief 6-month course of adjuvant chemotherapy with AC can significantly reduce the recurrence rate in women with stage II breast cancer.

Introduction

In 1974, we initiated a breast cancer adjuvant therapy program at the University of Arizona. Chemotherapy consisted of courses of adriamycin and cyclophosphamide (AC) at 3-week intervals. The choice of these agents was based upon our prior experience with advanced disease as summarized elsewhere [18] and evidence of drug synergism in animal tumors [9]. In 1975, we modified our trial to determine if comprehensive regional radiotherapy (RT) would improve the results of chemotherapy alone. Two years ago, we presented the preliminary results of this trial [19]. This report summarizes our current experience with adjuvant AC with or without RT for stage II breast cancer.

Patients and Methods

Since July, 1974, patients undergoing surgery for breast cancer who were potentially eligible for adjuvant treatment were referred for possible inclusion in the program.

* This work was supported by grants CA 17094 and CA 23074 from the National Cancer Institute, DHEW, Washington, DC (USA)

After referral, patients were evaluated for evidence of metastatic disease by means of a careful physical examination, routine laboratory work, chest radiograph, and bone scan. If the bone scan was abnormal, appropriate X-rays were obtained. Unless the X-rays confirmed overt metastatic disease, patients were eligible for adjuvant treatment. Additional laboratory, radiographic, or nuclear medicine studies were performed when clinically indicated. The eligibility criteria for this study included initiation of chemotherapy within 2 months after surgery for infiltrating ductal or infiltrating lobular adenocarcinoma of pathologic stages I, II, or III extent, no evidence of overt metastases, no prior breast cancer or heart disease, and informed written consent in accord with University of Arizona guidelines for protecting human subjects, as previously described [19]. In this report, we will focus only on those patients with stage II disease, as defined by the TNM classification using pathologic criteria [1]. For example, eligible patients were those whose maximum tumor diameter was 5.0 cm or less (T_1 or T_2) and who were found to have any number of positive axillary lymph nodes. The majority of patients with stage II cancer were randomized to receive either eight courses of AC at 3-week intervals or two courses of AC and comprehensive regional RT, followed by six more courses of AC at 3-week intervals. A group of patients was not randomized if they were unable to stay in Tucson for 5 weeks of RT. In addition, for purposes of analysis, a group of 18 patients, treated during 1974–1975 with postoperative RT followed by chemotherapy with AC, is included with the group of patients randomized to AC plus RT. The schedule of chemotherapy used for all patients was as follows: i.v. adriamycin (30 mg/m^2) was administered on day 1 of each 21-day cycle. Oral cyclophosphamide (150 mg/m^2) was administered for 4 days (days 3–6). Doses were reduced only due to serious nausea or vomiting or for serious leucopenia. RT was administered at least 1 week after the second dose of adriamycin. Radiation was given to the internal mammary lymph nodes with 12 MeV electrons; the chest wall and supraclavicular and axillary lymph nodes received 4 MeV X-rays at 200 rad per fraction, five fractions per week, to a total of 4,400 rad. Within 1–2 weeks after completion of RT, chemotherapy was reinstituted and continued without interruption for the remaining six cycles. Following completion of adjuvant treatment as described, patients were followed-up and careful clinical and laboratory reexamination was carried out every 3 months. Bone scans were repeated at 6-month intervals for the first year, and annually thereafter unless the scan was initially abnormal or had changed with time, in which case more frequent scans were obtained. Relapse was confirmed radiographically in all cases and histologically whenever possible. Comparison of various treatment groups was made to a large surgical control group. Identical data on important prognostic factors (e.g., tumor size, number of positive nodes, menopausel status, etc.) was used to match groups of treatment and control patients for comparison of relapse-free survival (RFS) from the time of surgery. RFS curves were plotted according to the method of Kaplan and Meier [14]. Tests of difference between groups of patients included the Breslow test [6], the Gehan-Wilcoxon test [11], and the log-rank test [17]. *P* values are based on the log-rank test.

Results

During 1974–1980, 138 patients with stage II breast cancer entered this study and are evaluable as shown in Table I. Eighty-two patients received AC and 56 received AC

Table 1. Clinical and pathologic features of 138 patients with stage II breast cancer treated with adriamycin plus cyclophosphamide (AC) plus radiotherapy (RT)

	AC	AC + RT	Totals
Patients	82	56	138
Age (years)			
< 40	13	11	24
40–50	16	10	26
50–60	20	23	43
> 60	33	12	45
Menopausal status			
Premenopausal	23	19	42
Perimenopausal	2	3	5
Postmenopausal	57	34	91
Nodal status			
1–3 positive	56	22	78
> 3 positive	26	34	60
Dose of AC			
≥ 85%	66	41	107 (78%)
< 85%	16	15	31

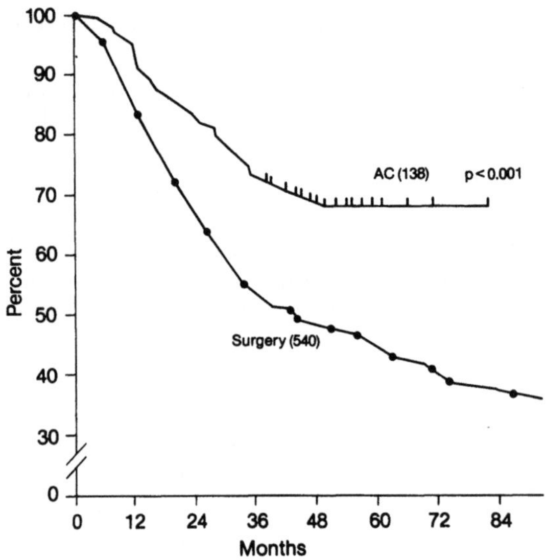

Fig. 1. Relapse-free survival (RFS) for 138 patients treated with or without with AC XRT compared to surgery alone ($P < 0{,}001$)

plus RT. Age distributions were similar (AC 31–75 and AC plus RT 24–79 years). There were slightly more older patients in the AC group (nine patients 70 years of age or older) compared to one patient in the AC plus RT group. Of the entire group 66% were postmenopausal, 4% perimenopausal (within 1 year of last menses), and 30% premenopausal. Menopausal status was well balanced according to treatment. Forty-four percent of patients had more than three involved axillary nodes and the

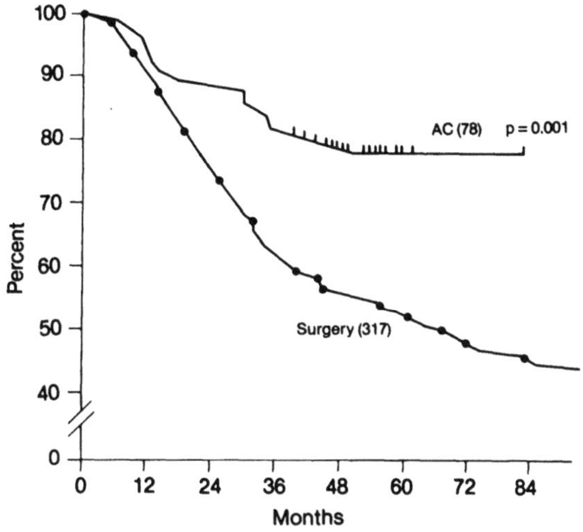

Fig. 2. Comparison of RFS for 78 patients with one to three positive nodes and 317 matched controls

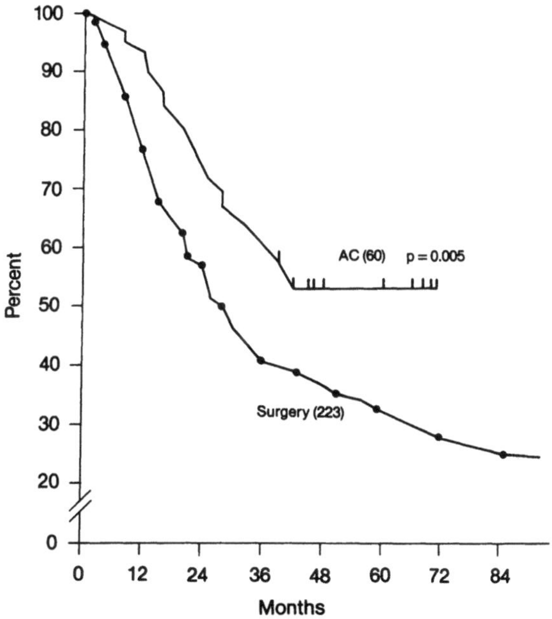

Fig. 3. Comparison of RFS for 60 patients with more than three positive nodes and 223 matched controls ($P = 0.005$)

distribution of these patients by treatment was similar. However, 70% of the patients with one to three positive nodes received AC without RT.

Overall RFS for the 138 patients compared to a carefully matched group of 540 surgical controls is shown in Fig. 1. The difference is highly significant ($P < 0.001$). This significant improvement in RFS was present in all major subgroups of patients (Figs. 2–5).

We next examined the influence of treatment on RFS. Both treatments produced RFS rates superior to surgery alone ($P < 0.01$). More importantly, there was no significant difference in outcome between AC and AC plus RT (Fig. 6). Furthermore, there was

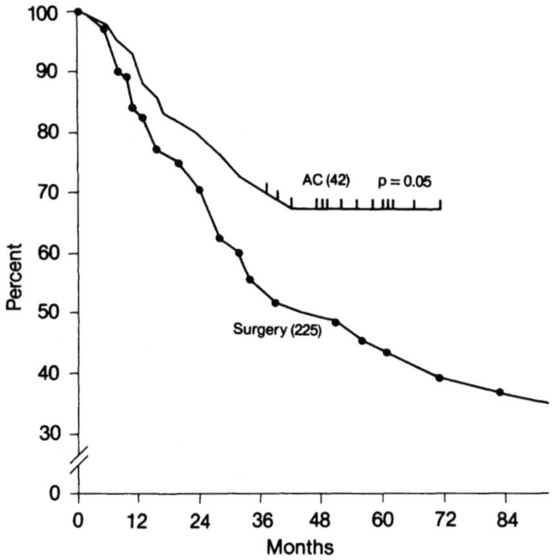

Fig. 4. Comparison of RFS for 42 premenopausal patients and 225 matched controls ($P = 0.05$)

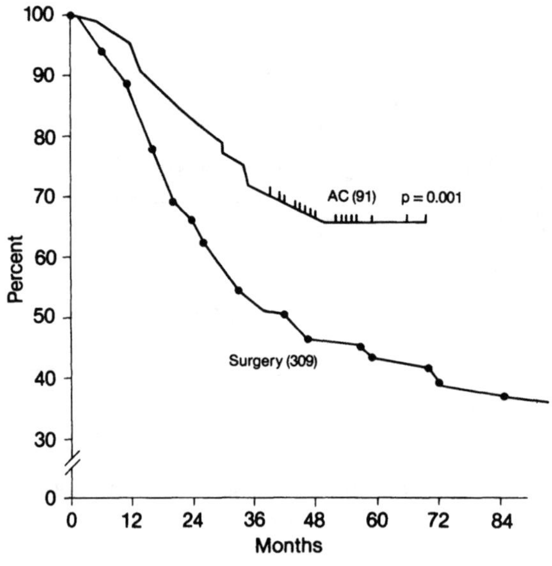

Fig. 5. Comparison of RFS for 91 postmenopausal patients (five perimenopausal patients are excluded) and 309 matched controls ($P < 0.001$)

no detectable difference in RFS for any subgroup according to treatment (AC versus AC plus RT for patients with one to three positive nodes, more than three positive nodes, premenopausal status, or postmenopausal status).

Discussion

In this study, we have demonstrated that a brief 6-month course of adjuvant chemotherapy with two synergistic agents significantly reduces the recurrence rate in

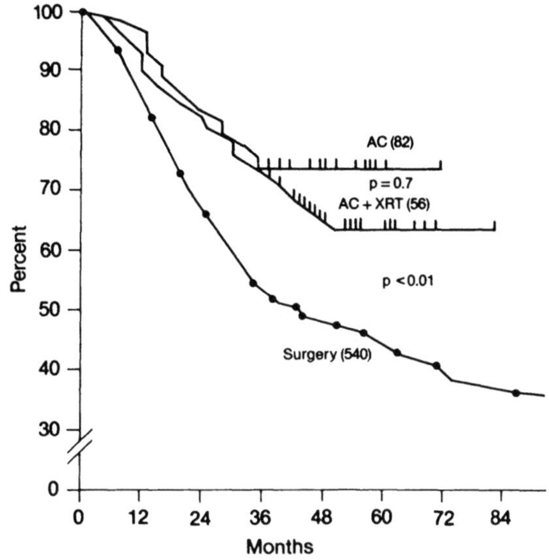

Fig. 6. Comparison of overall RFS for 82 patients who received AC with RFS of 56 who received AC plus XRT ($P = 0.7$). Comparison of AC-treated patients with 540 matched controls was significantly different ($P < 0.001$) as was the difference between AC plus XRT and controls ($P = 0.006$)

Table 2. Adjuvant breast cancer studies showing equal benefit in postmenopausal compared to premenopausal patients

Study	Regimen[a]
Arizona trial [20, present analysis]	AC plus RT
Anderson trial [7]	FAC plus BCG
British Multicentre Study [21]	CMFV
Buffalo [8]	CMFVP
SWOG Study [12]	CMFVP
Oslo [16]	C
Milan trials [3, 5]	CMF (85% of protocol doses)

[a] A, adriamycin; C, cyclophosphamide; RT, radiotherapy; F, 5-fluorouracil; V, vincristine, and P, prednisone

women with node-positive (stage II) breast cancer. This effect of adjuvant treatment is clearly manifest in all groups of women irrespective of nodal involvement or menopausal status. This treatment program is well tolerated and free from dose-limiting side effects [20]. To date, no patient has developed cardiac toxicity from adriamycin. This is not surprising, since the maximum total dose is 240 mg/m^2 and below the limits for likelihood of early cardiac toxicity. However, we also have not seen evidence of late cardiac toxicity during 3–5 years. The most frequent and disturbing side effect to patients has been hair loss. Recently, we reported a simple, inexpensive, and effective method of reducing adriamycin-induced hair loss [10]. Indeed, scalp hypothermia results in an overall frequency of hair loss with AC adjuvant chemotherapy similar to that with conventional CMF adjuvant chemotherapy [4].

We have consistently observed that AC chemotherapy worked as well in postmenopausal women as premenopausal [19, 20]. Although the initial reports of cyclophosphamide methotrexate and 5-fluorouracil (CMF) in the original Milan trial appeared to be promising in postmenopausal women, subsequent follow-up showed less benefit [3–5]. Indeed, this led many oncologists to the erroneous conclusion that adjuvant therapy was ineffective in postmenopausal women [13]. The notion that adjuvant treatment is ineffective in postmenopausal women appears to be disproven. Not only is our AC trial quite positive in postmenopausal patients (Fig. 5), but at least six other major adjuvant trials also show positive results in postmenopausal women (including the Milan trials) (Table 2). Reanalysis of the Milan data reveals that the adjuvant effect is strongly dependent on the dose of chemotherapy employed [2, 5]. Indeed, in the most recent report, postmenopausal patients who received more than 85% of the calculated full doses had equal benefit to equivalently dosed premenopausal patients [2]. One advantage of AC adjuvant chemotherapy is that more than 75% of patients received more than 85% of the calculated drug doses. This fact probably accounts for our early and consistent observation of equivalent benefit in postmenopausal women [19, 20]. Thus, the reassessment of the original Milan trial, in terms of dose response, results from our study, and data from other trials [7, 8, 12, 16, 21], should prove that adjuvant therapy is effective in postmenopausal women. Finally, our study provides a preliminary answer to the question of whether RT improves the results of adjuvant chemotherapy. There is no evidence to date that AC or AC plus RT differ in RFS rates. A report by Cooper et al. [8] suggested that postoperative RT prior to adjuvant chemotherapy was a significant factor in adverse outcome. Another trial also suggested a slightly higher recurrence rate in women randomized to receive postoperative RT followed by 24 months of adjuvant CMF treatment, compared to chemotherapy alone [15]. Our study fails to show any effect of RT on the results of treatment to date. We have not yet analyzed patterns of relapse in patients receiving combined therapy versus AC alone and this will be necessary before finally concluding that there is no role for routine postoperative RT in conjunction with adjuvant chemotherapy.

It must be recognized that adjuvant therapy for women with stage II breast cancer with four or more positive lymph nodes still represents a significant developmental problem. While the adjuvant effect can clearly be discerned from the survival curves, a significant relapse rate is still projected. More intensive adjuvant regimens, adding additional agents to AC or the use of alternating noncross-resistant combinations, should be considered for these high-risk patients.

References

1. American Joint Committee for Cancer Staging and End-Results Reporting (1977) Manual for staging of cancer. Chicago, pp 101–107
2. Bonadonna G, Valagussa P (1981) Dose-response effect of adjuvant chemotherapy in breast cancer. N Engl J Med 304: 10–15
3. Bonadonna G, Brusamolino E, Valagussa P, Rossi A, Brugnatelli L, Brambilla C, DeLena M, Tancini G, Bajetta E, Musumeci R, Veronesi V (1976) Combination chemotherapy as an adjuvant treatment in operable breast cancer. N Engl J Med 294: 405–410
4. Bonadonna G, Valagussa P, Rossi A, Zucali R, Tancini G, Bajetta E, Brambilla C, DeLena M, DiFranzo G, Banfi A, Rilke F, Veronesi V (1978) Are surgical adjuvant trials altering the course of breast cancer? Semin Oncol 5: 450–464

5. Bonadonna G, Valagussa P, Rossi A, Tancini G, Bajetta E, Marchini S, Veronesi V (1979) CMF adjuvant chemotherapy in operable breast cancer. In: Jones SE, Salmon SE (eds) Adjuvant therapy of cancer II. Grune & Stratton, New York, pp 227–235
6. Breslow N (1970) A generalized Kruskal-Wallis test for comparing K samples subject to unequal patterns of censorship. Biometrika 57: 579–594
7. Buzdar AU, Blumenschein CR, Gutterman JU et al. (1979) Postoperative adjuvant chemotherapy with fluorouracil, doxorubicin, cyclophosphamide, and BCG vaccine. JAMA 242: 1509–1513
8. Cooper RG, Holland JF, Glidewell O (1979) Adjuvant chemotherapy of breast cancer. Cancer 44: 793–798
9. Corbett T, Griswold D, Mayo J et al. (1975) Cyclophosphamide-adriamycin combination chemotherapy of transplantable murine tumors. Cancer Res 35: 1568–1573
10. Dean JC, Salmon SE, Griffith KS (1979) Prevention of doxorubicin-induced hair loss with scalp hypothermia. N Engl J Med 301: 1427–1429
11. Gehan EA (1965) A generalized Wilcoxon test for comparing arbitrarily single-censored samples. Biometrika 52: 203–223
12. Glucksberg H, Rivkin SE, Rasmussen S (1979) Adjuvant chemotherapy for stage II breast cancer: A comparison of CMFVP versus L-PAM. In: Jones SE, Salmon SE (eds) Adjuvant therapy of cancer II. Grune & Stratton, New York, pp 261–268
13. Henderson C, Canellos GP (1980) Cancer of the breast: The past decade. N Engl J Med 302: 17–30, 77–90
14. Kaplan E, Meier P (1958) Non-parametric estimations from incomplete observations. J Am Stat Assoc 53: 457–481
15. Muss H, Cooper MR, Ferree C, Richards F, Stuart J, White D, Rhyne L, Spurr C (1980) A randomized adjuvant study of CMF with and without radiation therapy for stage II breast cancer. Proc Am Soc Clin Oncol 21: 399
16. Nissen-Meyer R (1979) One short chemotherapy course in primary breast cancer: 12-Year follow-up in series 1 of the Scandinavian adjuvant chemotherapy study group. In: Jones SE, Salmon SE (eds) Adjuvant therapy of cancer II. Grune & Stratton, New York, pp 207–213
17. Peto R, Pike MC, Armitage P, Breslow NE, Cox BR, Howard SV, Mantel N, McPherson K, Peto J, Smith PG (1977) Design and analysis of randomized clinical trials requiring prolonged observation of each patient. Br J Cancer 35: 1–39
18. Salmon SE, Jones SE (1979) Studies of the combination of adriamycin and cyclophosphamide (alone or with other agents) for the treatment of breast cancer. Oncology 36: 40–47
19. Salmon SE, Wendt A, Jones SE, Jackson R, Giordano G, Miller R, Heusinkveld R, Moon TE (1979) Treatment of early breast cancer with adriamycin-cyclophosphamide with or without radiation therapy: Initial results of a brief and effective adjuvant program. In: Bonadonna G, Mathe G, Salmon SE (eds) Recent results in cancer research. Springer, Berlin Heidelberg New York, pp 98–104
20. Wendt AG, Jones SE, Salmon SE, Giordano GF, Jackson RA, Miller RS, Heusinkveld RS, Moon TE (1979) Adjuvant chemotherapy of breast cancer with adriamycin-cyclophosphamide with or without radiation therapy. In: Jones SE, Salmon SE (eds) Adjuvant therapy of cancer II. Grune & Stratton, New York, pp 285–293
21. Wheeler TK, Edelystyn GA, Bates TS et al. (1979) Four-drug combination chemotherapy following surgery for breast cancer. In: Jones SE, Salmon SE (eds) Adjuvant therapy of cancer II. Grune & Stratton, New York, pp 269–276

28. *A Randomized Trial of Postoperative Five-Versus Three-Drug Chemotherapy After Mastectomy: A Cancer and Leukemia Group B (CALGB) Study**

R. B. Weiss, D. C. Tormey, F. Holland, V. E. Weinberg, G. Lesnick, M. Perloff, G. Falkson, and O. J. Glidewell**

National Cancer Institute, Clinical Investigations Branch, Bethesda, MD 20205, USA

Summary

The Cancer and Leukemia Group B (CALB) has conducted a randomized study of adjuvant chemotherapy in patients with breast cancer who have involved axillary nodes at the time of mastectomy. Five-drug treatment (CMFVP) was compared with three-drug treatment (CMF). For patients with more than three involved nodes, the CMFVP regimen produced a significantly prolonged disease-free survival in comparison to the CMF regimen.

Introduction

In May, 1975, the Cancer and Leukemia Group B (CALB) initiated a randomized study of multimodality therapy for stage II breast carcinoma. The objective of this study in women with involved axillary nodes was to compare the disease-free survival after mastectomy produced by three different treatment regimens: cyclophosphamide (C), methotrexate (M), 5-fluorouracil (F), vincristine (V), and prednisone (P) (CMFVP); CMF; or CMF plus methanol extraction residue (MER) of bacillus Calmette-Guérin (BCG).

The rationale for this CALGB study was based upon three previous observations. a Cooper et al. [4] reported that treatment with CMFVP after mastectomy produced a markedly superior disease-free survival in patients with more than three involved nodes. No concurrent controls were used in this study, but the survival of these patients was significantly superior to that of 21,000 women from several large series with at least one positive node who did not receive postoperative chemotherapy [4]. Bonadonna et al. [2, 3] reported that treatment with CMF after mastectomy produced a longer disease-free and overall survival in patients with involved axillary nodes than a randomized comparable group treated with mastectomy alone. The subset of patients in this trial with more than three involved nodes, the one having the worst prognosis,

* This work was supported by grants CA 04457 and CA 16118 from the Division of Cancer Treatment, National Cancer Institute, Bethesda, MD (USA)

** The authors thank Mrs. Barbara B. Shepherd for her valuable assistance in the preparation of this manuscript

also showed a highly significant adjuvant chemotherapeutic effect. Work conducted by Weiss suggested the possible benefit of MER as an immunostimulant for the treatment of human cancer, particularly when minimal residual disease was present [6].

Patients and Methods

Women with operable breast cancer who had a radical or modified radical mastectomy and at least one involved axillary node were randomized to one of the three treatment regimens. Patients were stratified by age (greater or less than 50 years) and primary tumor size (greater or less than 3 cm). Although the protocol allowed postoperative radiotherapy to be administered to the chest wall and regional lymph nodes before chemotherapy to those patients whose physicians chose it, it was discouraged. Drug doses and schedules for the three regimens are outlined in Fig. 1. The induction treatment of 6 weeks consisted of daily oral C (80 mg/m^2), weekly i.v. F (500 mg/m^2), and i.v. M (30 or 40 mg/m^2, depending on whether the patient was over or under 60 years of age, respectively). In addition, patients randomized to five drugs received i.v. V (1 mg/m^2 weekly) and oral P (40 mg/m^2 daily for 21 days). The patients randomized to MER received, in addition to CMF, 1 mg of MER divided into five intradermal injection sites in weeks 1, 3, and 5. Monthly courses of chemotherapy to complete 1 year of treatment were then administered with the same induction combinations at the same doses of F, M, and V on days 1 and 8, daily C (100 mg/m^2) for 14 days, and P (40 mg/m^2), also for 14 days. MER was given on day 8. For all regimens, year 2 of treatment consisted of CMF courses at 8-week intervals. Chemotherapy was then stopped and the patients were followed for recurrence. Standard drug dose-attechenuation schedules for hematologic and other side effects were used. The two chemotherapy-only regimens are nearly identical to those described by Cooper et al.

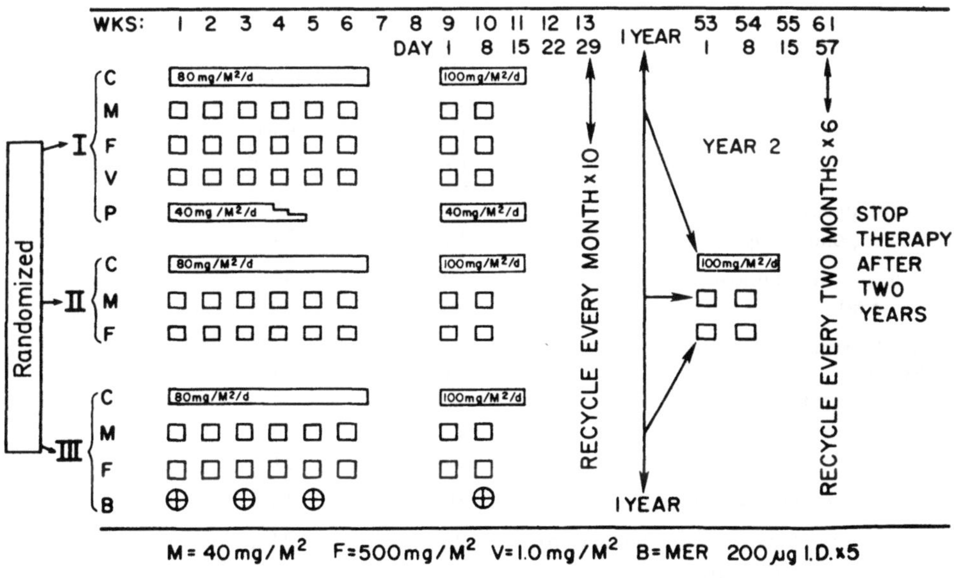

Fig. 1. The drug doses and schedules for the three treatment regimens

[4] and Bonadonna et al. [2], except that the Milan study [2] did not employ the 6-week induction schedule. Also, both of these original regimens were administered for only 9 months and 1 year, respectively.

Results

From 28 institutions, 552 evaluable patients in North America, Europa, and South Africa have been randomized prior to October, 1979, the cutoff for this analysis, to receive, chemotherapy alone. An additional 62 patients have received postoperative irradiation plus chemotherapy. Accural to the MER regimen was discontinued in October, 1978, when a previous preliminary analysis demonstrated a lack of disease-free survival benefit plus a large percentage of intolerable side effects [5]. After this data, patients were randomized only to one of the other two regimens. In this preliminary analysis, we will not present the results of the entire study, but will nodes confine the report to those patients who had more than three involved axillary nodes and who did not receive MER or radiotherapy.

A total of 234 evaluable patients with more than three positive nodes entered the study prior to October, 1979, and prospectively randomized to either CMFVP or CMF. The median observation time is 25.3 months with 4.3 years of patient entry. The 122 patients who received CMFVP and the 112 who received CMF were found to be comparable in their menopausal status, age, size of the breast tumor, number of positive nodes, and median time from mastectomy to start of chemotherapy (Table 1).

As depicted in Fig. 2, CMFVP is statistically ($P = 0.01$) superior to CMF in prolonging the disease-free interval (DFI) in all women with more than three metastatic axillary nodes. CMFVP is superior to CMF throughout the entire observation period, and at 36 months, using life-table estimates, 72% of the women treated with CMFVP were disease-free compared to 61% treated with CMF.

Table 1. Comparability of therapy groups for patients at highest risk

	CMFVP (n = 122)	CMF (n = 112)
Percent premenopausal	48	46
Percent postmenopausal	52	54
Mean age at diagnosis	50.7	49.9
% ⩾ 60	19	16
Size of primary tumor		
Mean	3.5	3.6
% ⩽ 2 CM	31	27
% > 2 and < 5	47	52
% ⩾ 5	22	21
Mean no. of metastatic axillary nodes	10.0	10.5
Median no. of days from mastectomy to onset chemotherapy	22.9	24.6

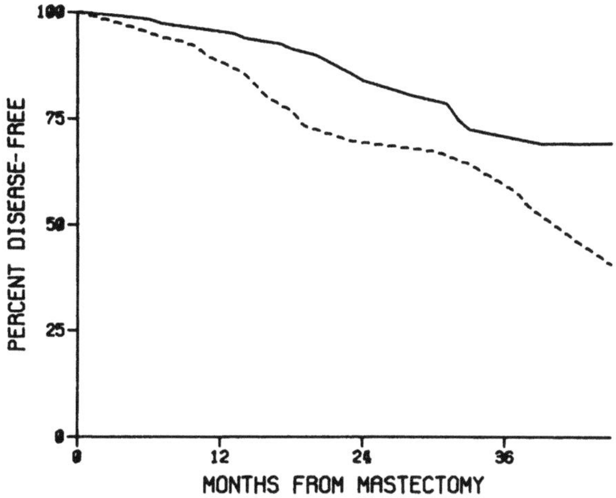

Fig. 2. The disease-free interval for patients with more than three involved nodes. ———, CMFVP 20/122; – – –, CMF 30/112 $P = 0.11$

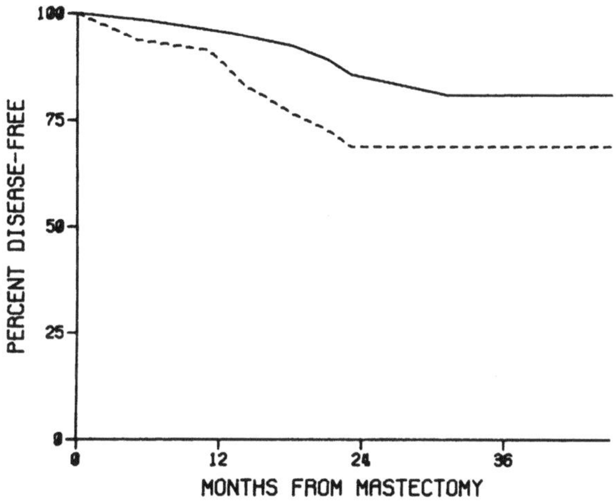

Fig. 3. The disease-free interval for premenopausal patients with more than three involved nodes. ———, CMFVP 6/58; – – –, CMF 11/51 $P = 0.05$

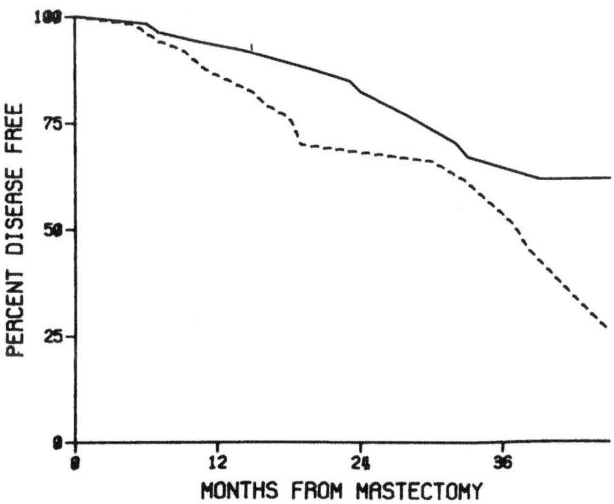

Fig. 4. The disease-free interval for postmenopausal patients with more than three involved nodes. ———, CMFVP 14/63; – – –, CMF 19/60 $P = 0.11$

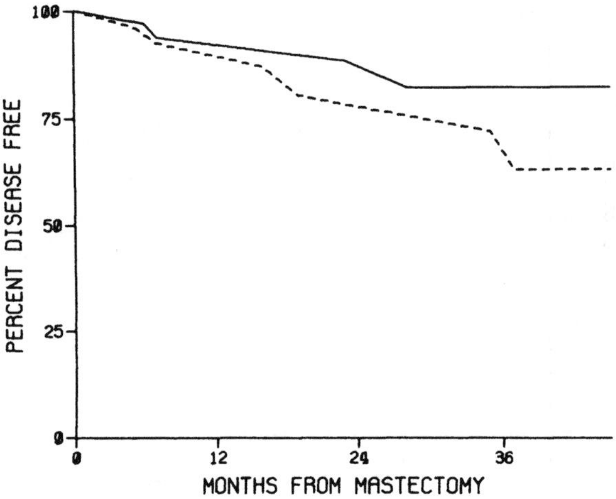

Fig. 5. The disease-free interval for patients with tumor size of 2 cm diameter or less and more than three involved nodes. ———, CMFVP 4/35; – – –, CMF 6/28

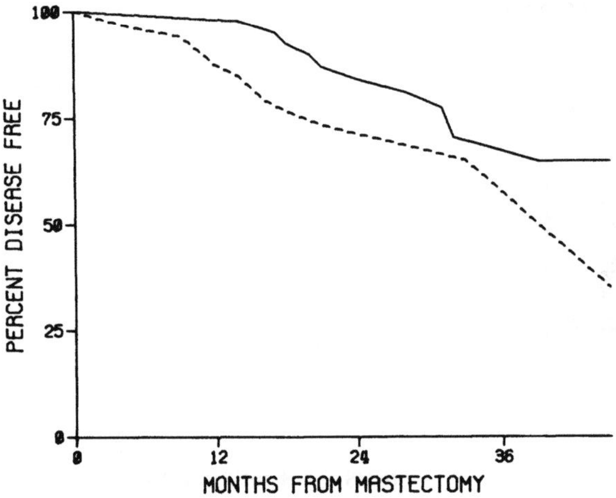

Fig. 6. The disease-free interval for patients with tumor size of more than 2 cm and less than 5 cm, with more than three involved nodes. ———, CMFVP 11/54; – – –, CMF 14/53 $P = 0.07$

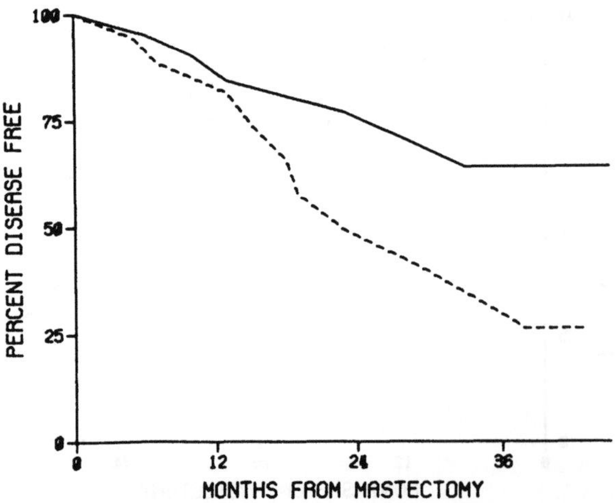

Fig. 7. The disease-free interval for patients with tumor size greater than 5 cm, with more than three involved nodes. ———, CMFVP 5/25; – – –, CMF 9/22 $P = 0.16$

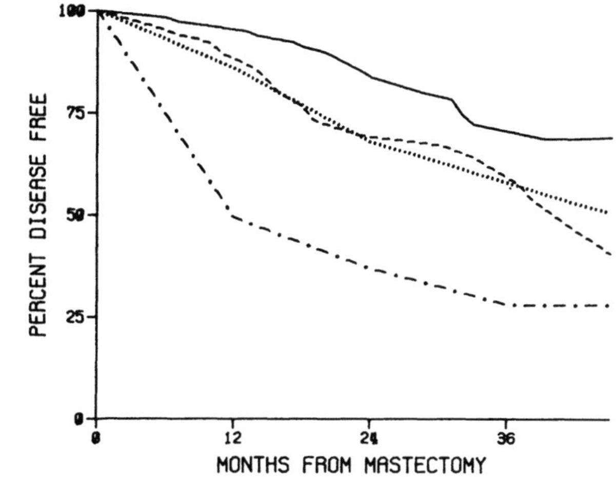

Fig. 8. The disease-free interval of patients with more than three involved nodes, comparing the two CALGB drug regimens with the Milan trial of no chemotherapy versus CMF [6]. ———, CALGB CMFVP; – – –, CALGB CMF; · · · · Milan CMF; – · – · –, Milan controls

When the two treatment groups are compared based on menopausal status, there is a significant advantage ($P = 0.05$) in DFI for CMFVP therapy in premenopausal women with more than three involved nodes (Fig. 3). A similar trend is seen for postmenopausal women in Fig. 4. These two graphs indicate that postmenopausal women continue to recur for a longer period of time than premenopausal women.

The effectiveness of the two treatments in terms of DFI has been compared in patients with tumors of different sizes, all of whom had more than three metastatic axillary nodes (Fig. 5–7). It can be observed that tumor diameter has prognostic significance and that the observable distinction between the two therapies, with CMFVP being consistently superior, appears to increase the more adverse the prognosis. With the small number of patients in each group, these observations are not statistically significant.

The toxicity of CMFVP is tolerable and, aside from specific side effects related to V and P, nearly identical to that of CMF.

The DFI of patients treated with CMFVP and CMF, according to the CALGB protocol, is compared with the CMF and control patients from Bonadonna's series [1] in Fig. 8, all patients having more than three involved axillary nodes. There are some differences in the CALGB and Bonadonna's CMF regimens, including the induction course and the longer treatment duration in the CALGB study. Also there is relative homogeneity of the Milan patients and investigators, as contrasted to the diversity of CALGB patients and investigators. Therefore, we can only make observations about trends rather than precise comparisons. The advantage of adjuvant chemotherapy, and specifically CMFVP therapy, for these patients is evident (Fig. 8). Noteworthy also is the fact that the DFI for the CALGB CMF-treated patients is very similar to that of the Milan CMF-treated patients at this time.

Discussion

A prospective randomized study comparing different drug regimens after mastectomy was conducted. The CMF regimen, as originally promulgated by Bonadonna [2], was compared with the five-drug CMFVP regimen, as devised by Cooper et al. [4], each with some modification. This CALGB study included an intensive 6-week induction course followed by intermittent therapy, for a total of 2 years of treatment. This study has shown that for comparable groups of patients with breast cancer who are at high risk of recurrence after mastectomy, namely, those with more than three involved axillary nodes, CMFVP given as an intensive induction followed by maintenance courses is significantly superior to CMF given by an identical schedule. The activity of CMFVP is demonstrable in premenopausal women and indicated in postmenopausal women. It is independent of tumor size. At this time these data are applicable only to patients with more than three positive axillary nodes.

References

1. Bonadonna G, Valagussa P (to be published) Adjuvant therapy of primary breast cancer. In: Carter SK, Glatstein E, Livingston RB (eds) Principles of cancer treatment. McGraw-Hill, New York
2. Bonadonna G, Brusamolino E, Valagussa P, et al. (1976) Combination chemotherapy as an adjuvant treatment in operable breast cancer. N Engl J Med 294: 405–410
3. Bonadonna G, Valagussa P, Rossi A, et al. (1978) Are surgical adjuvant trials altering the course of breast cancer? Semin Oncol 5: 450–464
4. Cooper RG, Holland JF, Glidewell O (1979) Adjuvant chemotherapy of breast cancer. Cancer 44: 793–798
5. Tormey D, Falkson G, Weiss R, Perloff M, Glidewell I, Holland JF (1979) Postoperative chemotherapy with/without immunotherapy for mammary carcinoma: A preliminary report. In: Jones SE, Salmon SE (eds) Adjuvant therapy of cancer II. Grune & Stratton, New York, pp 253–260
6. Weiss DW (1976) MER and other mycobacterial fractions in the immunotherapy of cancer. Med Clin North Am 60: 473–497

29. *Adjuvant Chemoimmunotherapy with LMF Plus BCG in Node-Negative and Node-Positive Breast Cancer – Intermediate Report at 4 Years**

H. J. Senn, R. Amgwerd, W. F. Jungi, R. Hochuli, J. Ammann, G. Engelhart, C. Heinz, A. Wick, F. Enderlin, G. Creux, B. Simon, R. Lanz, R. Bigler, and S. Seiler**

Kantonsspital, Oncology Center, CH-9007 St. Gallen, Switzerland

Summary

A randomized surgical adjuvant trial in 242 evaluable patients with T_{1-3a}, N_{0-1}, and M_0 breast cancer was initiated 4 years ago. The well-tolerated, oral combination chemotherapy with six cycles of Leukeran plus methotrexate plus fluorouracil (LMF) plus repeated BCG skin scarifications was used. After 4 years, the following results were seen: (1) significant increase of relapse-free (RFS) and also overall survival (S) in both pre- and postmenopausal node-negative patients versus surgical controls (RFS 91.1 vs. 70.1%, $P = 0.003$; S 96 vs. 88%, $P = 0.03$); (2) no significant increase of RFS or S in pre- and postmenopausal node-positive patients versus surgical controls (RFS 50.1 versus 44%, $P = 0.49$; S 70 versus 68%, $P = 0.9$, respectively); (3) Patients receiving greater than 90% of the planned LMF dose showed significantly better survival after 4 years; and (4) Nonrandomized comparison with concurrent Swiss adjuvant studies with LMF alone indicate no beneficial or harmful effect of BCG skin scarifications in addition to the six-cycle LMF.

Introduction

Since medium- to long-term survival expectancy and mortality in operable breast cancer have remained essentially unchanged during the past 40 years, the traditional surgical approach and the role of routine adjuvant radiotherapy have been seriously challenged [1, 6]. While early attempts involving short-term intra- or postoperative adjuvant chemotherapy have either failed or yielded inconclusive results, the crucial problem of occult disseminated micrometastases has prompted a new series of controlled adjuvant studies of operable breast cancer [3]. While most such investigations included only node-positive (N+) patients, we felt justified in Eastern Switzerland to include (on a stratified basis) also histologically node-negative (N−)

* This study was supported by the Swiss Cancer League, the Regional Cancer Leagues of St. Gallen, Appenzell, and Thurgau, as well as the E. E. Schellenberg Funds

** We greatly appreciate the skillful coordinating assistance of Miss Agnes Glaus, Head Nurse of the Departmnet of Medicine C, Kantonsspital St. Gallen, and of Dr. W. Berchtold, group statistician of OSAKO, Federal Technical University (ETH), Zürich

cases for two reasons: (1) a regionally lower relapse-free (RFS) and overall survival (S) in N− patients as reported (retrospectively) by Mutzner et al. [8]; and (2) the presumption that N− patients with truly "minimal tumor cell burden" after mastectomy would constitute an ideal and highly curable population to test the concept of adjuvant systemic therapy, since to date at least 25−30% of N− patients present recurrent, usually incurable breast cancer within 5 years of initial surgery.

The present analysis reports the 4-year results of a previously reported randomized trial with surgical controls, investigating the comparative influence of a relatively short-term oral Leukeran plus methotrexate plus fluorouracil (LMF) chemotherapy with low toxicity, which was supplemented later by repeated BCG skin scarifications [10]. Immunostimulation with BCG was added to the adjuvant chemotherapy due to its earlier claims to counterbalance immunodepressive side effects of cytotoxic treatment and to potentially prolong disease-free survival.

Patients and Design

A total of 254 women with proven breast cancer of clinical stages T_{1-3a}, N_{0-1}, and M_0 were stratified as to nodal stage (N− of N+) or the homolateral axilla and then randomized to receive no further treatment after modified radical mastectomy or six monthly 14-day cycles of oral LMF. This 6-month adjuvant chemotherapy phase was followed by monthly BCG skin scarifications for up to 2 years or recurrence, using rotating proximal extremity sites and Glaxo-strain BCG. Details of the procedure have been published [9, 10].

On March 1, 1980, 242 patients (95.3% of all randomized) were evaluable for a median follow-up of 49 months in both treatment arms (38−70 months). The treatment groups are well balanced regarding all known risk factors (Table 1).

Results

Table 2 summarizes comparative 4-year RFS rates of the various patient subgroups and the two treatment approaches. While there is a constant strong tendency towards

Table 1. Prognostic factor distribution in breast cancer chemoimmunotherapy study (Osako 06/74). Twelve of 254 patients were not evaluable due to staging errors, initial second neoplasm, or lost to follow-up

Subgroup	Surgical controls	LMF + BCG	All patients
N− and N+	125	117	242
N−	67	58	125
N+	58	59	117
N+ (1−3)	37	42	79
N+ (≥4)	21	18	39
T_{1-2a}	112	103	215
T_{3a}	13	14	27
Pre- and perimenopausal	63	64	127
Postmenopausal	62	53	115
Mean age at surgery (years)	56.7	53.0	55.3

Table 2. Four-year relapse-free survival (March 1, 1980)

Subgroup	Surgical controls (%)	LMF + BCG (%)	*P*
All N−	70.1	91.1	0.003
N− pre- and perimenopausal	75.9	93.6	0.048
N− postmenopausal	66.7	88.5	0.034
All N+	44.0	50.1	0.493
N+ pre- and perimenopausal	34.5	38.8	0.808
N+ postmenopausal	56.0	62.5	0.488
N+ (1−3)	48.7	53.9	0.526
N+ (≥ 4)	35.0	41.2	0.468

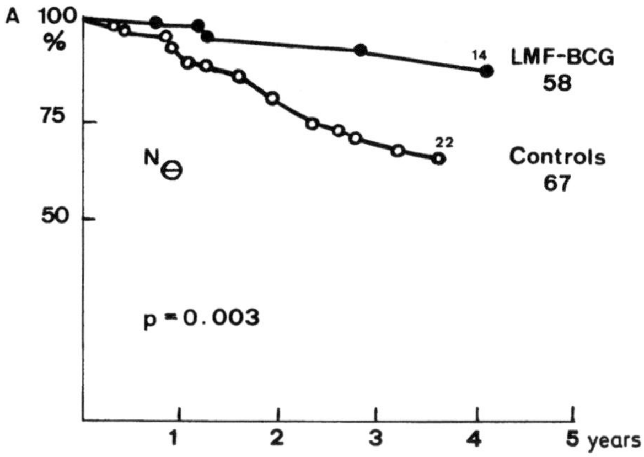

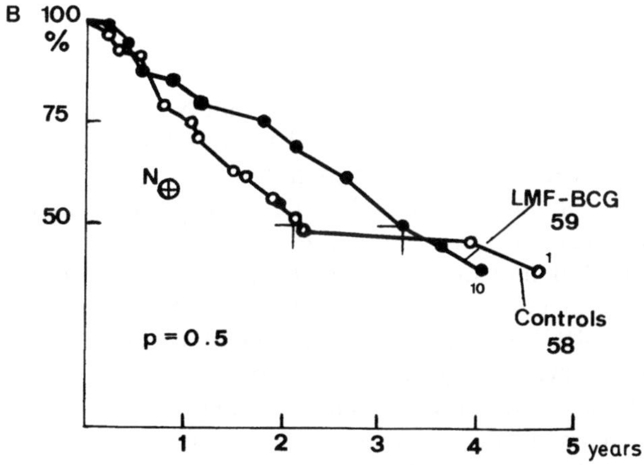

Fig. 1. Probability of disease-free survival at 4 years median postoperative observation time for **A** node-negative and **B** node-positive breast cancer patients. Comparison of surgical controls (○) versus adjuvant LMF plus BCG (●)

higher RFS rates in the whole group, it is clearly evident that mainly N− women really profit from the adjuvant chemoimmunotherapy with LMF-BCG (91.1% vs. 70.1% after 4 years, $P = 0.001$). Pre-, peri-, as well as postmenopausal N− patients also seem to profit, with a fairly constant gain of roughly 20% of higher RFS rates, 4 years after mastectomy.

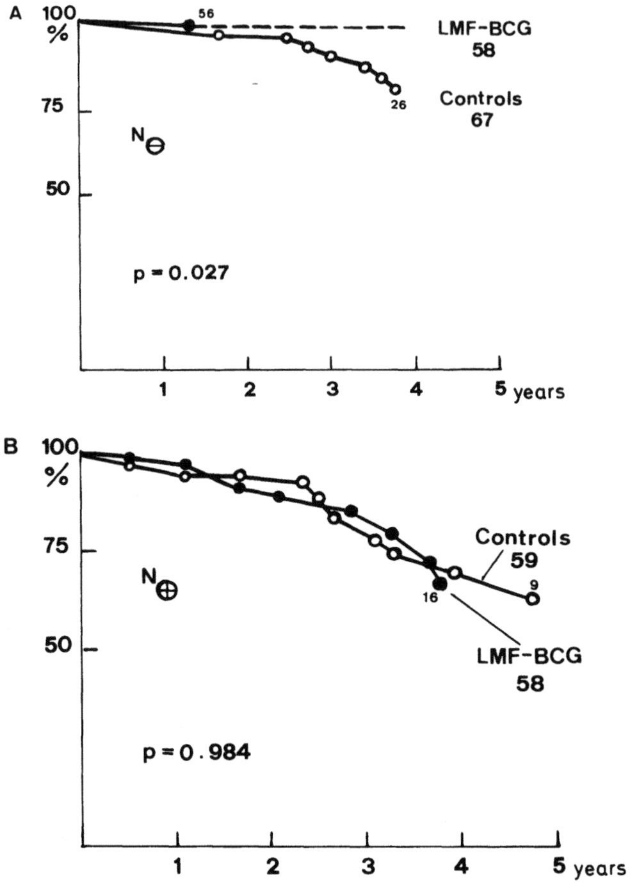

Fig. 2. Probability of overall survival at 4 years median postoperative observation time for **A** node-negative and **B** node-positive patients

It is, however, shown in Table 2 that N+ breast cancer patients treated with the same moderately intense and well-tolerated LMF-BCG regimen showed no significant improvement, as previously noted in 2- and 3-year interim reports [9, 10]. This holds true for all subsets of N+ cases, regarding menopausal status, degree of axillary involvement, and tumor size.

Fig. 1 demonstrates the marked and continuing difference of the RFS curves for surgical controls and LMF-BCG in N− patients, while N+ women treated with LMF-BCG experienced at best a temporary delay of about 1 year to relapse. But both N+ curves merge and even cross at 4 year ($P = 0.49$).

The same situation exists for overall survival (Fig. 2). For the first time we observe, at 4 years from mastectomy, a significant difference in survival expectancy for LMF-BCG-treated N− patients ($P = 0.03$). There is virtually no such tendency in N+ cases using the same adjuvant regimen.

Regarding the relatively low RFS expectancy of our group of surgically treated N− control patients we must emphasize previous similar experience at the local level [8]. All N− cases in this study have been subjected to a careful axillary node reanalysis, and among 125 N− cases one micrometastatis in one node was detected in two patients.

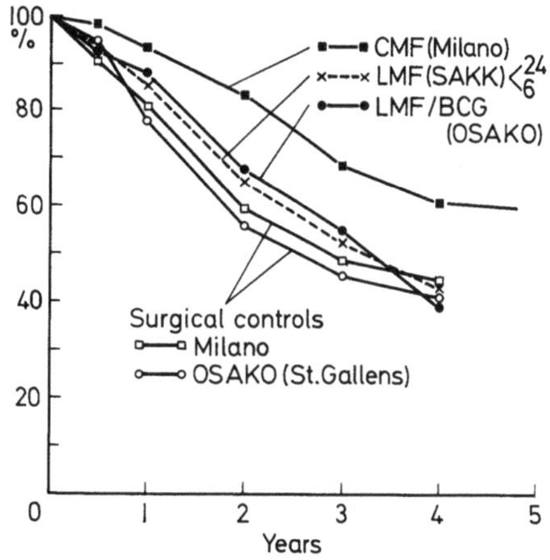

Fig. 3. Comparative probability of relapse-free survival in node-positive breast cancer in different surgical adjuvant trials: Milano surgical controls (□) versus CMF × 12 (■); OSAKO surgical controls (○) versus LMF × 6 plus BCG (●), and SAKK LMF × 6 versus LMF × 24 (*both)

Table 3. Site of first detected recurrence (4 years)

Subgroup site	Regimen A (surgical controls)	Regimen C (LMF-BCG)
N− ($n = 124$)		
Local	6/67 (8.9%)	2/58 (3.4%)
Regional	2/67 (3.0%)	0/58 (0%)
Distant and combined	11/67 (16.4%)	3/58 (5.1%)
All N−	19/67 (28.4%)	5/58 (8.6%)
N− ($n = 117$)		
Local	11/57 (19.2%)	8/59 (13.5%)
Regional	5/57 (8.7%)	3/59 (5.1%)
Distant and combined	16/57 (28.1%)	14/59 (23.7%)
All N−	32/57 (56.1%)	25/59 (42.4%)

There seems to exist, as in the Milano trial with CMF [2, 3], a strong relationship between total dose of LMF applied and RFS rates, and especially overall survival rates (Fig. 3). However, the two groups of treatment intensity are very imbalanced, since 75% patients completed their six monthy LMF chemotherapy cycles with total drug doses of more than 90%, due to excellent subjective and objective tolerance to the adjuvant regimen.

Late toxicity of the adjuvant LMF-BCG regimen used was not exceptional up to 4 years of median follow-up. No case of secondary acute leukemia has been observed in the patients receiving adjuvant therapy ($n = 116$).

Second (or concomitant?) solid neoplasms occurred in two cases each in the control as well as the LMF-BCG study group. The distribution and relative frequency of first detected recurrence of breast cancer manifestations are summarized in Table 3. After 4 years, 81 of 242 patients have relapsed. Of all relapses detected, 45% occurred first at locoregional and 55% primarily at distant or combined sites (hematogenous metastases).

Table 4. Treatment results of relapses (N– and N+)

Primary adjuvant treatment	Complete and partial remission	Median duration (months)
Surgical controls	38/50 (76%)	11.6 + (2–33)
LMF-BCG	20/31 (65%)	8.5 + (2–27)

Treatment at time of relapse was locoregional (surgery and/or radiotherapy plus hormonotherapy) or systemic (chemohormonotherapy containing adriamycin)

As demonstrated in Table 3, N– patients treated with LMF-BCG experienced significantly lower recurrences at all sites (local, regional, and distant), while no significant change in distribution or frequency was observed in N+ patients. In patients with initial locoregional relapse, LMF-BCG delayed the subsequent tumor-free interval to systemic disease by approximately 1 year in the N– and N+ population (22 months vs. 12 months in surgical controls, $P = 0.04$).
The remission rate and median duration of relapsing patients with (partially standardized) chemohormonotherapy, supplemented individually by local or CNS radiotherapy, are shown in Table 4. Objective rates of complete and partial remission are in the expected range of 65–76% and do not seem to differ from common experience in patients not receiving prior, temporary adjuvant chemotherapy. The median remission duration of 8 (surgical controls) to 11.5 months (prior to LMF-BCG) also does not seem to differ from generally published values [4].

Discussion

Based on animal tumor models and recent clinical experience, postoperative adjuvant chemotherapy (eventually combined with other modalities, such as immuno- or hormonotherapy) has emerged as a promising way to overcome the stagnation of cure rates in some types of common neoplasias, such as breast cancer [2, 3, 7].
Whereas in two similar, controlled adjuvant studies, a RFS and hopefully overall survival benefit by either L-phenylalanine mustard (L-PAM) (plus 5-FU) or cyclophosphamide + methotrexate + fluorouracil (CMF) was shown in high-risk premenopausal N+ patients at 4–5 years postmastectomy, no such lasting influence was observed in our corresponding subgroup of N+ patients.
A marginal delay of the disease-free interval (approximately 1 year) was of a transitory nature (1–3 years postmastectomy). There seems to be no difference in patient selection or initial surgery of N+ women between the Milano CMF trial and our OSAKO study with LMF-BCG, as their surgical control arms show virtually identical RFS curves (Fig. 3).
Consequently, we must conclude that our six cycles of oral LMF were less efficient in clearing the greater residual tumor cell burden after modified radical mastectomy in N+ patients than the more aggressive CMF regimen used by Bonadonna et al. [2, 3]. However, the data of the Milano trial have not yet been fully confirmed by others and a direct randomized comparison of CMF versus LMF is lacking. The duration of adjuvant treatment seems to be less critical than its biologic intensity.
That this is important for future adjuvant studies is stressed by the following findings: (1) RFS and overall survival (up to 3 years) are similar in the Milano studies with 12 or

only six cycles of CMF [11]; (2) The same is true (on a less effective basis) of 6 versus 24 months of oral LMF in the randomized SAKK study 27/76 (unpublished data); and (3) The Milano CMF trial [3, 11], as well as this and possibly other studies, disclose a significant survival benefit at 4–5 years for patients receiving the full dose of chemotherapy.

In contrast to the disappointing results with oral LMF in our N+ cases, we have clearly extended our earlier findings [9, 10], that the same well-tolerated and relatively short adjuvant regimen with LMF (followed by BCG) significantly increases RFS and overall survival in N− patients.

Pre-, peri-, and postmenopausal N− cases benefit from "soft" LMF (plus BCG), as well as all types of relapse sites (locoregional, systemic, and combined). To our knowledge, we report the first prospective (randomized) trial of adjuvant chemo-immunotherapy in N− breast cancer. Our results are comparable to similar data of a retrospective (nonrandomized) investigation which reports increased 10-year survival in N− but not N+ patients who had received a 4–6 month course of i.v. cyclophosphamide as compared to their own historical controls [5].

Since, possibly depending on staging and regional differences, 25–35% of so-called N− low-risk patients are still in relapse 5–8 years after initial surgery, we feel justified to expand our encouraging findings in a new N− breast cancer study comparing a surgical control arm with six cycles of our present LMF without BCG ("soft and long") and three cycles of CMF ("hard and short").

It is difficult to assess the potential impact of the nonspecific immunostimulation by repeated BCG skin scarifications in our adjuvant regimen, since we lack a randomized regimen with six-cycle LMF alone. However, both treatment arms (6- vs. 24-cycle LMF) without BCG in a concurrent Swiss national adjuvant study (SAKK 27/76) show virtually identical RFS and overall survival (up to 4 years) as compared to LMF-BCG. This renders a "negative", or even "positive", effect of BCG in addition to standard chemoadjuvant regimens in N+ patients highly unlikely. No other data or comparisons exist at present for N− breast cancer patients.

References

1. Baum M (1976) The curability of breast cancer. Br Med J 1: 439–444
2. Bonadonna G, Rossi A, Valagussa P, et al. (1977) The CMF program for operable breast cancer with positive axillary nodes: Updated analysis. Cancer 39: 2904–2915
3. Bonadonna G, Valagussa P, Rossi A, et al. (1978) Are surgical adjuvant trials going to alter the course of operable breast cancer? Semin Oncol 5: 450–464
4. Brunner KW, Martz G, Senn HJ, et al. (1975) A controlled study in the use of combined drug therapy in metastatic breast cancer. Cancer 36: 1208–1219
5. Donovan A, Powell J, Waterhouse JAH, et al. (1976) A prolonged course of cyclophosphamide as an adjunct to mastectomy in primary treatment of breast carcinoma. Br J Surg 63: 817–819
6. Fisher B, Wolmark N (1975) New concepts in the management of primary breast cancer. Cancer [Suppl 2] 36: 627–637
7. Huber H, Falkensammer M, Senn HJ (1978) Adjuvante zytostatische Chemotherapie. Springer, Berlin Heidelberg New York
8. Mutzner F, Amgwerd R, Gessner U (1977) Prognose des lokalen primären Mammakarzinoms unter der bisherigen Therapie. Schweiz Med Wochenschr 107: 992–995

9. Senn HJ, Mayr AC (1979) Adjuvant chemotherapy in breast cancer: Swiss cooperative studies. Cancer Treat Rev [Suppl] 6: 79–85
10. Senn HJ, Jungi WF, Amgwerd R, et al. (1978) Adjuvant chemoimmunotherapy with LMF+BCG in node-negative and node-positive breast cancer patients. Antibiot Chemother 24: 213–228
11. Tancini G, Bojetta E, Marchini S (1979) Preliminary 3-year results of 12 vs. 6 cycles of surgical adjuvant CMF in premenopausal breast cancer. Cancer Clin Trials 2: 285–292

30. *Adjuvant Intermittent Chemoimmunotherapy for Primary Breast Cancer: A Prospective Study with Immunologic Follow-Up*

M. Betzler, W. Schreml, M. Lang, H. P. Lohrmann, H. D. Flad, P. Schlag, C. Herfarth, and H. Heimpel

Universität Ulm, Department für Chirurgie, Steinhövelstrasse 9, D-7900 Ulm, Germany

Summary

In an interdisciplinary prospective study 50 patients surgically treated for breast cancer were treated with six monthly courses of aggressive adjuvant chemotherapy (adriamycin and cyclophosphamide) and were randomized to receive either immunotherapy with levamisole or no additional therapy. Probability of disease-free survival for the whole group is 54.9% at 42 months. There was no noticeable difference in disease-free survival for either pre- and postmenopausal women or for patients treated with or without levamisole. The addition of levamisole had no effect on the depression of in vitro immunologic functions during chemotherapy.

Introduction

An interdisciplinary study on adjuvant chemotherapy of primary breast cancer was started in June, 1976, when the first data on adjuvant chemotherapy of breast cancer were published [3, 5], with the following aims: (1) To test, in a phase II study, the feasibility of a short-term (6 months) highly aggressive chemotherapy regimen of adriamycin (ADM) and cyclophosphamide in breast cancer patients; (2) to study, in a phase III setting, the influence of additional immunotherapy with levamisole on the clinical and pathophysiologic effects of adjuvant chemotherapy; and (3) to perform thorough laboratory investigations on the influence of the chosen chemotherapeutic regimen on the immune status and on the hemopoietic system of the treated patients.

In this paper, the clinical and immunologic data of the study are summarized. An account of the effect of types of adjuvant chemo-immuno-therapy on granulopoiesis is given in the following article (Chap. 31, p. 192).

Patients and Methods

Fifty-two patients under the age of 65 years (34 premenopausal, 18 postmenopausal), who had received surgical treatment for primary breast cancer (modified radical mastectomy), were free of recognizable metastases, but were considered to be high

Recent Results in Cancer Research, Vol. 80

risks for recurrence (positive axillary lymph nodes or large primary tumor, i.e., T_3 in lateral location or T_2 in medial or central location). Nine patients were treated for large primary tumors only, 27 had one to three involved lymph nodes, and 14 had four or more positive nodes (Fig. 1).

All patients received six courses of ADM (50 mg/m^2 i.v.) and cyclophosphamide (500 mg/m^2) in 250 ml glucose as single doses at monthly intervals (Fig. 1). The patients were randomly assigned by the Department of Clinical Documentation to receive either no additional therapy or additional immunotherapy (levamisole, 150 mg orally on days 14, 15, 21, and 22 of each course and on 2 consecutive days every week for 1.5 year after completion of chemotherapy).

Clinical and laboratory studies were done every month during the chemotherapy period and every 3 months thereafter according to the guidelines established in our group [1]. Side effects were noted on a questionnaire. Before beginning chemoimmunotherapy, prior to the third and sixth infusion and again at 3-month intervals, the following immune parameters were tested: (1) Lymphocyte count; (2) relative distribution and absolute number of T and B lymphocytes in the peripheral blood as determined by rosette techniques; (3) stimulation of lymphocytes with the lectins phytohemagglutinin, concanavalin A (Con A), pokeweed mitogen, and with a pool of frozen-thawed irradiated allogeneic lymphocytes; and (4) antibody-dependent cell-mediated cytotoxicity (ADCC) using the mouse L1210 lymphoma line as target cells and a rabbit anti-L1210 IgG antibody at a final dilution of 1 : 4000. The special laboratory techniques have been previously published [2, 6].

The probability of disease-free survival was estimated at 3-month intervals by the actuarial method [7]. The observation period has now reached 42 months. The data calculated at 36 months were compared with the corresponding data of Bonadonna after the same period of time [4].

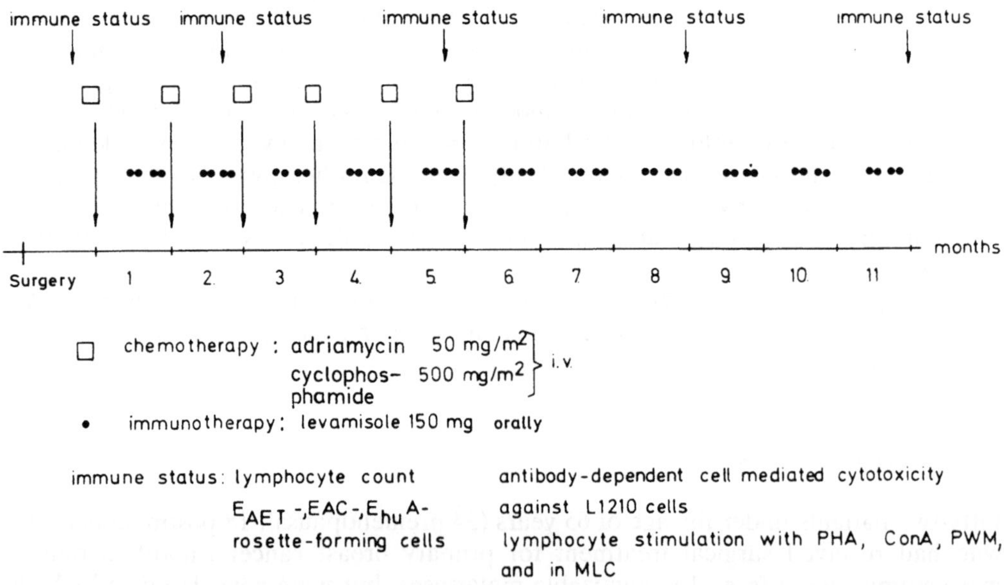

Fig. 1. Design of an adjuvant intermittent chemo-immunotherapy in primary breast cancer with an immunologic follow-up

Results

Patient Compliance

Two patients were taken off the study during the first course of chemotherapy, one for severe bone marrow depression with leukopenia, thrombopenia, and consequent sepsis and bleeding complications; the patient recovered and is free of disease up to now. The second patient refused further chemotherapy because of side effects and did not return for follow-up. Of the remaining 50 patients all have completed chemotherapy with a total of 300 courses. In ten instances a delay for leukopenia, in one for intercurrent infection, and , in six, for the performance of diagnostic biopsy to evaluate suspected locoregional recurrence of a suspicious finding in the contralateral breast. In one patient a delay and dose reduction was necessary in two courses because of severe stomatitis. Levamisole had to be discontinued in 6 of 24 patients before the scheduled completion of 2 years due to side effects.

Probability of Disease-Free Survival and Survival

The data at 36 months are compared with the corresponding data from the Bonadonna study (Figs. 2, 3, Table 1), comparing cyclophosphamide, methotrexate, 5-fluorouracil

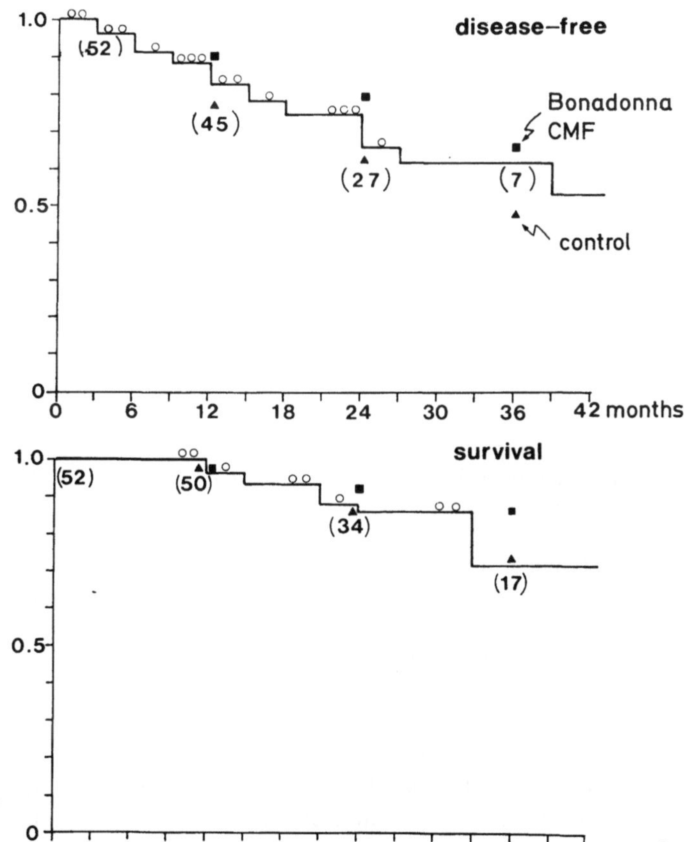

Fig. 2. Probability of disease-free survival and survival with the corresponding data from Bonadonna [4] (▲ = control, ■ = CMF) as determined by the actuarial method

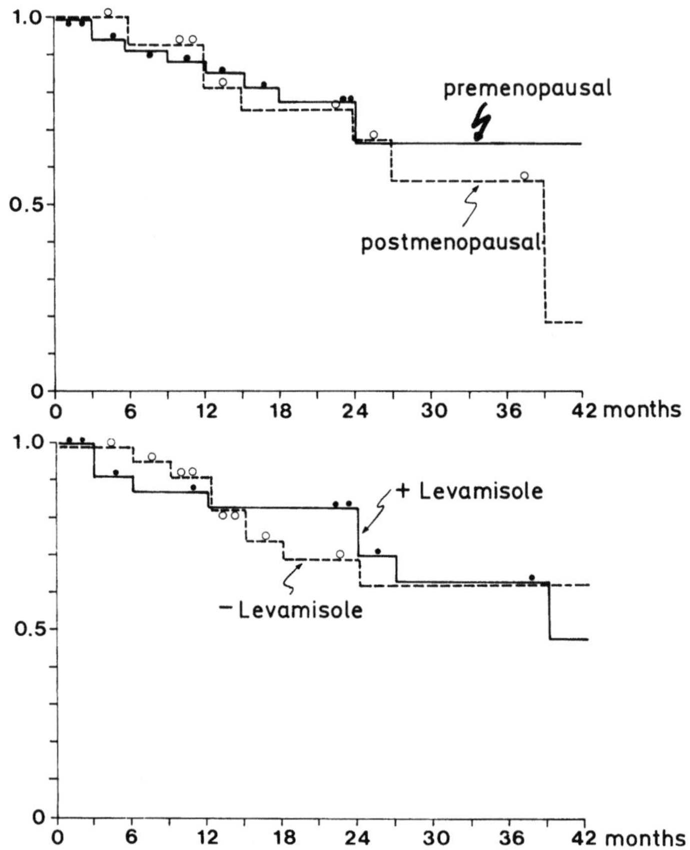

Fig. 3. Probability of disease-free survival for pre- and postmenopausal subgroups and for patients with and without levamisole determined by the actuarial method

Table 1. Probability of disease-free survival[a] A and survival[a] B at 36 months determined by the actuarial method with the corresponding data from Bonadonna [4]

		Ulm	Bonadonna [4]	
			Control	CMF
A	Total group	61%	51%	69.3%
	Premenopausal	65.4%	46.6%	77.4%
	Postmenopausal	53.8%	56.6%	61.9%
	With levamisole	58.2%	–	–
	Without levamisole	61.0%	–	–
B	Total group	86.7%	80.6%	88.3%

[a] At 36 months, actuarial method

(CMF) with a control group (no adjuvant therapy). The evaluation at this time indicates that the results for disease-free survival and survival fall between the control and CMF data of Bonadonna. The probability of disease-free survival for the subgroups of pre- and postmenopausal patients again fall between the control and the CMF data of Bonadonna. At 42 months the probability of disease-free survival for the

Table 2. Type and time of recurrences in correlation with the tumor stage

	Without recurrences	With recurrences	Postoperative (months)	Localization
T_2N_0	6	0		
T_3N_0	1	4	24	Lung
			15/21	Local/bone
			26	Lung
			1	Axillary LN → now disease-free
$T_1N_{1<4}$	7	0		
$T_1N_{1\geq 4}$	3	0		
$T_2N_{+<4}$	8	3	11	Contralateral breast → bone
			13	Lung
			22	Supraclavicular LN
$T_2N_{+\geq 4}$	3	4	24	Local
			11/13	Lung/brain[a]
			7	Supraclavicular LN
			10/12	Brain[a]
T_3N_+	3	4	5/21	Brain → liver[a]
			18/22	Supraclavicular LN, bone[a]
			1/5/12	Local/brain, liver[a]
			6	Lung, bone

[a] Patient died

whole group is 54.9%, for premenopausal, 67.9%, and, for postmenopausal, 18.8%. At this time the probability of survival for the whole group is 77.2%. The addition of levamisole to the adjuvant chemotherapy did not influence the results compared to chemotherapy alone; at 36 months, 58.2 and 61.0%, and at 42 months, 47.8 and 64.4%, respectively.

Type and Time of Recurrence

Five of 15 patients with a tumor recurrence have died (Table 2). In four of these cases CNS metastases led to the terminal complications. Up to now there has been no recurrence in the T_2-group without nodal involvement, whereas in the T_3-group without nodal involvement, four of five patients developed recurrent tumors. In the group with a small primary tumor (T_1) but with nodal involvement, all ten patients were free of recurrence. The fact that 8 of 12 patients with a large primary tumor (T_3) showed recurrences can be taken as an indication that the size of the primary tumor is an important prognostic sign and that adjuvant chemotherapy is especially efficient in patients with initially small tumor loading.

Clinical Side Effects

To evaluate clinical side effects, a questionnaire comprising ten items was completed by patients at the end of each course and the severity of side effects was rated on an

Table 3. Clinical side effects of an adjuvant intermittent chemoimmunotherapy in primary breast cancer

1. Due to chemotherapy
Alopecia (~ 100%)
Nausea, vomiting, anorexia
(severe to moderate, 75–100%)
Hemorrhagis cystitis (< 10%)
2. Due to levamisole
Rheumatoid joint pain (~ 10%)
Disturbed sense of taste (~ 5%)
3. General
Psychological stress and depression (~ 80%)

arbitrary scale by the attending physician. For those items for which more than occasional entries were made, the evaluation is demonstrated in Table 3. As was expected for this type of chemotherapy, gastrointestinal side effects were prominent (rated moderate to severe by most of the patients). Alopecia occurred in all patients while hemorrhagic cystitis was rarely observed. One important complaint during the study was psychological stress and depression in nearly 80% of the patients, with severe depression necessitating the consultation of a psychiatrist in three patients.

Side effects occurring under levamisole after discontinuation of chemotherapy were rheumatoid joint and muscle pain, edematous swelling of hands and feet, abnormal sense of taste, and general malaise which necessitated the discontinuation of levamisole in six patients.

Immunological Side Effects

T and B lymphocytes and their in vitro functions were reduced by intermittent combination chemotherapy with ADM and cyclophosphamide. Levamisole was not found to influence immunoparameters when given between chemotherapy or when given after chemotherapy. Lymphocytes showing Fc-receptors and mediating ADCC were less affected and were found even elevated in some patients prior to initiation of therapy [2, 6].

Discussion

The probability of survival and of disease-free survival for the whole group and for pre- and postmenopausal patients in our study fall between those of the control and the CMF group of Bonadonna. In contrast to a recently published phase II study on adjuvant therapy with ADM and cyclophosphamide [9], these data do not indicate any superiority of this more aggressive combination. Pre- and postmenopausal patients do not show different behavior in this study. This may be due to the fact that our age limit was 65 years of age, which made it possible to adhere to the planned dose schedule in most cases.

This phase II study indicates that a 6-month aggressive adjuvant chemotherapy regimen can be administered with high patient compliance when patient care is given high attention. There were only 2 of 52 patients lost from the study, both during the early phase.

The addition of levamisole to the adjuvant chemotherapy in 24 of 50 patients did not influence the clinical results as compared to chemotherapy alone, and was without any effect on the depression of in vitro immunologic functions. A potential additional effect on disease-free survival, described by Rojas for stage III breast cancer after local irradiation [8], was not detected during the observation period.

References

1. Betzler M, Schlag P, Schreml W, Herfarth C (1978) Mammakarzinom: Stadieneinteilung, Therapie und Nachsorge. Med Klin 73:633
2. Betzler M, Flad HD, Schreml W, et al. (1979) Quantitative and functional studies of lymphocyte subpopulations during adjuvant chemo(immuno)therapy in patients with breast cancer. In: Flad HD, Herfarth Ch, Betzler M (eds) Immunodiagnosis and immunotherapy of malignant tumors. Springer, Berlin Heidelberg New York
3. Bonadonna G, Brusamolino E, Valagussa P, et al. (1976) Combination chemotherapy as an adjuvant treatment in operable breast cancer. N Engl J Med 294:405
4. Bonadonna G, Valagussa P, Rossi A, et al. (1978) Are adjuvant trials altering the course of breast cancer? Semin Oncol 5:450–464
5. Fisher B, Carbone P, Economon SG, et al. (1975) L-Phenylalanine mustard (L-PAM) in the management of primary breast cancer: A report of early findings. N Engl J Med 292:117
6. Flad HD, Betzler M, Schreml W, et al. (1978) Verhalten lymphatischer Subpopulationen unter zytostatischer Therapie. In: Huber H, Senn HJ, Falkensammer M (eds) Adjuvante zytostatische Chemotherapie. Zytostatische Therapie als Rezidivprophylaxe? Hämatologie und Bluttransfusion, vol 22. Springer, Berlin Heidelberg New York, S 25
7. Immich H (1977) Medizinische Statistik. Schattauer, Stuttgart
8. Rojas AF, Mickiewicz E, Feierstein JN, Glait H, Olivari AJ (1976) Levamisole in advanced human breast cancer. Lancet 1:211
9. Wendt AG, Jones SE, Salmon SE, et al. (1979) Adjuvant treatment of breast cancer with adriamycin-cyclophosphamide with or without radiation therapy. In: Jones SE, Salmon SE (eds) Adjuvant therapy of cancer II. Grune & Stratton, New York, pp 63–70

31. Short-Term and Long-Term Effects of Chemoimmunotherapy on Granulopoiesis: Adjuvant Therapy of Breast Cancer*

H. P. Lohrmann, W. Schreml, and M. Lang

Universität Ulm, Department für Innere Medizin, Abteilung Innere Medizin III (Haematologie-Onkologie), Steinhövelstrasse 9, D-7900 Ulm, Germany

Summary

The effect of adjuvant chemoimmunotherapy on normal human granulopoiesis has been studied. The short-term pattern of hemopoietic depletion and regeneration confirms that human bone marrow shows reaction to cytotoxic agents similarly to that observed in animal experiments. A regenerative response to the drug-induced depletion of the committed stem cell compartment occurs very early, thus suggesting local CFUC population size control of negative feedback from the early granulocytic compartments. Levamisole in that particular regimen did not influence the reaction pattern of granulopoiesis following cytotoxic drug exposure. A model of quantitative evaluation leads to a description of compartment changes which is compatible with the concepts of hemopoietic reaction to cytotoxic drugs. Of particular importance to the planning of adjuvant therapy is the observation of a long-term defect of granulopoiesis after discontinuation of chemotherapy. Studies like those presented here should be performed on any regimen of adjuvant therapy to select the least toxic regimen when several cytotoxic combinations with similar activities are available.

Introduction

Since systemic adjuvant therapy is given to potentially cured patients, toxic side effects require particular consideration. In addition, adjuvant chemoimmunotherapy provides an opportunity to observe the reaction of normal human hematopoiesis to cytotoxic drugs and/or immunomodulators. In the patients of an interdisciplinary clinical study described in the previous paper, the pattern of reaction of the granulopoietic system during and after adjuvant chemoimmunotherapy was studied. The following points were of particular interest: (1) A description of the acute granulopoietic reaction to cytotoxic agents and the elucidation of regulatory mechanisms possibly involved in human granulopoiesis; (2) a definition of possible long-term defects persisting after completion of adjuvant chemotherapy; (3) an evaluation of possible modulations of the reaction of granulopoiesis to chemotherapy

* Supported by Deutsche Forschungsgemeinschaft (SFB 112) Projekt A6

by additional immunotherapy; and (4) an attempt to quantitatively describe human bone marrow compartments during chemotherapy-induced perturbation.

Patients and Methods

The characteristics of the 52 patients receiving adjuvant chemoimmunotherapy are detailed in the preceding article (Chap. 30, p. 185).

Hematologic Studies

Routine hematologic techniques were used for counting the peripheral blood (PB) polymorphonuclear cells (PMN) and to establish bone marrow (BM) differentials. Functional BM PMN reserve was defined as the maximum increment of PB PMN after rapid i.v. infusion of 200 mg hydrocortisone. Stem cells committed to granulopoiesis-monocytopoiesis (CFUC) were assayed in PB and BM in a single layer agar culture system with human placenta-conditioned medium as a source of stimulating activity; proliferative activity of BM CFUC was determined by ^{3}H-thymidine suicide [6, 8].

Quantitative Analysis of Bone Marrow Data

An attempt to quantitate BM data was performed by morphometric evaluation of methacrylate sections of BM spicules [9]. Evaluation was performed on microphotographs taken under standard conditions from representative areas of BM spicules. Areas of cellular marrow and of fat were cut out and the ratio determined by weighing. Cell number per volume was estimated according to the method of Aberchrombie [1].

Statistical Analysis

Statistical analysis was done using a computer program for a desk computer (Hewlett-Packard model 9830A), utilizing a two-sided Mann-Whitney U-test or Student's t-test as necessary. For comparison of the levamisole-treated and control groups, the confidence intervals for the mean were calculated, with P values of 0.04–0.3. Overlapping confidence intervals was interpreted as indication that no significant difference could be demostrated accepting a probability of error given by the P value [4].

Results

Short-Term Effects

Changes of PB PMN and PB CFUC pool size are shown in Fig. 1. Data for BM PMN reserve, BM differential counts, and the incidence of BM CFUC and their proliferative rate are shown in Table 1.

Table 1. Parameters of bone marrow changes after adjuvant chemotherapy (median values)

	First course						Sixth course						
	Day						Day						
	0	2	4	10	14	21	0	2	4	10	14	21	56
CFUC per 10^5 cells	38	12	18	37	74	55	39	7	24	31	53	50	24[a]
^{3}H-thymidine suicide	47	54	63	56	51	40	45	49	56	48	44	48	44
Δ PMN/μl	4,600		5,700	2,000	1,700	5,200	4,650		5,750	2,300	1,650	3,400	4,050
Proliferation (%)	10.6	6.9	7.0	11.2	16.0	13.0	8.2	6.6	6.4	5.5	10.0	11.0	7.7[b]
Maturation (%)	36.8	52.9	50.4	21.5	12.8	43.5	40.1	62.0	56.3	15.4	11.1	37.8	31.2
PMN (%)	11.7	17.4	23.1	9.4	1.7	5.2	10.4	22.6	21.1	3.4	1.7	4.2	7.1[c]

[a] $P < 0.05$
[b] $P < 0.01$
[c] $P < 0.001$

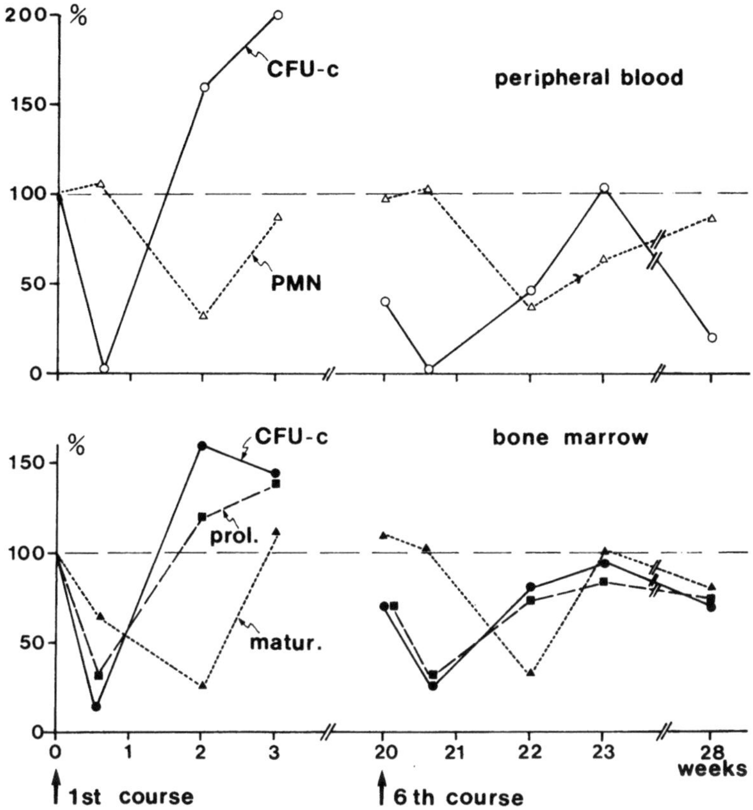

Fig. 1. *Top* Changes of CFUC/1 and PMN/μl peripheral blood (median values); *bottom* changes of the quantitative estimate of the bone pool size for CFUC, proliferative and maturation compartments (median values)

Long-Term Effects

At day 56 after cessation of chemotherapy, several parameters of granulopoiesis showed significant depression as compared to pretreatment values (Table 1). PB PMN are consistently below control values throughout the observation period, now extending up to 40 months after chemotherapy; statistical significance at the 0.05 level is reached at few time points (Table 2). The most prolonged effect was seen on the pool size of circulating CFUC which remains markedly depressed throughout the follow-up period (Table 2).

Influence of Additional Immune Modulation

Fig. 2 shows the course of PB PMN and CFUC analysed separately for the groups with chemotherapy only and with chemoimmunotherapy. No difference is seen between the two groups, according to our statistical criteria. Using the same statistical criteria, there was also no difference in BM PMN reserve and BM CFUC concentration during the sixth course of therapy [13].

Table 2. Long-term follow-up of peripheral blood parameters after cessation of chemotherapy. Ct. indicates pretreatment values of those patients studied at the specified time point

Days	56	100–150	151–200	201–250	251–300	301–350	351–450
PMN/μl							
n	44	40	18	22	22	14	30
Control	3,550	3,550	3,400	3,590	3,920	3,650	3,420
Post-therapy	3,050	2,635	2,750	2,855	3,250	2,770	2,980
P	< 0.02			< 0.05			
CFUC/l							
n	37	30	16	14	18	10	25
Control	25,500	25,750	20,150	30,400	17,000	24,300	19,500
Post-therapy	3,800	5,600	7,410	8,225	7,000	8,500	9,090
P	< 0.001	< 0.001	< 0.02	< 0.02	< 0.02	< 0.02	< 0.01

Days	451–550	551–650	651–750	751–850	851–1,050	1,051–1,250
PMN/μl						
n	32	22	16	14	14	10
Control	3,640	3,910	3,970	3,050	4,400	4,000
Post-therapy	3,150	2,880	3,070	3,130	2,870	2,930
P	< 0.01	< 0.05				
CFUC/l						
n	28	19	17	14	14	10
Control	25,150	26,400	25,500	27,450	34,400	33,500
Post-therapy	7,400	8,100	8,000	7,220	13,680	8,040
P	< 0.001	< 0.02	< 0.02	< 0.02		< 0.02

Quantitative Considerations

An attempt was made to establish a more quantitative parameter of BM changes by utilizing the morphometrically determined cellularity of BM spicules. From cellularity per centimeter of BM and the short-term data already presented, a quantitative value for the size of various BM compartments of granulopoiesis was calculated. The median values in percent of the pretreatment value are plotted in Fig. 1.

Discussion

Short-Term Effects

There is an almost immediate and severe damage to the early granulopoietic compartment following administration of the chemotherapeutic agents. CFUC in BM and PB, and the cells of the proliferating granulocytic pool have the lowest values from days 2–4. This damage proceeds in a wave-like fashion through the ensuing, increasingly differentiated compartments of granulopoiesis, with PMN in the BM and PB being maximally depleted around day 14. This pattern indicates a direct toxic effect

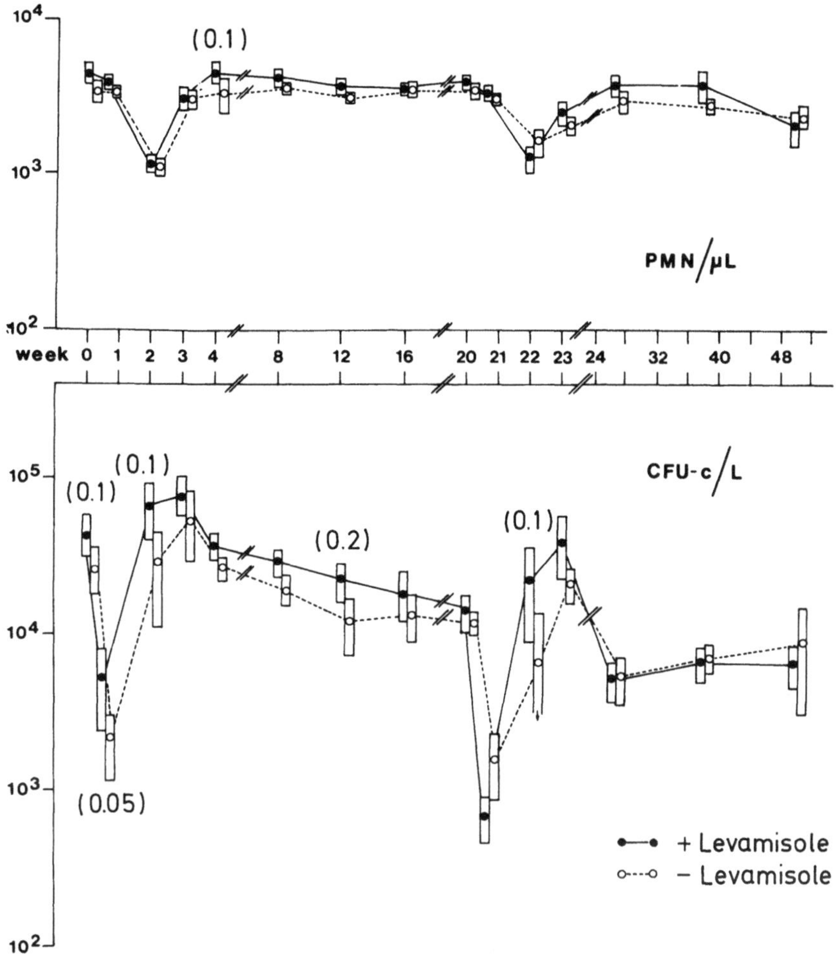

Fig. 2. *Top*, changes of peripheral blood PMN and *bottom* CFUC. ● Chemotherapy plus levamisole; ○ chemotherapy without levamisole; vertical bars indicate confidence interval at which overlap occurs; $P < 0.3$ are specified in parentheses

of cytotoxic treatment on the proliferating compartments of granulopoiesis, and an indirect effect on the maturing compartment, the latter probably caused by a decreased cellular influx from the primarily damaged cellular pools. Regeneration of granulopoiesis starts as early as days 2–4, and is first recognizable from the increased proliferative activity of BM CFUC. The mechanisms for cytotoxic action described in animal models [11] can thus be confirmed for human granulopoiesis.

It is evident that proliferation of CFUC starts early after chemotherapy, at a time when PMN in BM and PB are only little reduced. BM CFUC return to their original proliferative state at a time when PMN progressively decrease in BM and PB. With regard to regulation of the proliferation of BM CFUC, we conclude that mature granulocytic cells in BM and PB are no major factor in the regulation of CFUC proliferation by negative feedback control. Rather, local CFUC population size control or a negative feedback control from the early granulocytic compartments may be operative.

Long-Term Effects of Cytotoxic Drugs

Our data show a persisting defect at all levels of granulopoiesis after cessation of adjuvant chemotherapy with cyclophosphamide and adriamycin. This defect is most pronounced and most persistent in the PB CFUC pool. Animal experiments suggest the irreversibility of a cytotoxic drug-induced stem cell defect [2, 10], and also that such damage to stem cell pools may exist while PB cell counts are originally normal. The demonstration of a persisting stem cell defect after adjuvant chemotherapy is of particular concern, since long-term survival of these patients may allow development of late BM failure [7].

Influence of Additional Immune Modulation

The effect of cytotoxic agents on granulopoiesis can be influenced by unspecific factors like BCG [5], endotoxin [2], or *C. parvum* [3]. Depending on the time sequence of application, toxicity may be markedly aggravated or mitigated. It was of interest to see whether levamisole would modulate the pattern of cytotoxicity. Our data show that levamisole, given during the later phase of BM regeneration, does not exert any detectable influence on granulopoiesis.

Quantitative Considerations

One of the unsolved problems of reporting BM data in humans is the lack of a quantitative method which could be repeated serially at short intervals. Our attempt to arrive at a quantitative expression for the BM compartments can, as yet, not be ascertained by experimental methods. However, the data presented in Fig. 1 are at least compatible with the concepts of BM reaction to cytotoxic drugs as derived from animal experiments. The BM CFUC pool and the proliferative granulopoietic compartment follow a very similar pattern of depletion and regeneration. Also, the changes in the PB CFUC pool follow a similar time course. The reaction of the maturing granulocytic compartment is delayed, as well as the changes of PB PMN. It appears that the early granulopoietic compartments are somewhat depressed during the sixth course of chemotherapy, while the reaction of maturing BM compartments and PB PMN is not markedly different from that seen after the first course.

Reference

1. Abercrombie M (1946) Estimation of nuclear population from microtome sections. Anat Rec 94: 239–247
2. Botnik CE, Hannon EC, Hellman S (1978) Multisystem stem cell failure after apparent recovery from alkylating agents. Cancer Res 38: 1942–1947

3. Foster RS (1978) Altered toxicity of 5-fluorouracil following treatment with *Corynebacterium parvum.* Cancer Res 38: 850–858
4. Immich H (1977) Medizinische Statistik. Schattauer, Stuttgart
5. Ladisch S, Reaman G, Poplack DG (1979) Bacillus Calmette-Guérin enhancement of colony-stimulating activity and myeloid colony formation following administration of cyclophosphamide. Cancer Res 39: 2544–2546
6. Lohrmann HP (1978) Thymidine suicide of human granulocytic progenitor cells (CFUC). Biomedicine 28: 319–323
7. Lohrmann HP (1979) Tolerance of hemopoiesis for repeated cytotoxic drug therapy. Blut 39: 237–244
8. Lohrmann HP, Hansi W, Heimpel H (1978) Human placenta-conditioned medium for stimulation of human granulopoietic precursor cell (CFUC) colony growth in vitro. Blut 36: 81–88
9. Lohrmann HP, Neu G, Schreml W (1978) Methacrylate-embedded bone marrow particle histology. Klin Wochenschr 56: 727–729
10. Morley A, Trainor K, Blake J (1975) A primary stem cell lesion in experimental chronic hypoplastic marrow failure. Blood 45: 681–689
11. Page PL, Cook PA, Greenberg HM, Hartwell BL, Robinson SH (1978) Cytotoxic reduction of murine marrow stem cells and subsequent recovery. Exp Hematol [Suppl 3] 6: 68
12. Reissmann KR, Udupa KB, Okamura H (1970) Effect of endotoxin on normal and 5-fluorouracil-suppressed hematopoietic stem cells. J Lab Clin Med 67: 652–658
13. Schreml W, Lohrmann HP (1979) No effects of levamisole on cytotoxic drug-induced changes of human granulopoiesis. Blut 38: 331–336

32. *A New Adjuvant Treatment with Polyadenylic-Polyuridylic Acid in Operable Breast Cancer*

F. Lacour, J. Lacour, A. Spira, M. Michelson, G. Delage, J. Y. Petit, and J. Viguier

Institut Gustave-Roussy, Laboratoire d-Immunologie, 16 bis Avenue Paul Vaillant-Couturier, F-94800 Villejuif, France

Summary

Adjuvant treatment with polyadenylic-polyuridylic acid poly A-poly U was tested in 300 patients with operable breast cancer who had all received the same locoregional treatment. They were randomized into two groups; 155 patients receiving 30 mg poly A-poly U i.v. once a week for 6 weeks and 145 controls. Overall survival was significantly improved in the poly A-Poly U group ($P < 0.05$). The most striking difference ($P < 0.03$) was observed in the group of positive node patients, who had a 5-year relapse-free actuarial survival rate of 71% versus 47% in the controls.

Introduction

The aim of this study was to increase the resistance of the patient to malignancy after surgery by the use of an immunomodulator. The synthetic double-stranded complex of polyadenylic-polyuridylic acid (poly A-poly U) was chosen because of its defined chemical composition and its well-known structure. It was shown by Braun and Nakano in 1967 [4] to be a good immunostimulator and it has been successfully used as an adjunct to surgery in spontaneous or transplantable tumor [6, 10, 11]. Since it had not been shown to have any toxicity, enhancing effect, or other side effect, a prospective randomized trial was initiated in 1972 at the Institut Gustave-Roussy (IGR) using poly A-poly U as an adjuvant treatment in patients with operable breast cancer [12]. This 7-year study terminated in 1979 with a total number of 300 patients.

Protocol

Patient selection was based upon the following criteria: The tumor was an infiltrating carcinoma of medium size (2–7 cm at its greatest diameter without skin involvement and without complete fixation to the pectoralis major); there were no palpable nodes, or nodes were palpable but movable; and there was no detectable metastasis. According to the UICC classification using the TNM system, these patients corresponded to category T_2 and part of T_3, N_0 N_1, and M_0.

Recent Results in Cancer Research, Vol. 80

The locoregional treatment was the same for all the women. According to our protocol, conventional treatment (CVT) consisted of a modified radical or extended mastectomy without complementary treatment when the axillary nodes were negative (N−). Positive node patients (N+) received complementary cobalt therapy and radiotherapeutic castration if the woman still had menses or had entered menopause within 2 years.

The patients were randomly divided into two groups; an experimental group receiving poly A-poly U (one i.v. injection 30 mg per week for 6 weeks) starting 8 days after the operation, and a control group receiving a placebo (i.v. injections of normal saline on the same schedule).

Poly A-poly U was prepared by one of us as described elsewhere [9]. It was dissolved in NaCl 0.15 M and then filtered through a Millipore twin 90, 0.22 μm (Millipore). Sterility was verified by incubation in thioglycolate broth and trypease soy broth. The solution was stored at −20° C.

Patients were given a complete clinical examination every 3 months.

Results

The comparability of the two therapeutic groups was first verified and evaluated by χ^2 analysis and analysis of variance. There was no significant difference betweeen the groups in regard to primary clinical or histologic prognostic factors, hormonal status, site, and locoregional treatment (Table 1). However, they differed in terms of mortality and metastases. The percentage of deaths was 25% (36 cases) in the CVT group and 14% (21 cases) in the CVT plus poly A-poly U group. The incidence of metastases was 31% (43 cases) and 22% (32 cases), respectively. These differences are

Table 1. Comparability of the two therapeutic groups. CVT indicates conventional therapy and poly A-poly U indicates polyadenylic-polyuridylic acid

	CVT	CVT + poly A-poly U	
Number of patients	145	155	
Mean follow-up time (months)	54.8	52.6	NS
Postmenopause	52%	46%	NS
T1	6%	6%	NS
T2	88%	87%	NS
T3	6%	7%	NS
Internal of medial location	42%	43%	NS
Modified radical mastectomy	67%	76%	NS
Extended mastectomy	33%	24%	NS
Axillary node involvement	71%	66%	NS
Histological grading according to Bloom and Richardson			
Grade I	15%	16%	NS
Grade II	45%	52%	NS
Grade III	40%	32%	NS
Radiotherapeutic castration	33%	27%	NS

reflected in the survival curves (Fig. 1), which were compared using a Mantel-Haenszel procedure [13], with a significant difference ($P < 0.05$) in favor of the poly A-poly U group. The 5-year overall actuarial survival rate was 72% in the CT and 82% in the CVT plus poly A-poly U group. There was also a pronounced but not significant difference in relapse-free survival (Fig. 2) with a 5-year actuarial rate of 56% and 72%, respectively.

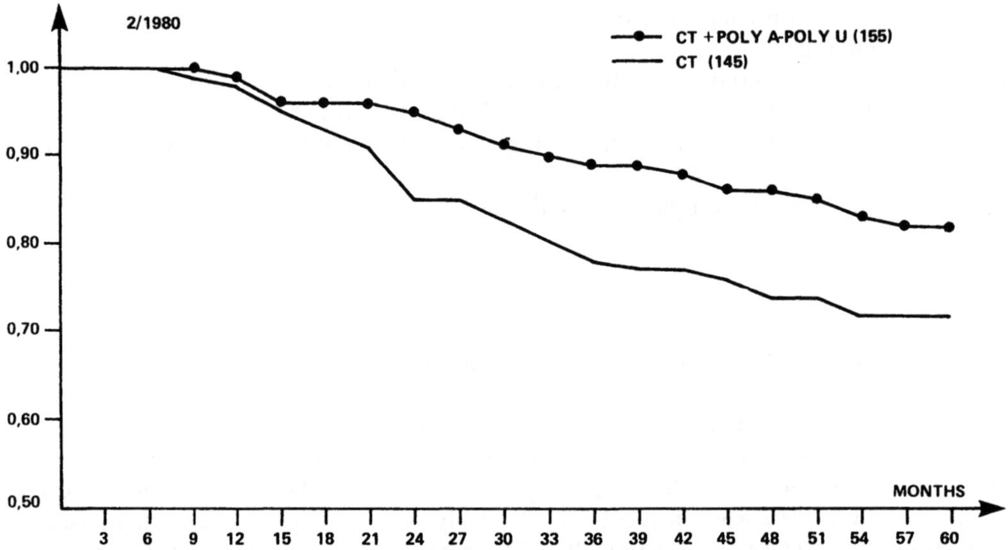

Fig. 1. Overall survival curves for the entire series of patients. CT indicates conventional therapy. $P \leq 0.05$ (Mantel-Haenszel method)

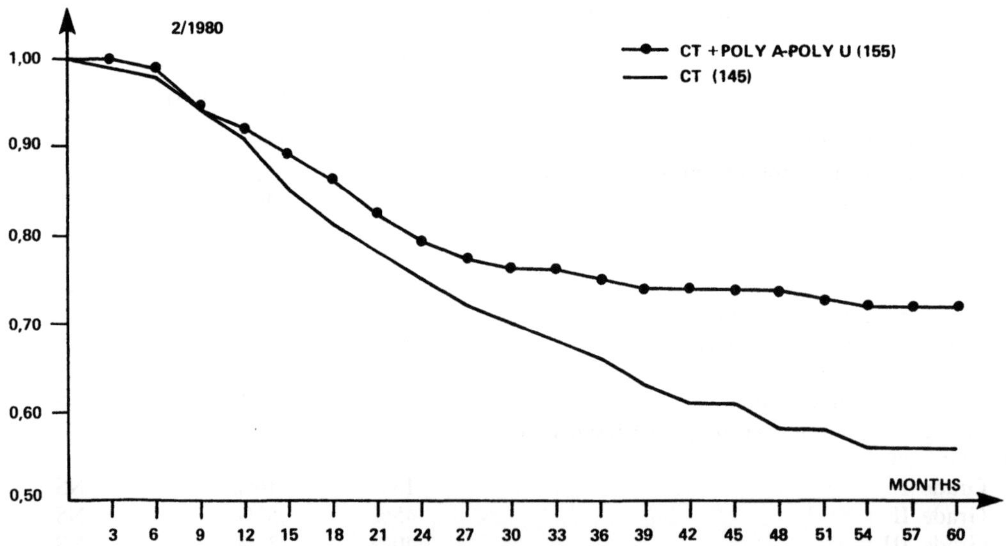

Fig. 2. Relapse-free survival curves for the entire series. CT indicates conventional therapy. $P = 0.11$ NS (Mantel-Haenszel method)

A separate analysis was made of the 205 N+ patients, who were numerically the largest; 102 were in the CVT group and 103 in the CVT plus poly A-poly U group. These patients have a higher risk of metastasis and would be expected to respond better to adjuvant therapy. Within this category, evaluation of the two therapeutic groups for comparability showed no significant difference. The percentage of deaths was 31% (32) in the CVT group and 18% (19) in the CVT poly A-poly U group. The

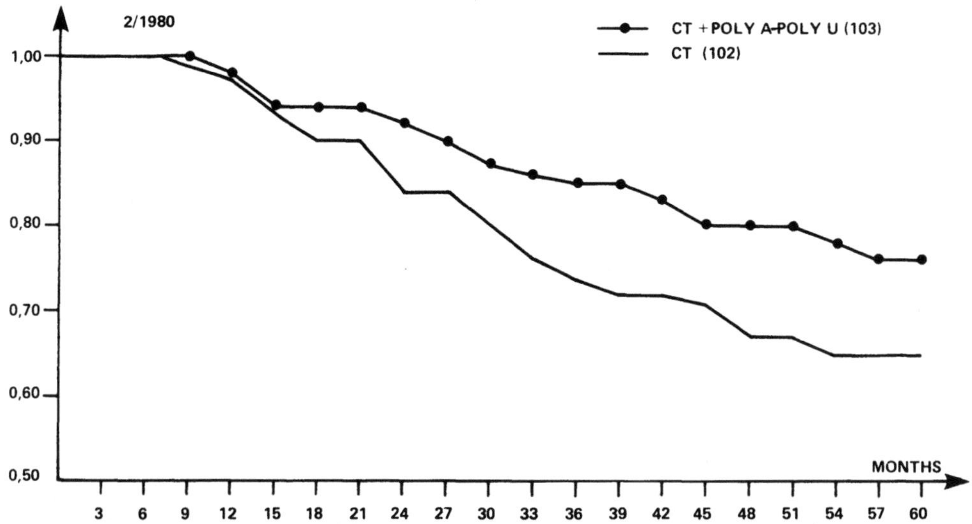

Fig. 3. Overall survival curves for positive node patients. CT indicates conventional therapy. $P \leqslant 0.07$ (Mantel-Haenszel method)

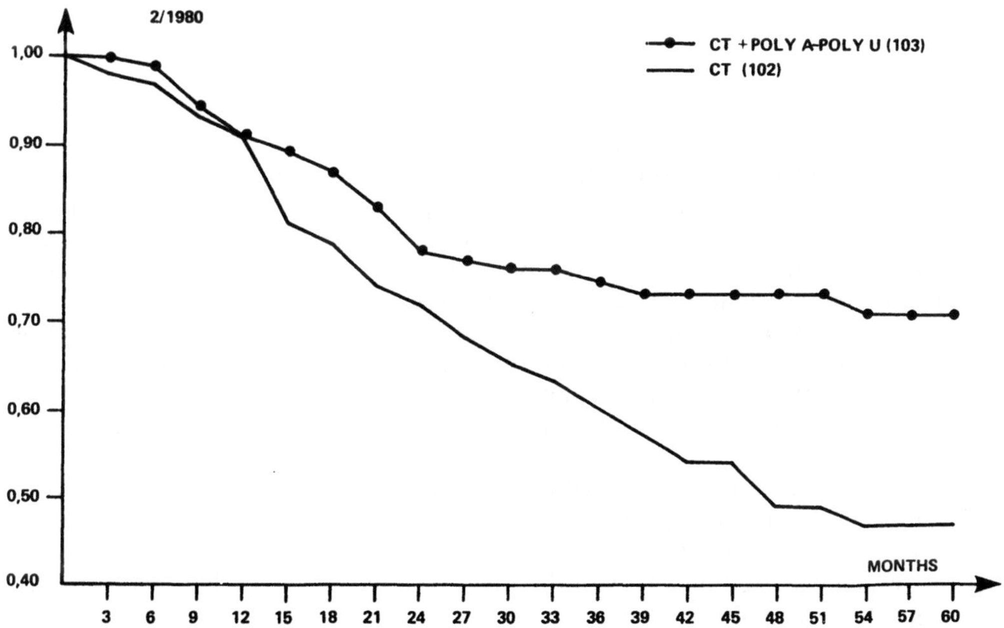

Fig. 4. Relapse-free survival curves for positive node patients. CT indicates conventional therapy. $P \leqslant 0.03$ (Mantel-Haenszel method)

Table 2. Survival according to the number of nodes involved. CVT indicates conventional therapy and poly A-poly U is polyadenylic-polyuridylic acid

	≤ 3 Nodes		≥ 4 Nodes		P
	CVT (52)	CVT + poly A-poly U (51)	CVT (48)	CVT + poly A-poly U (49)	
Overall survival	79% (41)	92% (47) 0.05	56% (27)	69% (34)	NS
Relapse-free survival	67% (35)	80% (41) 0.06	44% (21)	63% (31)	NS

incidence of treatment failures, including deaths, recurrences, and metastasis, was 43% (44 cases) in the first group versus 27% (28 cases) in the second. The overall survival curves presented in Fig. 3 differ, but not significantly ($P \leq 0.07$). The actuarial 5 year survival rate was 65% in the CVT group and 76% in the poly A-poly U group. The most striking difference ($P \leq 0.03$) is observed when comparing the two curves for relapse-free survival (Fig. 4). After 5 years, 47% of patients in the CVT group and 71% in the poly A-poly U group were relapse-free.

A more detailed analysis was then performed related to the number of nodes involved (Table 2). Survival was always higher in the poly A-poly U group, and this difference was statistically significant when three nodes or less were involved. It was also pronounced in patients with four or more positive nodes, but not significantly. The same comparison was made between pre- and postmenopausal patients. The results were similar to the preceding ones in that survival was still better for patients receiving poly A-poly U. It appears that the benefit was greater for post-menopausal patients, but this was only on the borderline of statistical significance ($P = 0.065$).

Discussion

There was a significant increase in the overall 5-year survival for patients treated with poly A-poly U and an even more striking and significant difference in the relapse-free survival with this drug in N+ patients. Thus, poly A-poly U as an adjuvant to locoregional treatment had a definite inhibitory effect on human breast cancer. These observations are in favor of our initial hypothesis that an appropriate immunologic stimulus can improve the success of local treatment when it is given at the most favorable time (when the tumor load confronting the host is minimal, as after surgical removal). They also confirm that the positive experimental results obtained with poly A-poly U in spontaneous mouse mammary carcinoma can be extrapolated to man, especially since poly A-poly U never revealed any toxic or systemic effect in mice.

Among the 155 patients treated with poly A-poly U, no signs of toxicity were observed. The blood cell count remained normal and treatment was well-tolerated, being painless and simple. The only adverse effect observed was a slight fever in 20 patients, which occurred mainly with the first two injections in early trials using the first preparation of poly A-poly U.

The mechanism of action of poly A-poly U is still unknown, and little information is available on its use in human cancers. Wanebo et al. [14] described only paradoxical immunologic effects of this complex in a limited series of cancer patients. Our clinical results strongly suggest that poly A-poly U can to completely suppress and cure microscopic distant metastases, or at least to reduce the number of neoplastic cells, thus partially controlling distant foci.

We know, from previous in vitro experiments, that poly A-poly U has no cytotoxic effect on cancer cells. On the contrary, it is able to penetrate into the cells and can stimulate both RNA and DNA synthesis in a normal human lymphocyte cell line [9]. We also know that these effects are not correlated with an increase of interferon synthesis, because poly A-poly U is a poor inducer of interferon. Serum determinations performed by I. Gresser (Institut de Recherches Scientifiques sur le Cancer, Villejuif) in several of our patients revealed no production of interferon at 6, 12, or 24 h after i.v. injection of 30 mg poly A-poly U.

The results obtained in this study with poly A-poly U were most likely the consequence of an immunomodulating effect. Numerous studies favor this hypothesis. For instance, it is known that poly A-poly U stimulates the cell immune response and it has been shown to markedly improve the capacity of neonatally thymectomized mice to respond to skin homografts [7]. Poly A-poly U, when injected in A/Sn mice (300–600 μg i.p.) markedly increased the proportion of spleen T lymphocytes, which rose to 80% of the total cell population [8]. In addition, poly A-poly U has been shown to restore responsiveness in aging C57 mice which normally display impaired antibody responses [5]. Its greater suggested effect in the older women of our series (postmenopausal) reinforces this interpretation. But other mechanisms cannot be excluded and further research is necessary.

There are trials in progress on operable breast cancer using immunotherapeutic agents such as BCG vaccine, levamisole, and *C. parvum,* or associating immuno- and chemotherapy as listed in the International Registry of Immunotherapy. But, to the best of our knowledge, they are not yet complete.

The results of this study seem important, since the immunotherapy with poly A-poly U may be another effective form of adjuvant therapy in breast cancer. In fact, the main question is whether this immunotherapy is as effective as chemotherapy. It is very difficult indeed to compare our study with the Milan study [2, 3] since its patient selection was not similar to ours. Even though all were in the operable category, patients did not receive the same primary treatment: Our N+ patients received surgery and cobalt therapy before receiving poly A-poly U, whereas the Milan patients had surgery first and then chemotherapy. Consequently, valid comparisons cannot be made. However, when looking at the 5-year results, the general impression is that the survival rates are in the same range.

Of course, a longer follow-up time and other comparative studies are needed to appreciate the long-term effects of both adjuvant therapies.

It should be stressed that adjuvant immunotherapy with poly A-poly U is a short and simple treatment which does not affect the quality of life of the patients. It will be of interest to determine its effectiveness in other types of tumors.

Acknowledgements. This work was supported by Cancer Research Institute (New York), the Centre National de la Recherche Scientifique, the Caisse Nationale d'Assurance Maladie des travailleurs salariés (Division ASS), and the Institut Gustave-Roussy. We wish to express our appreciation to Dr. O. J. Plescia for helpful discussions and for testing the stimulatory effect on humoral immunity of the poly A-poly U preparations, and to Thomas Huynh for expert technical assistance.

References

1. Bloom HJG, Richardson WW (1957) Histological grading and prognosis in breast cancer. Br J Cancer 11: 359–362
2. Bonadonna G (1980) Improved disease-free and overall survival in operable breast cancer (N+) by surgical adjuvant immunotherapy. International Congress on Semology (abstr), p 56
3. Bonadonna G, Brusamolino E, Valagussa P, et al (1976) Combination chemotherapy as an adjuvant treatment in operable breast cancer. N Engl J Med 294: 405–410
4. Braun W, Nakano M (1967) Antibody formation: Stimulation by polyadenylic and polycytidylic acids. Science 157: 819–821
5. Braun W, Ishizuka M, Yajima Y, Webb D, Winchurch R (1971) Spectrum and mode of action of poly A. poly U. in the stimulation of immune responses. In: Beers RF, Braun W (eds) Biological effects of polynucleotides. Springer, Berlin Heidelberg New York, pp 139–156
6. Braun W, Plescia OJ, Raskowa J, Webb D (1971) Basic proteins and synthetic polynucleotides as modifiers of immunogenicity of syngeneic tumor cells. Isr J Med Sci 7: 72–82
7. Cone ER, Johnson AG (1971) Regulation of the immune system by synthetic polynucleotides. III. Action an antigen reactive cells of thymic origin. J Exp Med 133: 665–676
8. Donner M, Vaillier D, Lacour F (1977) Changes in lymphocytes subpopulations in mice receiving a single injection of poly A. poly U. Ann Immunol (Paris) 128: 1039–1052
9. Fenster ED, Lacour F, Harel J (1975) Nuclear penetration and stimulation of nucleic acids synthesis by poly A. poly U. in mammalian cells. Exp Cell Res 94: 315–320
10. Lacour F, Spira A, Lacour J, Prade M (1972) Polyadenylic-polyuridylic acid an adjunct to surgery in the treatment of spontaneous mammary tumors in C_3H/He mice and transplantable melanoma in hamster. Cancer Res 32: 648–649
11. Lacour F, Delage G, Fenster E, Harel J (1975) Inhibitory action of poly A. poly U. on tumor growth. Enhancement of host immune response? In: Gotlieb AA, Plescia O, Bishop HL (eds) Fundamental aspects of neoplasia. Springer, Berlin Heidelberg New York, pp 123–138
12. Lacour J, Lacour F, Spira A, Delage G, Michelson AM (1974) Essai d'immunothérapie (poly A. poly U.) adjuvante dans le traitement du cancer du sein. Bull Cancer (Paris) 61: 275–280
13. Mantel N (1965) Evaluation of survival data and two new rank order statistics arising its consideration. Cancer Chemother Rep 50: 163–171
14. Wanebo HY, Kemeny M, Pinsky CM, Hirshaut Y, Oettgen HF (1976) Influence of poly A. poly U. on immune response in cancer patients. Ann NY Acad Sci 277: 288–298

V. Lung Carcinoma

33. Metastatic CNS Disease in Small Cell Carcinoma of the Bronchus: The Role of Radiotherapy and Chemotherapy

J. M. A. Whitehouse and C. J. Williams

CRC and Wessex Regional Medical Oncology Unit, Southampton, United Kingdom

Introduction

Improved survival frequently reveals new patterns in malignant disease. Control of central nervous system (CNS) disease in acute lymphoblastic leukaemia (ALL) is responsible for the profound improvement in prognosis for that disease [32] and is a stimulus to examine yet more closely specific features of the natural history of other cancers. Small cell cancer of the lung (SCBC) has some similarity to ALL: It is sensitive to some anticancer drugs; it is often widely disseminated; and without treatment it is rapidly fatal, and spreading to the CNS is now recognised to occur in a significant proportion of cases. Although only representing about 25% of lung cancers, it is of particular interest because of these characteristics.
Intensive pretherapy assessment has revealed a tendency to widespread metastases [14, 26]. This is reflected in the median survival of 7–11 weeks in untreated patients [6]. The introduction of more effective chemotherapy used in combination with selective radiotherapy (RT) has considerably increased survival. However, although the extent of disease can be defined at the outset using simple staging systems, for example 'localised' (hemithorax and ipsilateral supraclavicular lymph nodes) and 'extensive' disease (the remainder), or TNM stage I, II, and III disease, differences in overall survival tend to be marginal. This may imply that the disease in the majority of cases is widespread from the outset. Certainly metastasis to the brain is more common than previously appreciated. In view of the parallels with ALL, this complication has been the subject of a number of studies which have included an assessment of the role of prophylactic therapy to the CNS.

CNS Metastases

About 10% of patients have cerebral metastases at the time of presentation [1, 9, 10, 13, 27]. Using brain scan and lumbar puncture (LP), Nugent et al. [28] found CNS metastases in 8 of 68 asymptomatic patients. In a recent study of 81 asymptomatic patients who underwent computerized tomography (CT) scanning of the brain at presentation 6 (7.4%) were demonstrated to have cerebral metastases [20]. Brain metastases are frequently multiple in SCBC [12, 28]. Although the majority of patients having cerebral metastases become symptomatic, a small proportion having autopsy

Recent Results in Cancer Research, Vol. 80

evidence of CNS infiltration remain asymptomatic throughout the course of their disease. Newman and Hansen [27] reported that in 20 of 45 (40%) patients with lung cancer of various cell types, brain metastases were the cause of death. In a collected series of 478 patients [2, 15, 29], 38% had CNS involvement prior to death. Komaki et al. [22] treated 74 patients with either irradiation to the tumour alone or combined with chemotherapy. The median survival was 30 weeks and at 12 months the incidence of CNS metastases was 28% and by 24 months 58%. The increasing incidence of brain metastases with time has been clearly shown by Newman and Hansen [27].

Autopsy studies are inevitably biased by selection and thus the proportion of patients found to have CNS involvement may be artificially high. Nonetheless, many studies have found this to exceed 60%. Although Nugent et al. [28] found that the predominant site of CNS metastases was cerebral (91%), while the spinal cord was involved in 18%, leptomeninges in 24% and multiple sites of involvement occurred in 32%. Hirsch et al. [15] have reported on the distribution of CNS metastases within the cranium (72% were supratentorial, 53% infratentorial, 14% pituitary and 19% involved the intracranial meninges). The importance of the CNS as a focus of metastatic disease in SCBC is thus clearly established.

The sensitivity of SCBC to irradiation therapy [33] at the outset of treatment encouraged the belief that cerebral metastases might also be readily controlled. Unfortunately, experience has not supported this. Einhorn et al. [10] reported that the primary site of relapse in five remission patients with SCBC ended with the development of brain metastases and all died within 1 month, despite receiving whole brain irradiation. Similarly, Holoye et al. [16] reported that 8 of 45 (18%) patients had their first evidence of recurrence in the brain and that the median survival from that recurrence was only 10 weeks, again, despite whole brain irradiation. Newman and Hansen [27] found that doses of greater than 4,000 rad irradiation to the brain only improved survival of patients with SCBC with proven cerebral metastases by 30 days when compared with similar patients who did not receive cerebral irradiation.

Clearly, whole brain irradiation does not significantly improve the survival of patients with established brain relapse, for most of these patients have extensive metastatic disease involving other sites. The failure to control established cerebral metastases using whole brain irradiation is also emphasised by the fact that this approach may often fail to relieve neurological symptoms, distressing both the patient and relatives during the terminal phase of the illness.

Prophylactic Cranial Irradiation

There are a number of series in which prophylactic whole brain irradiation has been employed in a non-randomised fashion [3–5, 7, 11, 17, 22–24, 34] (Table 1). These ten reports involved a total of 677 patients, 25 of whom (3.7%) developed CNS metastases.

This collective incidence is markedly lower than what might be anticipated in patients not receiving prophylactic cranial irradiation. In the study by Komaki et al. [22], the incidence of cerebral metastases was 11% at 12 and 24 months in thoise receiving prophylactic therapy, compared with 28% at 12 months and 58% at 24 months in patients who did not receive prophylaxis. Several randomized studies of prophylactic cranial irradiation (3,000 rad mid-plane dose delivered by opposed lateral fields in ten fractions over 14 days) have now been reported and these indicate that the significant

Table 1. Prevention of brain metastases by prophylactic whole brain irradiation (non-randomised studies)

Author	No. of treatable patients	No. with brain metastases
Levitt et al. [23]	29	5 (17%)
Skarin et al. [34]	9	0
Hornback et al. [17]	29	0
Choi and Carey [7]	15	1 (7%)
Bereton et al. [5]	46	0
Einhorn et al. [11]	58	1 (2%)
Alexander et al. [3]	24	0
Livingston et al. [24]	358	9 (3%)
Bagley et al. [4]	52	3 (6%)
Komaki et al. [22]	57	6 (11%)
Total	677	25 (3.7%)

reduction in the incidence of brain metastases can be achieved using this method. Tulloh et al. [36] and Jackson et al. [198] demonstrated a significant reduction in the incidence of brain metastases from 20% in the untreated group to 2% in those receiving prophylactic whole brain irradiation.

Although there is substantial evidence from these studies indicating that prophylactic whole brain irradiation can effectively reduce the incidence of CNS relapse, there has not been a concomitant improvement in survival [19, 22, 36, 39]. A feature of SCBC is widespread multisystem relapse, so that control of CNS metastases might not alone be expected to improve survival in the majority of patients. Despite the failure to improve survival, the reduction of CNS relapse has markedly reduced the incidence of distressing neurological symptoms. In addition, short-term toxicity is minimal. In the majority of reported series longer-term toxicity has not been significant. However, Johnson et al. [21] reported a neurological syndrome of poor attention span, recent memory loss, action tremor, slurred speech and myoclonus. The symptoms developed 2–4 months after starting treatment and resolved spontaneously within 4 months in all affected patients. The treatment administered to these patients was, however, particulary intensive and involved concomitant chemotherapy and RT to both the whole brain and the primary tumour.

The extra-cranial incidence of CNS metastases involving the spinal cord and leptomeninges, identifies an additional shortcoming of prophylactic therapy to the whole brain only. Metastatic spread to these structures has been found to occur in 5–20% of patients [4, 5, 24, 28]. Irradiation of the neuroaxis and intrathecal chemotherapy have yet to be adequately evaluated, but inevitably the crucial factor determining long-term survival will be overall disease control.

Chemotherapy

Considerable interest has focused on those drugs which are known to cross the blood-brain barrier. It is assumed that drug access to the normal CNS and that containing metastases is identical. However, it is quite possible that the development of new vasculature to focal metastases creates conditions of altered permeability. Until these conditions are properly evaluated, it is inevitable that the principal attention concentrates on the consequences of the administration of those drugs known to cross the blood-brain barrier. The nitrosourea drugs are commonly used in the treatment of primary brain tumours, but are also effective in SCBC [38] and do cross the blood-brain barrier [31, 37]. Madajewicz et al. [25] used intracarotid or intravertebral artery infusion of BCNU every 4 weeks in the treatment of established CNS metastases from a variety of carcinomas of the lung and demonstrated an overall response in 13 of 26 (50%) patients and four of six patients with SCBC had a complete response. Oral or i.v. nitrosourea drugs have been used as attempted prophylaxis against brain metastases in SCBC [1, 3, 8, 18, 28, 40]. The nitrosoureas were included with other drug combinations and no formal trials have been undertaken. The combined results of non-randomized series suggests that there may be a reduction in the incidence of brain metastases [6]. Inevitably, where drugs are used in combination, overall survival may be modified so that the real effect of the inclusion of a nitrosourea in the combination, may be difficult to assess.

Another drug which is commonly included in combination chemotherapy for primary brain tumours is procarbazine. This does cross the blood-brain barrier [30] and is also an effective agent in SCBC [38]. In those randomised studies including procarbazine [1, 29], the overall incidence of brain metastases exceeded 30%. This parallels the incidence in patients who did not receive whole brain irradiation or chemotherapy with an agent anticipated to be active in the CNS. It is curious that where procarbazine and a nitrosourea were administered simultaneously, the incidence of cerebral metastases parallels that of patients receiving no prophylactic treatment.

Tattersall et al. [35] randomised 84 patients with limited disease SCBC to receive either high-dose methotrexate or intrathecal methotrexate with the first three courses of combination chemotherapy. Prophylactic brain irradiation was not given. Three of the 35 patients receiving high-dose methotrexate and 7 of 49 patients receiving intrathecal methotrexate relapsed in the CNS. There was no significant difference between the two groups and no definitive conclusions can yet be drawn concerning the value of either therapy in the control of CNS metastases.

Discussion

The advent of drugs active against SCBC has resulted in response rates of 60–80% when these are used in combination. The median survival in untreated patients of 7–11 weeks has been improved by combination chemotherapy to a median of about 12 months.

Intensive staging has indicated that, in many patients, disease is widespread at presentation and as many as 10% of patients have silent CNS metastases. About 40% of patients may subsequently develop CNS metastases during the course of their management and, in some, these result in distressing neurological complications. Not all these metastases are confined intracranially.

Despite the apparent sensitivity of SCBC to chemotherapy and RT at the outset, neither whole brain irradiation nor chemotherapy with agents believed to cross the blood-brain barrier appear very effective and the median survival from diagnosis of cerebral relapse to death is about 1 month. In those patients in whom the primary focus of disease (all identified metastases) are sufficiently responsive to therapy for complete remission to be achieved, it appears that whole brain irradiation administered prophylactically can significantly reduce the incidence of subsequent CNS relapse. It seems very unlikely that reseeding of disease occurs from the CNS as is postulated for ALL. Inability to detect minimal residual disease and limitations of therapy imposed by toxicity to normal tissues make the definition of complete remission a crude appreciation only.

Although combination chemotherapy has prolonged survival significantly, access by these drugs to the CNS appears inadequate since CNS relapse is a feature of patients receiving chemotherapy alone. When drugs crossing the blood-brain barrier are included, in particular the nitrosoureas, a significant reduction in the incidence of CNS metastases has not yet been clearly demonstrated. It might be anticipated that the improved access of these drugs to sites such as the CNS could be equated with improved penetration of similarly inaccessible, but extra-CNS deposits. Were this the case, combinations including the nitrosoureas, might be associated with improved survival. This does not appear to be the case. Indeed, high-dose methotrexate, for which excellent penetration might be predicted, has no obvious advantage over alternative chemotherapy.

Many studies, both randomised and non-randomised, indicate that CNS disease can be effectively controlled by prophylactic irradiation. The immediate problem is therefore to gain effective control of systemic but extra-CNS disease, since few patients survive beyond 2 years despite an initial high response to available therapy. New approaches to systemic therapy are required if further progress is to be achieved.

We draw the following conclusions concerning CNS involvement by SCBC: (1) At least 10% of patients at presentation and as many as 40% during the course of their management will have CNS metastases; (2) Therapy of established CNS metastases using RT rarely prolongs life significantly and may fail to palliate some; (3) Prophylactic whole brain irradiation substantially reduces the incidence of metastatic disease to the CNS; (4) The distribution of CNS metastases defined postmortem indicates that about 20% of these metastases occur extra-cranially and the place of RT to the neuroaxis or of intrathecal drugs is not yet established; (5) Chemotherapy using agents believed to cross the blood-brain barrier, i.e. high-dose methotrexate and the nitrosoureas, does not appear to reduce the incidence of cerebral metastases substantially; and (6) Though combination chemotherapy and prophylactic whole brain irradiation at the outset is associated with a high response rate and a temporary improvement in survival, few patients survive longer than 12 years. New approaches to achieve long term disease control are, therefore, required.

References

1. Abeloff M, Ettinger D, Baylin B, Hazra T (1976) Management of small cell carcinoma of the lung. Therapy, staging and biochemical markers. Cancer 38: 1394–1401
2. Aisner J, Ostrow S, Wiernik PH (1980) Leptomeningeal carcinomatosis in small cell carcinoma of the lung. Abstract II World Conference on Lung Cancer, Copenhagen
3. Alexander M, Glatstein G, Arnold C, Daniels J (1977) The role of radiation therapy in stage II and IV oat cell carcinoma of the lung. Proc Am Assoc Cancer Res Am Soc Clin Oncol 18: 316

4. Bagley C Jr, Rudolph R, Clarke E Jr (1978) CVM chemotherapy for small cell lung carcinoma. Am Assoc Cancer Res Am Soc Clin Oncol 19: 230
5. Bereton H, Kent C, Johnson RE (1977) Chemotherapy and radiotherapy for small cell lung cancer: A remedy for past therapeutic failures. Am Assoc Cancer Res Am Soc Clin Oncol 18: 275
6. Bunn P, Cohen M, Ihde D, Fossieck B Jr (1977) Advances in the small cell bronchochronic carcinoma. Cancer Treat Rep 81: 333–342
7. Choi C, Carey R (1976) Small cell anaplastic carcinoma of the lung. Reappraisal of current management. Cancer 37: 2651–2657
8. Donovan M, Baxter D, Sponzo R, Cunningham T, Horton J (1976) The rational for combined modality management in small cell cancer of the lung. Am Assoc Cancer Res Am Soc Clin Oncol
9. Eagen RT, Maurer LM, Forcier RJ, Tulloh M (1974) Small cell carcinoma of the lung: Staging, paraneoplastic syndromes, treatment and survival. Cancer 33: 527–532
10. Einhorn L, Fee W, Farber M, Livingston R, Gottlieb J (1976) Improved chemotherapy for small cell undifferentiated lung cancer. JAMA 235: 1225–1230
11. Einhorn L, Hornback N, Bond B (1977) Combination chemotherapy, radiotherapy and immunotherapy in small cell undifferentiated lung cancer. Am Assoc Cancer Res Am Soc Clin Oncol 18: 267
12. Fine DH, Deeley T (1971) The necropsy findings in carcinoma of the bronchus. Br J Dis Chest 65: 238–242
13. Hansen H (1973) Should initial treatment of small cell carcinoma induce systemic chemotherapy and brain irradiation. Cancer Chemother Rep Part 3 4: 239–241
14. Hansen H, Muggia F (1972) Staging of inoperable patients with bronchogenic carcinoma with special reference to bone marrow examination and peritoneoscopy. Cancer 30: 1395–1401
15. Hirsch FR, Paulson OB, Hansen HH, Vraa-Jensen J (1980) Brain metastases in small cell carcinoma of the lung. Abstract II World Conference on Lung Cancer, Copenhagen
16. Holoye P, Samuels M, Lanzotti V, Smith J, Barkley H Jr (1977) Combination chemotherapy and radiation therapy for small cell carcinoma. JAMA 237: 1221–1224
17. Hornback N, Einhorn L, Shidmia H, Joe BT, Krause M, Furnas B (1976) Oat cell carcinoma of the lung, early treatment results of combination radiation therapy and chemotherapy. Cancer 37: 2658–2664
18. Israel L, Delpierre A, Choffel C, Millerson B, Edelstein R (1977) Immunochemotherapy in 34 cases of oat cell carcinoma of the lung. Cancer Treat Rep 61: 343–348
19. Jackson DV, Cooper MR, Richards R III, Ferree C, Muss HB, White DR, Spurr CL (1977) The value of prophylactic cranial irradiation in small cell carcinoma of the lung. JAMA 237: 2730–2733
20. Jacobs J, Vincent RG (1980) Results of screening computerised tomography (CT) of the brain in lung carcinoma patients. Abstract II World Conference on Lung Cancer, Copenhagen
21. Johnson RE, Bereton H, Kent C (1976) Small cell carcinoma of the lung: An attempt to remedy causes of post-therapeutic failure. Lancet 2: 289–291
22. Komaki R, Cox J, Whitson W (1980) Risk of brain metastasis from small cell carcinoma of the lung related to length of survival and prophylactic irradiation. Abstract II World Conference on Lung Cancer, Copenhagen
23. Levitt M, Meikle A, Weinerman B (1976) Intensive combined modality therapy in oat cell carcinoma of the lung. Proc Am Assoc Cancer Res Am Soc Clin Oncol 17: 308
24. Livingston RB, Moore TN, Heilbrun L, Bottomley R, Lehane D, Rivkin S, Thigpen T (1978) Small cell carcinoma of the lung: Combined chemotherapy and irradiation: A southwest oncology group study. Ann Intern Med 88: 194–199
25. Madajewicz S, West CR, Takita H, Vincent Ra, Avellanosa A, Park HC, Caracandas J (1980) Chemotherapy of metastatic brain tumours. Abstract II World Conference on Lung Cancer, Copenhagen

26. Margolis R, Hansen H, Muggia F, Kanhouwa S (1974) Diagnosis of liver metastases in bronchogenic carcinoma: A comparative study of liver scans, function tests and peritoneoscopy with liver biopsy. Cancer 34: 1825–1829
27. Newman SJ, Hansen H (1974) Frequency diagnosis and treatment of brain metastases in 247 consecutive patients with bronchogenic carcinoma. Cancer 33: 492–496
28. Nugent JL, Bunn P, Ihde D, Matthews M, Cohen M, Devita V, Minna J (1978) Diagnosis and treatment of CNS complications of small cell bronchogenic carcinoma (SCBC). Am Assoc Cancer Res Am Soc Clin Oncol 19: 464
29. Nugent JL, Bunn P, Matthews M, Ihde D, Cohen M, Gazdar A, Minna J (1979) CNS metastases in small cell bronchogenic carcinoma. Cancer 44: 1885–1893
30. Oliverio VT (1971) Pharmacologic disposition of procarbazine. In: Carter SK (ed) Proceedings of the chemotherapy conference on procarbazine. (Matulane: NSC-77213) Development and application. US Government Printing Office, pp 19–28
31. Oliverio VT (1976) Pharmacology of the nitrosoureas: An overview. Cancer Treat Rep 60: 703–707
32. Pinkel D, Simone J, Hustu O, Rhomes JA (1972) Nine years' experience with "total therapy" of childhood acute lymphocytic leukaemia. Paediatrics 50: 246–251
33. Salazar O, Rubin P, Brown JC, Feldstein M, Keller MS (1976) Predictors of radiation response in lung cancer. Cancer 37: 2636–2650
34. Skarin A, Lokich J, Goodman R, Chaffey J, Frei E III (1975) Combination intensive chemotherapy and radiotherapy in oat cell carcinoma of the lung. Proc Am Assoc Cancer Res 16: 264
35. Tattersall MHN, Fox RM, Woods RL (1980) A randomised study of high dose methotrexate and intrathecal methotrexate in small cell lung cancer treated by combination chemotherapy. Abstract II World Conference on Lung Cancer, Copenhagen
36. Tulloh M, Maurer L, Forcier R (1977) A randomised trial of prophylactic whole brain irradiation in small cell carcinoma of the lung. Am Assoc Cancer Res Am Soc Clin Oncol 18: 319
37. Walker M, Hilton J (1976) Nitrosourea pharmacodynamics in relation to the central nervous system. Cancer Treat Rep 60: 725–728
38. Wasserman T, Comis R, Goldsmith M et al. (1975) Tabular analysis of the clinical chemotherapy of solid tumours. Cancer Chemother Rep Part 3 6: 399–419
39. Williams CJ, Alexander M, Glastein E, Daniels J (1977) Role of radiation therapy in combination with chemotherapy in extensive oat cell cancer of the lung: A randomised study. Cancer Treat Rep 61: 1427–1431
40. Williams CJ, Alexander M, Glatstein E, Daniels J (1977) The role of adjuvant radiation therapy in stage III and IV oat cell carcinoma of the lung. In: Salmon SE, Jones SE (eds) Adjuvant therapy of cancer. North Holland, Amsterdam, pp 237–244

34. Interim Results of EORTC Protocol 08742: Comparison, After Irradiation of Locally Advanced Squamous Cell Bronchial Carcinoma, of Abstention, Immunotherapy, Combination Chemotherapy, or Chemoimmunotherapy

L. Israel, A. Depiere, and O. Dalesio*

Hôpital Avicenne, Bobigny, France

Summary

After irradiation of locally unresectable epidermoid bronchial carcinoma, 1 year of chemotherapy is significantly superior in delaying both local recurrences and distant metastases and prolonging the disease-free interval. However, BCG immunotherapy alone seems to be superior in terms of survival to no therapy, chemotherapy, and immunochemotherapy. This could be due to a better tolerance to secondary treatments given at time of recurrence.

Patients and Methods

From September, 1974, to May, 1979, 238 patients with locally unresectable, documented squamous cell carcinoma of the lung confined to one side of the thorax have met the conditions of eligibility; that is, at least a partial radiologic and fiberoptic response to radiation therapy (RT) of the tumor and the mediastinum (respectively, 5,500 and 4,500 rad). Of these, 208 patients have been included in the present analysis.

At the completion of RT, the patients were randomized into four groups: (1) control; (2) 0.2 ml (2.10^6 organisms) intradermal lyophilized Pasteur BCG in four limbs every 4 weeks for 18 months; (3) monthly chemotherapy with CCNU (100 mg/m^2) methotrexate (MTX) (40 mg/m^2), and cytoxan (1 g/m^2) every 4 weeks for 1 year; and (4) a combination of BCG and chemotherapy at same doses and for the same periods of time as above. Analysis presented here was performed in May, 1980, by means of the generalized Wilcoxon test and the log rank test, comparing only global curves and making no attempt to seek time-related differences.

It must be stated that only 50% of the irradiated patients achieved partial or complete remission and were subsequently randomized.

---

* For the Lung Group of EORTC. Participating members: O. Mondo, Pr. Bignon, Dr. Blanchon, Dr. Choffel, Pr. Chretien, Pr. Dubois de Montreynaud, Pr. Germouty, Pr. Giroulle, Pr. Grassie, I.N.T. Milan, Pr. Kenis, Pr. Laval, Dr. Miech, Pr. Mostecky, Dr. Namer, Pr. Paramelle, Pr. Rimoldi, Pr. Rochemaure, Dr. Roviaro, Pr. Voisin

Recent Results in Cancer Research, Vol. 80

Results

Only a brief description will be given here of the results so far obtained, together with curves and figures that summarize the present data.

Projected median survival is shown in Table 1 and Fig. 1. To date, chemotherapy alone is superior to the control group ($P = 0.02$), whereas no other difference has reached any significance. There is a trend toward immunotherapy alone being also superior to control, whereas immunochemotherapy and the control group are very similar.

Concerning distant metastases, chemotherapy (median survival not yet reached) is significantly superior ($P > 0.04$) to the control and seems also to be superior to the other three arms (Table 2 and Fig. 2).

As could be guessed, chemotherapy, being the most effective in delaying both local recurrences and distant metastases, is significantly superior to other modalities in

Table 1. Local recurrence

Treatment	Median (weeks)
Immunotherapy	44.8
Chemotherapy	51.7
Immuno- plus chemotherapy	35.5
None	30.1

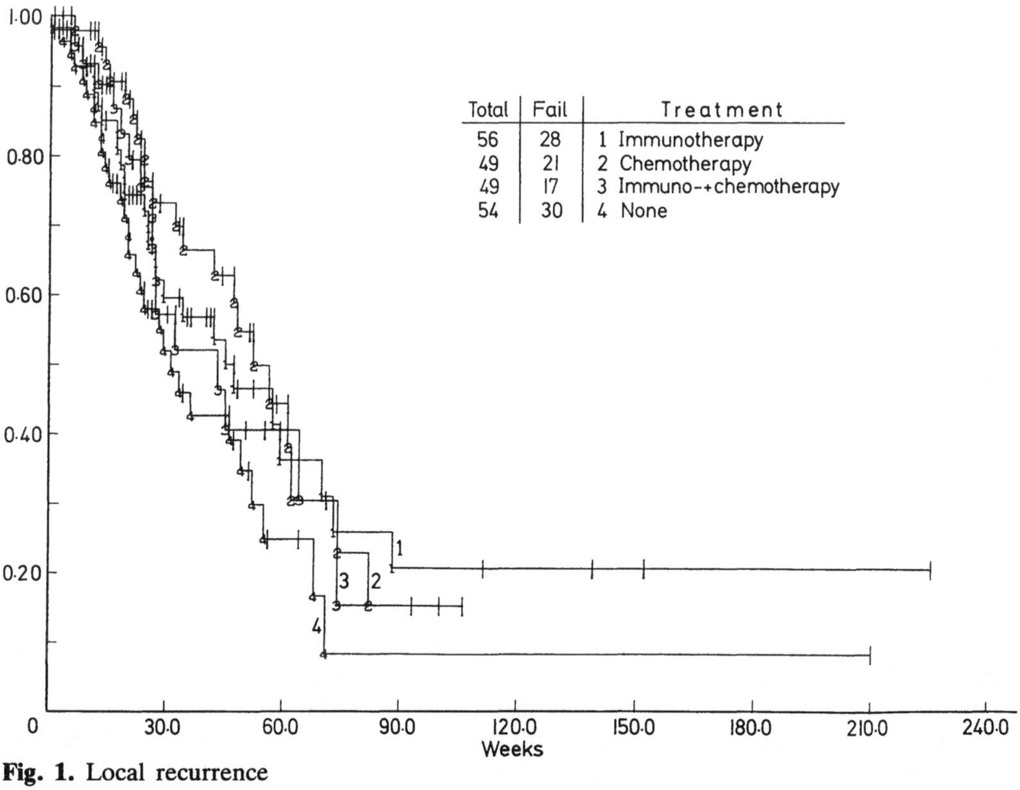

Fig. 1. Local recurrence

Table 2. Distant metastases

Treatment	Median (weeks)
Immunotherapy	49.7
Chemotherapy	Not est.
Immuno- plus chemotherapy	52.4
None	46.1

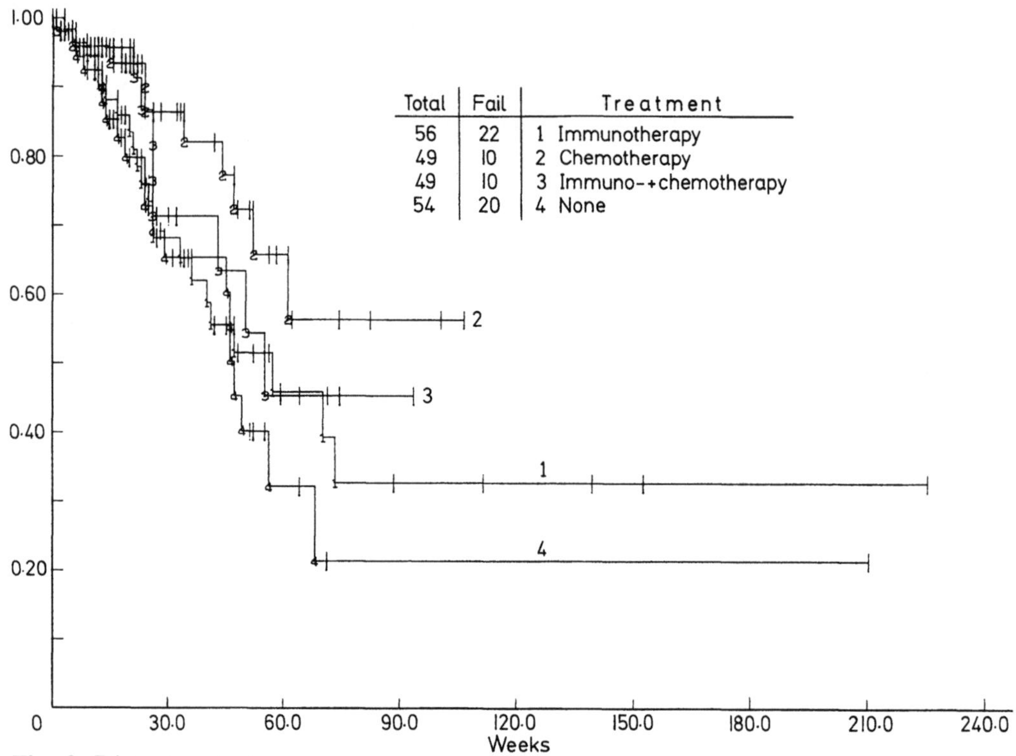

Fig. 2. Distant metastases

Table 3. Disease-free interval from time of randomization

Treatment	Median (weeks)
Immunotherapy	27.0
Chemotherapy	47.0
Immuno- plus chemotherapy	64.0
None	24.0

prolonging disease-free survival, whereas immunotherapy does no better than immunochemotherapy or the control group (Table 3 and Fig. 3).

The survival figures show no significant difference as yet, but there is a trend in favor of immunotherapy alone over all other modalities; 35% BCG patients have reached or will reach a 4-year survival time as compared to 0 for other modalities.

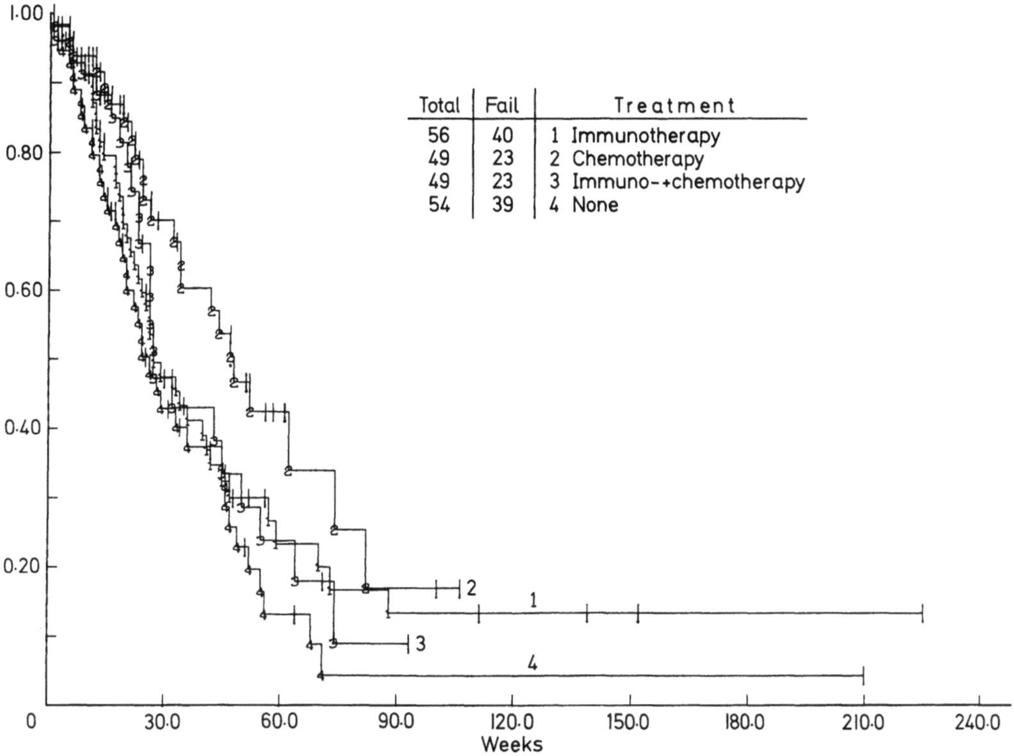

Fig. 3. Disease-free interval from randomization

Table 4. Survival from time of randomization

Treatment	Median (weeks)
Immunotherapy	84.5
Chemotherapy	62.4
Immuno- plus chemotherapy	64.6
None	69.1

Discussion

If all patients were to be treated by a single strategy, and if all of them were to die at the time of recurrence, chemotherapy would undoubtedly the treatment of choice. The only progress would be to improve the efficacy of present chemotherapy. This, incidentally, is the case now [1].

The fact that immunotherapy alone seems to be better in terms of survival means that patients are receiving new agents at the time of recurrence and that these new agents, whatever they are, are more effective in prolonging survival in patients not previously given chemotherapy. This also means that chemotherapy given at the time of recurrence is more effective in prolonging survival in patients having received systemic BCG than patients not treated at all.

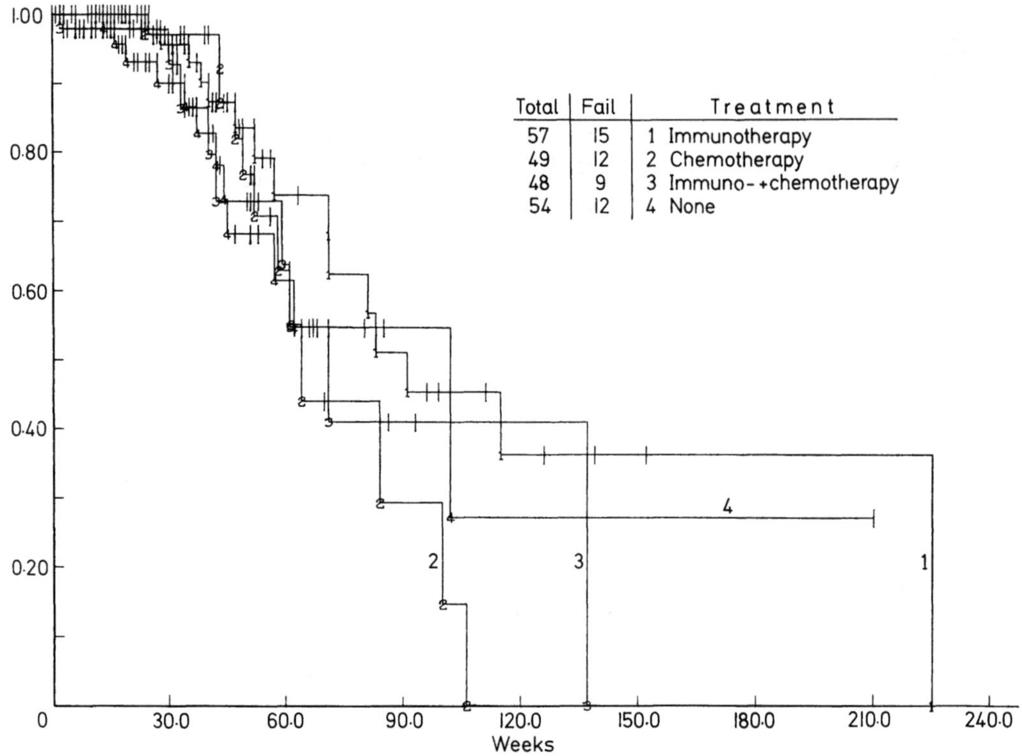

Fig. 4. Survival from time of randomization

It could be, if these trends are confirmed, that nonspecific stimulation via systemic BCG does not increase defenses against cancer, but merely increases response rates and tolerance to a subsequent chemotherapy, as well as benefitting the host in general. In such a case, though of benefit, this modality could not be called immunotherapy and the question is left open whether any agent or a specific route (intrapleural, intradermal etc.), can really enhance anticancer mechanisms.

Reference

1. Israël L, Breau JL, Aguilera J (to be published) Successful phase II trial of 6 days continuous infusions of cis-DD-platinum and bleomycin in squamous cell carcinoma of the lung. European Symposium on Lung Cancer. September, 1980, Haldiki, Porto Carras, Greece

35. *Immunologically Defined Prognostic Subgroups as Predictors of Response to BCG Immunotherapy**

J. W. Reid, G. B. Cannon, E. Perlin, J. Blom, R. Connor, and R. B. Herberman**

Naval Regional Medical Center, Box 666, Portsmouth, VA 23708, USA

Summary

Fifty-two stage I and II patients with nonsmall cell lung cancer were randomized after resection to no further therapy, BCG, or BCG plus allogeneic tumor cells. Patients have been observed for 16–65 months (mean 39.5). When the two immunotherapy arms were combined and plotted against controls, trend analysis suggested ($P = 0.088$) an increase in disease-free interval (DFI) only for stage I patients. The one-way mixed lymphocyte culture (MLC) values were depressed in some patients prior to any immune stimulation. Immunotherapy significantly benefited DFI among patients with a depressed MLC.

Introduction

The general tenor of cancer immunotherapy in the last decade and a half has been one of repeated disappointments and tantalizingly near misses.

Before most of these trials were undertaken, animal experiments had clearly defined certain situations where immunotherapy was uniformly unsuccessful, the most important being even a moderate tumor burden. Administration of BCG to stage I or II lung cancer patients, after complete resection of all detectable tumor, embodies the principle of minimal tumor burden in a malignancy of demonstrated antigenicity and high relapse rate. This would appear to maximize the chance of demonstrating an effect of BCG on survival. Nevertheless, results continue to be marginal. Immunologic assays could be used to crudely infer tumor burden size and thus refine the principle of minimal tumor burden beyond what is possible with pathologic staging. If so, it may be

* The opinions or assertions contained herein are those of the authors and do not necessarily reflect those of the various United States Government Agencies represented. This study is supported in part by the Navy Bureau of Medicine and Surgery, Clinical Investigation Program CI 8-08-1182PS

** The authors wish to thank Mrs. Joyce Siwarsky of Litton Bionetics, Bethesda, Maryland, for data collection, storage, and retrieval; Mr. Bill Taylor, Mrs. Ruth Taylor, and Mrs. Beckie Combs of Portsmouth, Virginia, for their help in manuscript preparation, and Drs. William Heim, Sidney Ballinger, Mitchell Mills, and Charles Miller for referral of patients

possible to demonstrate an effect of BCG on more narrowly defined subgroups. In 1974 we began a clinical trial of systemic immunotherapy in postresection lung cancer. The patients were followed-up with a number of immune assays which, in general, did not detect significant immunostimulation, but did identify a subgroup of patients that remained immunosuppressed after extirpation of all detectable tumor. Partial results of this study have been reported elsewhere [9, 10]. This paper will be a summary of survival as related to the mixed lymphocyte culture (MLC) and pathologic stage.

Patients and Methods

The patient population was 52 patients with lung cancer histologically classified as epidermoid, large-cell undifferentiated, and adenocarcinoma. After thoracotomy patients were staged according to the method of Carr and Mountain [2]. Within 1 month after resection patients were randomized by drawing a card to one of the three groups; no further therapy, BCG, or BCG plus allogeneic tumor cells.

That patients were free of disease was confirmed by a complete evaluation which included appropriate radionuclide scans, bone marrow biopsy, and 12 channel serum chemistry. These were repeated every 3–6 months or as clinically indicated. The date

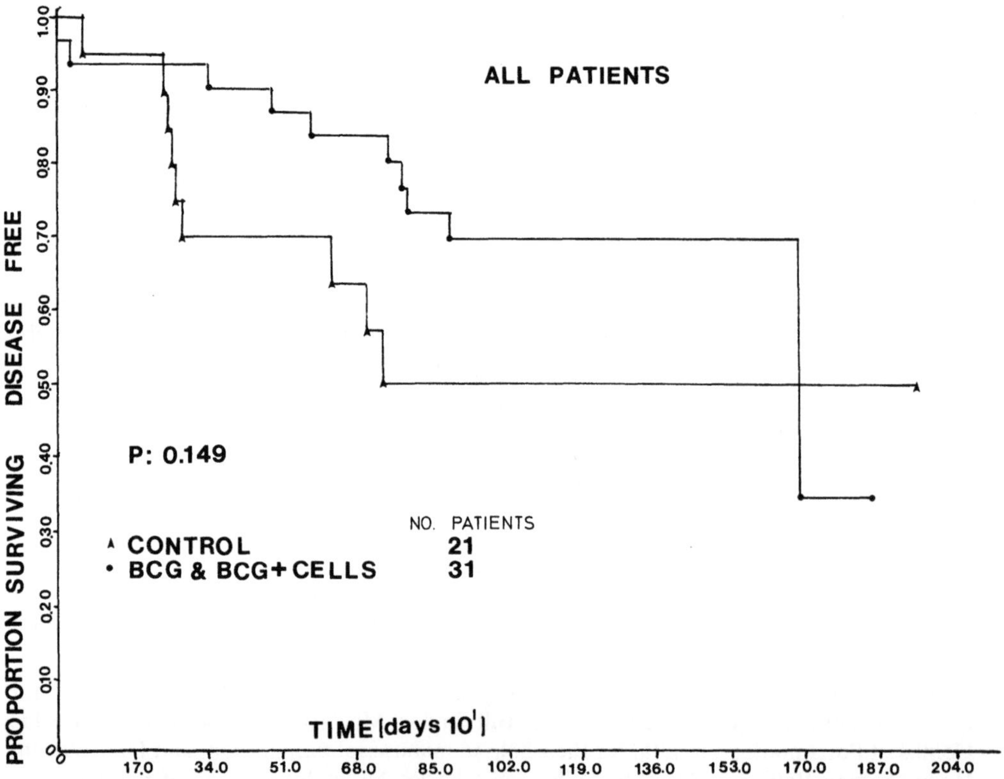

Fig. 1. Disease-free interval (DFI) of stage I and II lung cancer patients comparing no treatment to immunotherapy

of relapse was determined by the appearance of objective criteria, such as a new lesion on X-ray, positive-node biopsy, or unequivocal and persistently positive radionuclide scan.

Within 2 months postoperatively and prior to any immune stimulation, blood was drawn for a MLC [3]. The stimulating population in the MLC was a cryopreserved mitomycin-C-treated pool of allogeneic lymphocytes.

The results of the MLC are reported as the relative proliferation index (RPI), a technique which compares the patient's values with the mean of three normal controls done the same day, thereby reducing variability [4]. Using this approach, an RPI of less than 0.50 is depressed and an RPI greater than 0.50 is in the normal range. Those patients randomized to BCG received 150 mg Pasteur Institute BCG ($3-5 \times 10^8$ organisms) using the multiple puncture technique with a 20-point sterneedle (Heaf gun). Patients were given BCG twice monthly beginning 14–28 days after thoracotomy. Twenty-four months of treatment were planned.

Patients randomized to BCG plus cells received BCG as above and in addition were given approximately 10^8 histologically matched allogeneic tumor cells intradermally at the site of the previous BCG inoculation 2 weeks earlier. The allogeneic tumor cells were obtained at thoracotomy, single-cell suspensions prepared, irradiated, then cryopreserved until use. At the time of administration 10^8 cells were suspended in 1 ml saline.

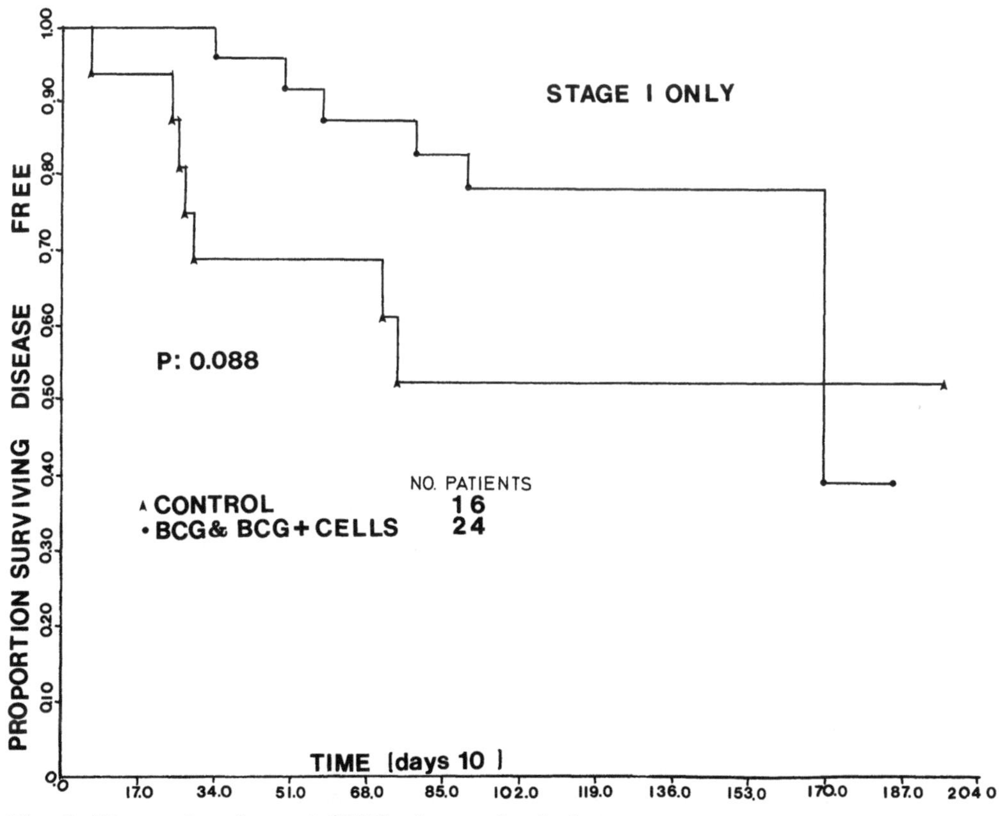

Fig. 2. Disease free interval (DFI) of stage I-only lung cancer

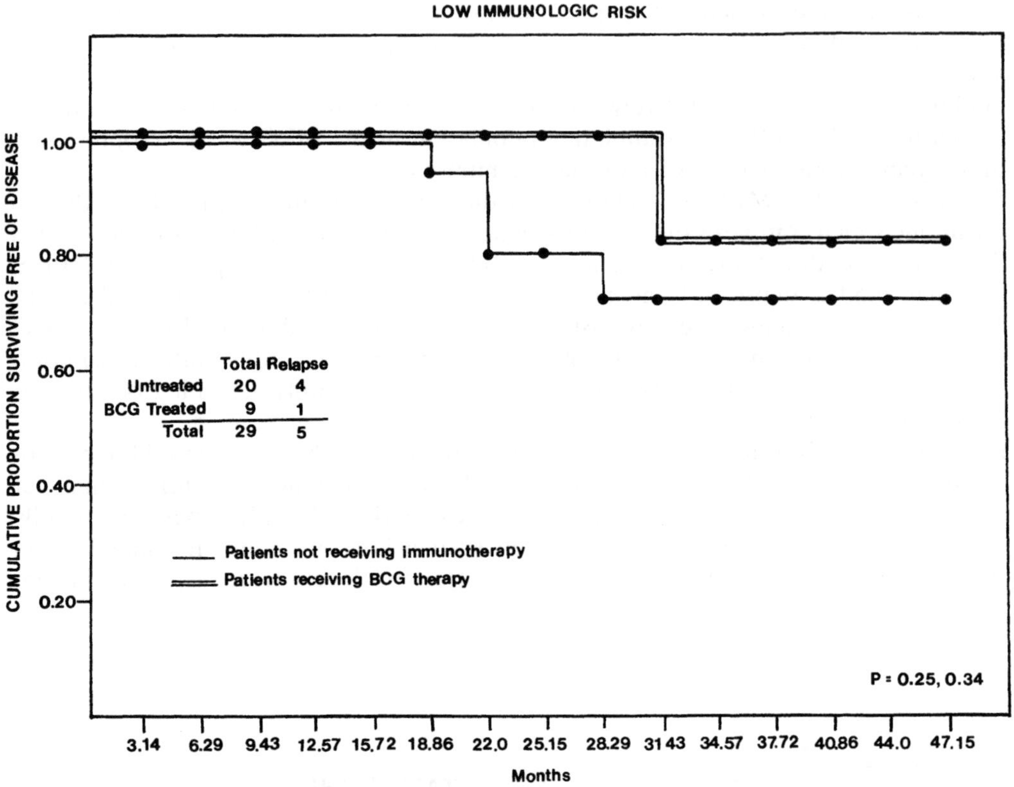

Fig. 3. Disease free interval (DFI) in low-risk (normal MLC) lung cancer patients. BCG did not improve the DFI

For statistical analysis of differences in disease-free interval (DFI) or survival, the Kaplan-Meier method was employed [8]. These differences were tested both with Cox's log rank test and Breslow's censored rank test, and trends in survival from control to immunotherapy were tested using Tarone's trend tests [11].

Results

After approximately 3 years, no further patients were randomized to the BCG plus cells arm. At that time there was no difference in the survival of the two immunotherapy arms. Twenty-one patients, all males, were randomized to no further therapy (control), and 31 patients, including seven females, were randomized to receive immunotherapy, of which 18 received BCG alone and 13 received BCG plus cells. The age of the patients and the histologic type of the tumors were both distributed uniformly among the three randomization arms.

Fig. 1 depicts DFI for all patients. There is no statistically significant difference at approximately 5.5 years between control and the combined immunotherapy arms. When only stage I patients are considered (Fig. 2), the difference in the curves approaches more closely but still does not reach significance.

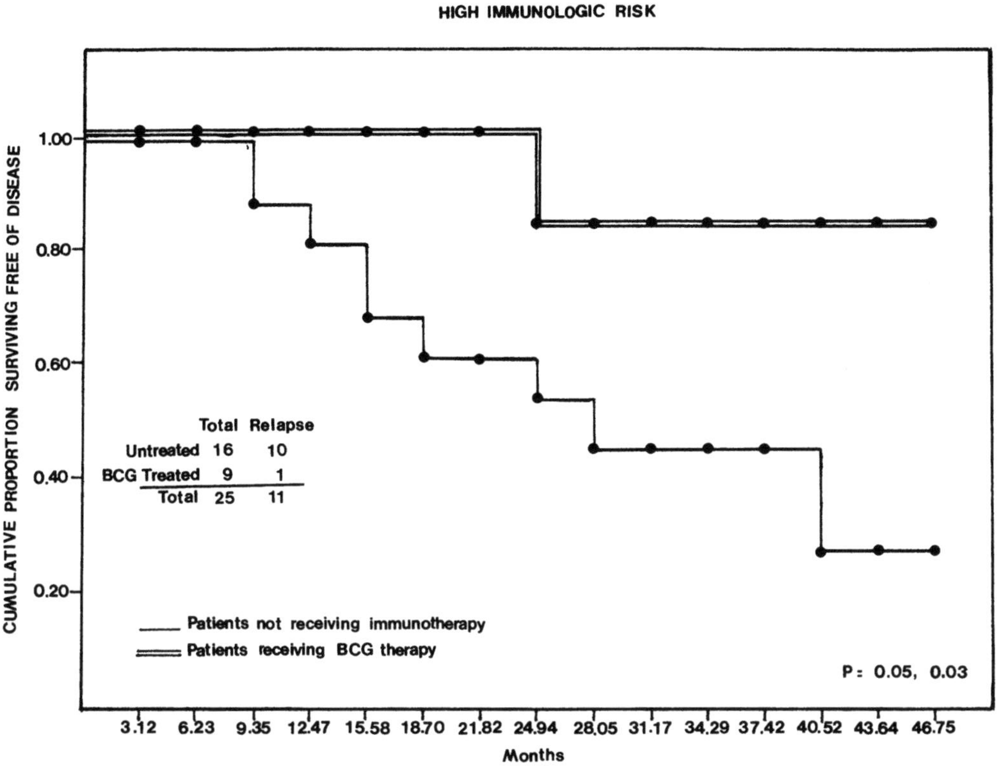

Fig. 4. BCG produced a significant benefit in disease-free interval (DFI) of high-risk (depressed MLC) lung cancer patients

It would be desirable to define a subgroup of lung cancer patients who are at high risk of relapse in whom adjuvant immunotherapy could be tested. The possibility that an in vitro immunologic assay would correlate with relapse was intriguing, and we found that the MLC could be used to define such a prognostic subgroup.

On the basis of the first postoperative MLC, patients were divided into two troups; those with RPI greater than 0.50 were considered normal and those with RPI less than 0.50 depressed. Of the 54 patients so tested, 29 were normal and considered to be at low risk for recurrence and 25 were depressed and considered to be at higher risk. When the normal and depressed groups are compared irrespective of treatment (Fig. 5) there was a highly significant difference ($P = 0.005$ and 0.003, respectively) in DFI in favor of the normal group. Fig. 3 shows the relapse rate of the low-risk group and demonstrates no difference within this group of the controls and BCG-treated patients ($P = 0.25$ and 0.34, respectively). In the high-risk group (Fig. 4), there was a significant difference ($P = 0.05$ and 0.03, respectively) in the two arms.

Discussion

In stage I alone and in combined stage I and II there was no significant difference in the trend analysis in this trial. The closest approach to significance occurred in the DFI of

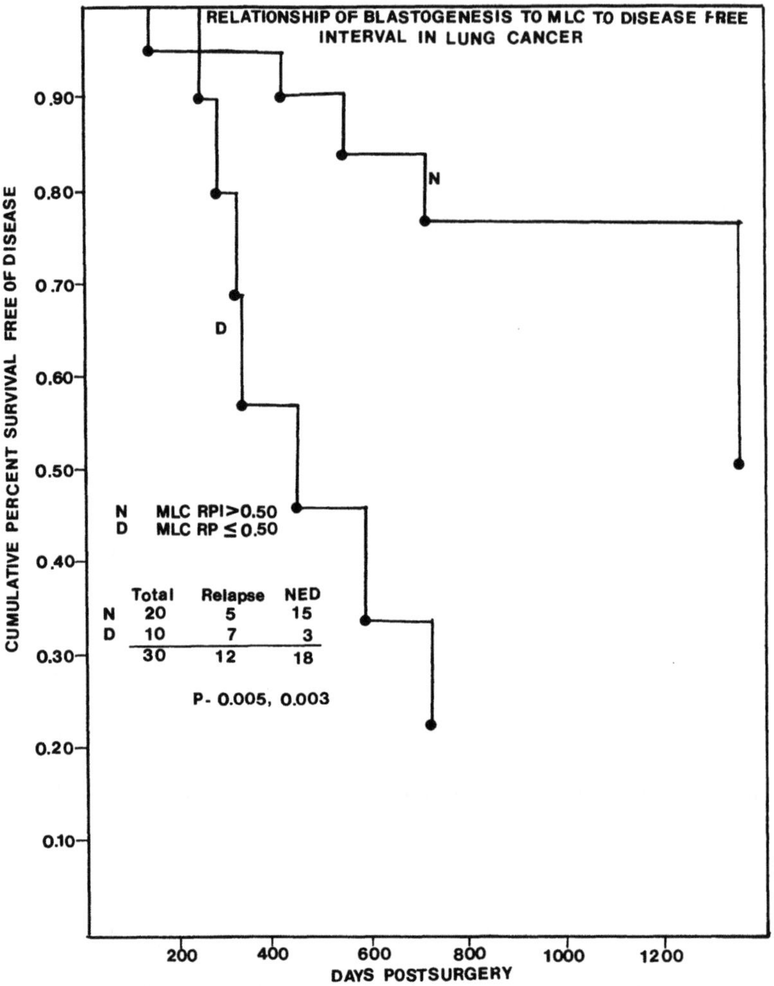

Fig. 5. Disease free interval (DFI) of lung cancer patients with normal MLC (N) was significantly better than those with depressed (D) MLC

stage I patients ($P = 0.088$). This is as expected, since this group has the smallest tumor burden and, thus, avoids the variability of postrelapse survival. In a previous report of this series in which the two immunotherapy arms were not combined, the DFI of stage I patients did reach significance in the trend analysis ($P = 0.031$), favoring the immunotherapy arm [10]. This, as well as the divergence of the curves in this group, is encouraging since in spite of small numbers it does suggest that there exists a subgroup of postthoractomy lung cancer patients who may benefit from adjuvant immunotherapy.

Depressed MLC responses in cancer patients have been described a number of times [1, 5]. How reliably a depressed postoperative MLC reflects the continued presence of tumor is unclear. This study demonstrates a significantly more rapid relapse rate in the subgroup with depressed MLC. The wide divergence of the curves suggests that the MLC identifies a subgroup at high risk for relapse. In a larger study, Cannon et al. [1]

found that the MLC could identify a high-risk subgroup within the $T_1 N_0 M_0$ stage, the lowest risk group definable by current clinical and pathologic staging. It thus appears that the MLC may be a more sensitive discriminator of prognosis than current clinical staging methods.

BCG did not prolong the DFI in the subgroup with normal MLC. This may have been because the effect of BCG is too small to detect in a good prognosis group. On the other hand, it is probably the group with the smallest tumor burden, thus, the effect of BCG should be greatest.

BCG did prolong the DFI in the high-risk subgroup identified by a depressed MLC. One may infer that the MLC-depressed group had a heavier postoperative tumor burden, but present techniques do not allow direct confirmation of this. Jerrells found that 40% of lung and breast cancer patients with depressed lymphoproliferative responses had suppressor cells, the majority of which were adherent and, therefore, probably monocytes or macrophages [6]. The MLC was followed longitudinally in most patients in this series. The MLC of the high-risk group (depressed MLC) continued to be depressed in those patients who received BCG. There is evidence, therefore, that BCG does not restore a depressed MLC to normal. The salubrious effect of BCG is not, therefore, via any mechanism involving the MLC or by altering suppressor cell activity.

The use of an immunologic assay to extend clinical staging by defining high-risk subgroups amenable to adjuvant therapy is of obvious importance. The concept of defining prognostic subgroups on the basis of immunologic assays and then applying adjuvant immunotherapy on that basis is a new one which is potentially useful both to clinicians and immunologists. This area is worthy of vigorous investigation.

Conclusion

BCG and BCG plus allogeneic tumor cells are only marginally effective as adjuvant therapy in stage I and II lung cancer. The value of adjuvant immunotherapy may be increased by using in vitro assays, such as the MLC to define prognostic subsets. The MLC done in the perioperative period may be used to define a subset of patients as high risk of recurrence. Intradermal BCG may prolong the DFI in this high-risk subset, and further study should be done in this area.

References

1. Cannon GB, Dean JH, Herberman RB, Reid JW, Miller C, Lang NP (1980) Association of depressed postoperative lymphoproliferative responses to alloantigens with poor prognosis in patients with stage I lung cancer. Int J Cancer 25: 9–17
2. Carr DT, Mountain CF (1974) The staging of lung cancer. Semin Oncol 1: 229–234
3. Cannon GB, Weese JL, Oldham RK, Herberman RB, Dean JH, McCoy JL (1978) Lymphocyte proliferation responses of patients with carcinoma of the breast or lung to mitogens, alloantigens, and tumor-associated antigens. In: Nieburgs HE (ed) Proceedings of third international symposium for detection and prevention of cancer, vol 1. Mt. Sinai School of Medicine, City University of New York. New York, pp 425–446
4. Dean JH, Cannon R, Herberman RB, Silva J, McCoy JL, Oldham RK (1977) The relative proliferation index as a more sensitive parameter for evaluating lymphoproliferative responses of cancer patients to mitogens and alloantigens. Int J Cancer 20: 359–370

5. Jerrells TR, Dean JH, Herberman RB (1978) Relationships between T lymphocyte levels and lymphoproliferative responses to mitogens and alloantigens in lung and breast cancer patients. Int J Cancer 21: 282–290
6. Jerrells TR, Dean JH, McCoy JL, Richardson GL, Herberman RB (1978) Role of suppressor cells in depression of in vitro lymphoproliferative responses of lung and breast cancer patients. J Natl Cancer Inst 61: 1001–1009
7. Jerrells TR, Dean JH, Richardson G, Cannon GB, Herberman RB (1979) Increased monocyte medicated cytostasis of lymphoid cells lines in breast and lung cancer patients. Int J Cancer 23: 768–776
8. Kaplan EL, Meier P (1958) Nonparametric estimates from incomplete observation. J Am Stat Assoc 35: 457–481
9. Oldham RK, Weese JL, Herberman RB, Perlin E, Mills M, Heim W, Blom J, Green D, Reid J, Ballinger S, Law I, McCoy JL, Dean JH, Cannon GB, Djeu J (1976) Immunologic monitoring and immunotherapy in carcinoma of the lung. Int J Cancer 18: 739–749
10. Reid JW, Perlin E, Oldham RK, Weese JL, Heim W, Mills M, Miller C, Blom J, Green D, Ballinger S, Cannon BG, Law I, Connor R, Herberman RB (to be published) Immunotherapy of carcinoma of the lung with intradermal BCG and allogeneic tumor cells: A clinical trial. Elsevier North-Holland, New York
11. Thomas DG, Breslow N, Gart JJ (1977) Trend and homogeneity analyses of proportions and life-table data. Comput Biomed Res 10: 373–381

36. *Intrapleural BCG Immunotherapy of Lung Cancer Patients**

C. Maver, H. Kausel, L. Lininger, and M. McKneally

Albany Medical College, Medical Education Building, Room 514,
Albany, NY 12208, USA

Summary

Stage I lung cancer patients were benefited by intrapleural treatment with 10^7 colony-forming units of Tice-strain BCG. This improvement was dependent upon a negative tuberculin test prior to therapy.

Introduction

The intrapleural administration of BCG following surgery seems to benefit a group of patients with stage I lung cancer. This observation, first reported in 1976 [5], is based on randomized clinical trials conducted at affiliated hospitals of the Albany Medical College: 191 patients are currently enrolled in these trials. BCG is most effective in stage I patients who are capable of a primary immune response to BCG.

Patients and Methods

All patients with surgically resectable primary lung cancer admitted to the Division of Thoracic Surgery at affiliated hospitals of the Albany Medical College were eligible for entry. Routine preoperative and diagnostic assessment included pulmonary function studies, complete blood count, biochemical blood screening, and chest radiograph. Organ-specific scans were performed only when clinical symptoms or biochemical tests suggested the possibility of metastatic disease. Delayed hypersensitivity responses to tuberculin antigens [old tuberculin (10 units) and purified protein derivative (PPD) (5 units)] and to phytohemagglutinin (PHA) (0.1 mg) were assessed at least 48 h prior to surgery. A positive skin test was defined as more than 10 mm induration with or without accompanying erythema recorded 48 h after test.

---

* The research for this study was supported in part by the New York State Kidney Disease Institute, Division of Laboratories and Research, an agency of the New York State Department of Health, National Cancer Institute grant R01-CA-27039, and contract N01-CB-53940

Following surgical resection, all patients were staged according to American Joint Committee for Cancer Staging and End Results Reporting guidelines [8] and were stratified by histologic cell type [5]. Patients with oat cell carcinoma were excluded from the study. Patients were randomly assigned by closed envelope technique to receive a single dose of BCG given intrapleurally or to enter the control group. The technique of the administration of BCG and/or isoniazid are described elsewhere [6, 7]. Test patients received 10^7 colony-forming units of Tice-strain BCG intrapleurally. Fourteen days after BCG, a 90-day course of oral isoniazid (300 mg/day) was initiated. Control patients received isoniazid, but no BCG. From 1973–1978, mediastinal node biopsy was not a requirement for staging and was not routinely performed. All patients were followed as outpatients by physical examination, chest radiograph, and routine blood tests at regular intervals after surgery. Skin tests were repeated in those patients who were preoperatively negative.

Recurrences were defined as clinical or pathologically proven evidence of local or distant progression of cancer. New solitary lung tumors were included as recurrences. New primary cancers were identified by typical clinical signs of a distinctly different tumor (colon, rectum, breast, or prostate) and were generally confirmed by biopsy or excision.

Statistical review of patient status was carried out a 4-month intervals and was based upon data collected at regular follow-up visits and from telephone contact with the patient and the referring physician. Comparisons were made using the Gehan generalization of Wilcoxon's test [1].

In 1977 it became clear that the 30 patients with stage I disease treated with intrapleural BCG had a higher survival rate than the 36 patients in the control group. After careful statistical review, this randomized trial was closed to further patient entry. Subsequently, all new stage I patients were entered into a second trial wherein half were randomized to receive intrapleural BCG, and half received intrapleural BCG augmented with cutaneous BCG restimulation by tine-test technique. Restimulation was performed at 1, 2, 3, 6, and 12 months after surgery and at 6-month intervals thereafter. As in the previous study, all patients were given oral isoniazid (300 mg/day) for a period of 3 months beginning 14 days after BCG instillation.

A distinctive feature of the new trial was that mediastinal node biopsy became a regular practice to exclude patients with micrometastases to mediastinal nodes from the stage I protocol. This requirement was introduced because the survival rate of the stage I control group in the first study was lower than expected, based on the results of Anderson [8] and Memorial Sloan Kettering [4].

Results

One-hundred ninety-one patients with resected lung cancer entered study protocols since 1973. The median duration of follow-up for these patients is 46 months and the longest period of observation is 83 months.

There has been a reduction in the recurrence rate among stage I patients treated with intrapleural BCG. Among 30 stage I patients treated with BCG during 1973–1977, there have been 11 recurrences of lung cancer, one new primary cancer, and three unrelated deaths. Among 36 simultaneously randomized control patients, 20 recurrences of lung cancer, three new primary neoplams, and one noncancer death have been recorded. The survival curves for patients in these two groups are reported

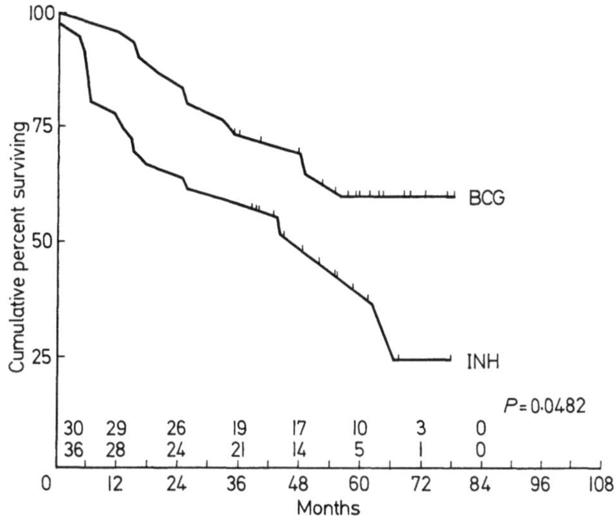

Fig. 1. Deaths: Stage I, all causes

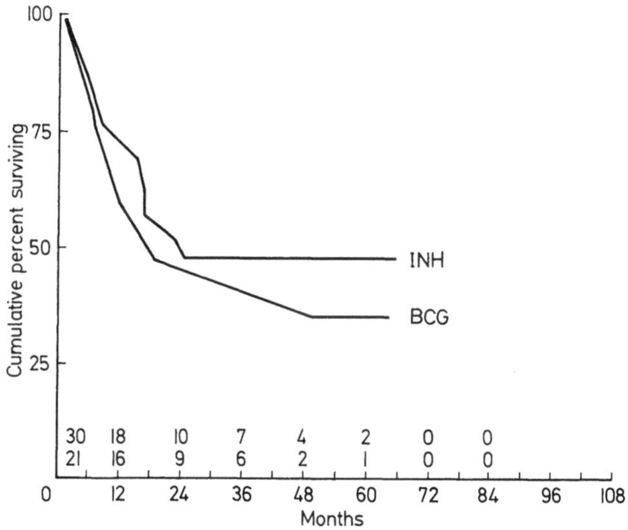

Fig. 2. Deaths: Stages II and III, all causes

in Fig. 1 and the difference betweeen groups is statistically significant ($P = 0.048$).

From 1978–1979, an additional 52 state I patients have been treated by surgical resection followed by intrapleural BCG, either given as a single treatment (30 patients) or augmented by repeated cutaneous restimulation (22 patients). Among these 52 patients there have been five recurrences, two new primary cancers, and one noncancer death. It is too early to speculate on the therapeutic efficacy of cutaneous restimulation and no significant difference in recurrence rates between these treatment groups is demonstrable at the time of this report.

BCG as administered in this program did not benefit patients with stage II or III lung cancer (Fig. 2). Patients who were PPD-positive (PPD+) during the preoperative period had a greater febrile response following BCG therapy than patients who were PPD-negative (PPD–). The average maximum temperature elevation for PPD+

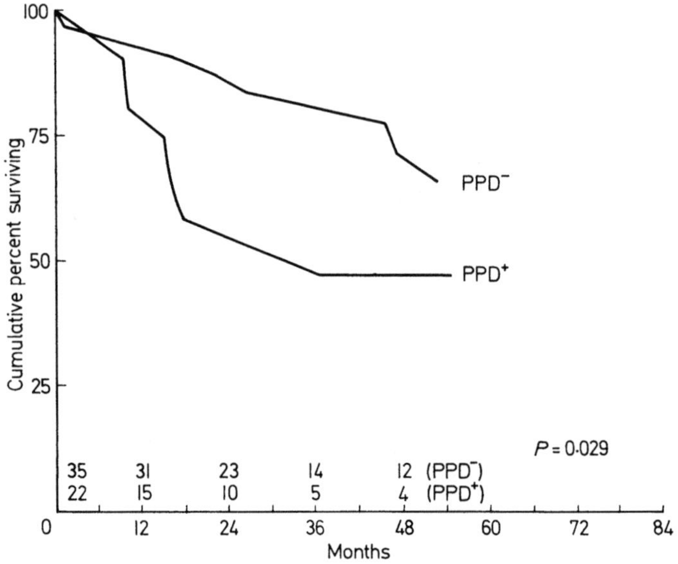

Fig. 3. Recurrences: BCG stage I

patients was 102.5° F (102.5° F = 39.2° C) ± 0.4 compared with 101.2 F (101.2° C = 38.4° C) ± 0.1 for patients ($P = 0.01$).

Actuarial survival analysis for stage I BCG-treated patients relative to tuberculin status shows that patients who were PPD− preoperatively have a higher disease-free survival rate following BCG than patients who were PPD+. This difference (Fig. 3) cannot be explained by an imbalance in prognostic factors favoring PPD− patients. A similar but smaller trend toward improved survival was observed in PPD− control patients. Among the control patients, this trend may be explained in part by an imbalance in prognostic factors, since 96% of stage I PPD− control patients had no tumor evident in hilar lymph nodes at the time of surgery whereas only 60% of PPD+ control patients had negative lymph nodes.

Patients who were PPD− prior to surgery were retested several times during the first 12 postoperative months. Ninety percent of patients treated with BCG and 45% of controls converted from PPD− to PPD+ within 12 months of surgery.

Discussion

Our data continues to suggest that intrapleural BCG administered as an immunotherapeutic adjuvant following stage I lung cancer surgery can lead to improved survival times. This observation is based on a small group of patients and is undermined by the fact that the failure rate in control patients is somewhat higher than expected. Because of the configuration of the survival curves and the time elapsed since the initiation of our study, it is unlikely that the statistical significance of the difference observed here will be lost. Recently Lowe et al. [3] reported that no benefit was observed from the intrapleural administration of 10^7 colony-forming units of Glaxo-strain BCG in a small trial. They indicate that febrile responses to BCG were not often observed in their trial. The majority of patients treated in our BCG trial experienced temperature elevations. The difference in the strains of BCG employed, and the tuberculin status of the two series may be responsible for the discrepancies. The validity of the biologic observations suggested by our small trial will be determined by other larger cooperative trials now in progress.

Wright et al. [9] recently reported that the conversion of a preoperatively negative tuberculin test to positive following BCG therapy is a potentially important predictor of successful therapy. Patients who were PPD+ prior to BCG therapy did not experience an improvement in survival over control patients in his experience. Our data are in agreement with Wright's. The majority (68%) of our patients were PPD− during the preoperative period. Following BCG therapy, 90% of PPD− patients converted to positive. The survival of these patients was significantly higher than patients who failed to convert this test or who were positive to the test prior to therapy.

It is of interest that a larger number of control patients converted preoperatively negative tuberculin tests to positive following surgery and repeated skin testing. While it could be postulated that this conversion might be due to the removal of an immunosuppressive tumor burden, it is more likely that repeated skin testing with tuberculin antigens (PPD and old tuberculin) may have led to sensitization via the cutaneous route. This phenomenon has been previously reported by other investigators [2]. No survival advantage was observed among control patients who converted to positive. We conclude from our experience that intrapleural BCG was associated with a small but definite survival advantage for tuberculin-negative stage I patients. This observation awaits confirmation. We stress that intrapleural BCG should not be administered as standard care outside the limits of controlled clinical trials until the question of its efficacy is resolved.

References

1. Gehan E (1965) A generalized two-sample Wilcoxon test for doubly censored data. Biometrika 52: 650–653
2. Israel L, Mugica J, Chahinian PH (1973) Prognosis of early bronchogenic carcinoma. Survival curves of 451 patients after resection of lung cancer in relation to the results of preoperative tuberculin skin test. Biomedicine 19: 68–72
3. Lowe J, Shore DF, Iles PB, Langman MJS, Baldwin RW (1980) Intrapleural BCG in operable lung cancer. Lancet 1: 11–14
4. Martini N, Beattie EJ Jr (1977) Results of surgical treatment in stage I lung cancer. J Thorac Cardiovasc Surg 74: 499–505
5. McKneally MF, Payne WS (1978) Pulmonary neoplasms: Malignant and benign. In: Effler DB (ed) Blades' surgical diseases of the chest, 4th edn. Mosby, St. Louis, pp 117–144
6. McKneally MF, Maver C, Kausel HW (1976) Regional immunotherapy of lung cancer with intrapleural BCG. Lancet 1: 377–379
7. McKneally MF, Maver C, Kausel HW, Alley RD (1976) Regional immunotherapy with intrapleural BCG for lung cancer. J Thorac Cardiovasc Surg 72: 333–338
8. Mountain CF (1977) Assessment of the role of surgery for control of lung cancer. Ann Thorac Surg 24: 365–373
9. Wright PW, Hill LD, Peterson AV, Bernstein ID (1980) Host response to purified protein derivative of tuberculin predicts outcome in patients receiving intrapleural bacillus Calmette-Guerin and levamisole for resectable, non-small cell lung cancer. Proc Am Assoc Cancer Res 21: 230

37. *Specific Active Immunotherapy in Lung Cancer: The Induction of Long-Lasting Cellular Responses to Tumour-Associated Antigens*

T. H. M. Stewart, A. C. Hollinshead, J. E. Harris, and S. Raman

University of Ottawa, School of Medicine, Ottawa, Ontario, Canada

Introduction

In this report we give details of skin tests with soluble tumour-associated antigens in patients entered into the phase II trial of stage I lung cancer patients in Ottawa. We show that in non-immunized patients a weak positive reaction to such antigens following surgery is a favourable sign. Strong reactions in the group which received immunochemotherapy are associated with fewer failures than in the group which received immunization alone which had weak to moderate reactions. Strong delayed hypersensitivity reactions can be induced that endure more than 5 years. If such reactions indicate resistance to tumour growth, as in animal systems, then prophylactic immunization of healthy adults who are at high risk of developing lung cancer would be expected to reduce the incidence of the disease.
Survival of the non-immunized and immunized patients was reported 2 years ago in the last publication of this plenary session of the EORTC [8]. We again report on the survival of these two groups of patients, as of March 1, 1980.

Patients and Methods

Full details of patient selection, TNM staging and all relevant characteristics have already been presented in previous publications as has the preparation of soluble antigens, immunization procedures and the use of methotrexate (MTX) [6, 7].

Results

Late Skin Testing

Following surgical resection of the lung, cancer patients were skin tested with soluble tumour-associated antigen, derived in most instances from allogeneic tumours, matched as closely as possible with the histology of the resected tumour. The usual skin test dose was 100 µg in 0.1 ml. Not all patients could be tested in the later months after surgery; some died, some refused and for others the distance from Ottawa made such testing impractical.

Recent Results in Cancer Research, Vol. 80

Table 1. Late testing of stage I patients with tumour-associated antigens (TAA) matched for histology of the primary tumour. Non-immunized: control or methotrexate-treated (MTX) patients

Patient	Controls				
	Tested (months post-operatively)	Recall antigen	TAA	DHR[a]	Status (months)
1.	4		Adeno	5 × 5	Alive (37)
2.	15		Large cell anaplastic	10 × 8	Died (22)
3.	31		Squamous	8 × 8	Alive (65)
4.	32	+	Squamous	Negative	Died (39)
5.	42		Squamous	5 × 5	Alive (77)
	MTX				
6.	3		Squamous	16 × 16	Alive (56)
7.	4	+	Alveolar	Negative	Died (27)
8.	6	+	Squamous	Negative	Died (24)
9.	12	+	Squamous	Negative	Alive (52)
10.	12		Adeno	16 × 16	Alive (53)
11.	20	+	Adeno	Negative	Died (22)
12.	30 (mean 17.36 months)		Adeno	9 × 9	Alive (70)

[a] DHR = mm induration at 48 h (mean 5.75 mm); DHR positive (1 of 7 dead) and DHR negative to soluble cancer antigen (4 of 5 dead)

Non-Immunized Stage I Group

Twelve patients were tested. Seven patients showed weak to moderate reactions to tumour antigen; one of these patients died of lung cancer 7 months later. Five patients showed no reaction to tumour antigen, yet gave a positive reaction to at least one recall bacterial antigen; thus they were not completely anergic. Four of these patients died of lung cancer at 2, 7, 18, and 23 months after testing. Details of these skin tests are given in Table 1.

Immunized Group

Eleven patients were tested at varying intervals following surgery with 13 skin tests. All patients showed positive reactions and two died of lung cancer 13 and 32 months later. The mean strength of these reactions was three-times greater than those in the non-immunized group. Details are given in Table 2.

Immunochemotherapy Group

Nine patients were tested following surgery with a total of 16 tests. One patient died of cerebral metastases 4 months after testing. A second patient died of staphylococcal

Table 2. Late testing of stage I patients with TAA

Patient	Immunized patients			
	Tested (months post-operatively)	TAA	DHR[a]	Status (months)
1.	4	Squamous	11 × 11	
	40	Squamous	40 × 35	Alive (44)[b]
2.	5	Alveolar	18 × 15	Alive (32)
3.	6	Adeno	13 × 11	Alive (35)
4.	8	Squamous	36 × 27	Alive (41)
5.	10	Squamous	12 × 12	Died (42)
6.	13	Autologous (10 μg)	16 × 15	
	36	Autologous (20 μg)	43 × 36	Alive (45)[b]
7.	17	Adeno (autologous)	7 × 7	Alive (57)
8.	18	Squamous	7 × 5	Alive (57)
9.	25	Anaplastic	13 × 13	Alive (67)
10.	27	Squamous	16 × 16	Died (40)
11.	29	Squamous	8 × 7	Alive (55)
	(mean 17 months)			

[a] DHR = mm induration at 48 h (mean 17.9 mm); 2 of 11 positive patients died of lung cancer
[b] Note the increase of reactivity of antigen over a period of 3 years

septicemia 26 months after testing, at 71 years of age, while clinically free of disease. Much stronger reactions are seen in this group, earlier and maintaining strength with time (Table 3). Patient 4 was tested 5.5 years following immunization and showed 20 × 20 mm induration to 100 μg autologous antigen that had been stored at −80° C. The mean diameter of these delayed hypersensitivity reactions was 32 mm, double that of the immunized group and six-times as strong as the mean reaction in the control non-immunized group.

Survival

The non-immunized group consisted of 24 patients; 16 concomitant control patients and eight who received MTX. Eight control patients died of lung cancer at 8, 14, 17, 22, 30, 32, 46, and 65 months respectively. Of those who received MTX, four have died of lung cancer at 6, 22, 24, and 26 months respectively.

The immunized group consisted of 15 patients who received allogeneic antigen and Freund's complete adjuvant and 13 patients who received immunochemotherapy. Of the 15 who were immunized four have died of lung cancer at 27, 40, 42, and 43 months respectively. One patient had inoperable recurrence of squamous carcinoma in his trachea in November, 1977, and is alive as of April, 1980. One patient had a stump

Table 3. Late testing of stage I patients with TAA: immunochemotherapy patients

Patient	Immunized patients			
	Tested (months) (postoperatively)	TAA	DHR[a]	Status (months)
1.	3	Squamous	77 × 63	
	4		10 × 10	
	36		45 × 31	Alive (44)[b]
2.	3	Squamous	9 × 8	
	20	Squamous	20 × 19	
		Adeno	22 × 21	Alive (29)[c]
3.	10	Squamous	11 × 11	Died (14)
4.	3	Squamous	40 × 40	
	16	Anaplastic (autol.)[d]	40 × 40	
	47	Anaplastic (autol.)	30 × 30	Alive (56)[b]
5.	18	Adeno (autol.)	14 × 12	Alive (58)
6.	22	Squamous	18 × 16	Alive (62)
7.	23	Adeno	10 × 10	Alive (62)
8.	24	Squamous	25 × 33	Died (50) (non-cancer death)
9.	25	Adeno	55 × 55	
	56	Adeno	27 × 22	Alive (65)
	(mean 19 months)			

[a] 1 of 9 positive patients died of lung cancer
[b] Note the strong reactivity relatively early following the combination of MTX and immunization
[c] This patient had a primary squamous adenocarcinoma and was late tested for each antigen
[d] Autologous antigen

recurrence, after 20 months, of her large cell carcinoma, received cobalt treatment and died 4 years later of respiratory failure, free of disease. A third patient had recurrence of his squamous cell carcinoma at 12 months. A total pneumonectomy was performed and he died of respiratory failure and pneumonia 3.5 years later, at 73 years of age. At necropsy, foci of squamous cell carcinoma were found at the stump of his pneumonectomy, surrounded by a dense desmoplastic reaction with a moderate lymphocytic infiltrate. Thus there have been seven failures in this group, four deaths as well as and remarkable longevity following local recurrence in three patients.

Of the 13 patients who received immunochemotherapy, one died of cerebral metastases, after 14 months, of large cell carcinoma. A second patient developed a stump recurrence of squamous cell carcinoma, after 3 years, and died 3 years later of disseminated cancer. Two patients were free of disease at the time of their death; one of cardiac arrest 39 months after surgery, the other of staphylococcal septicemia 51 months after surgery, at 71 years of age. In this group, two have died of lung cancer. Details are shown in Fig. 1.

a

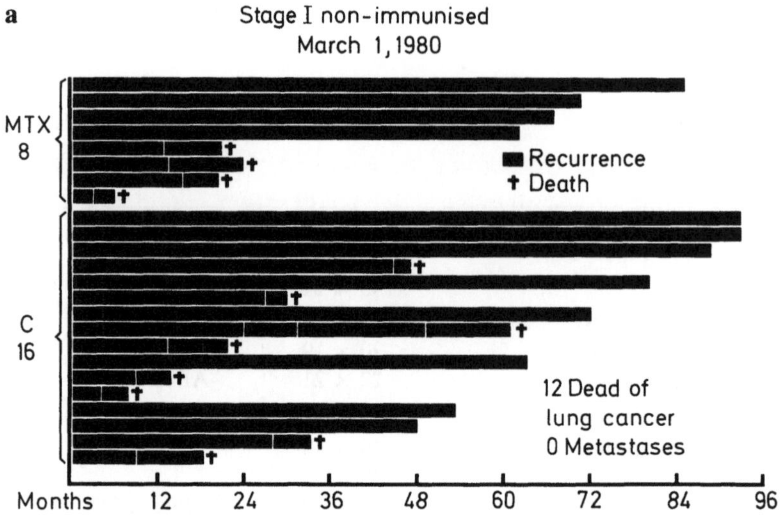

b

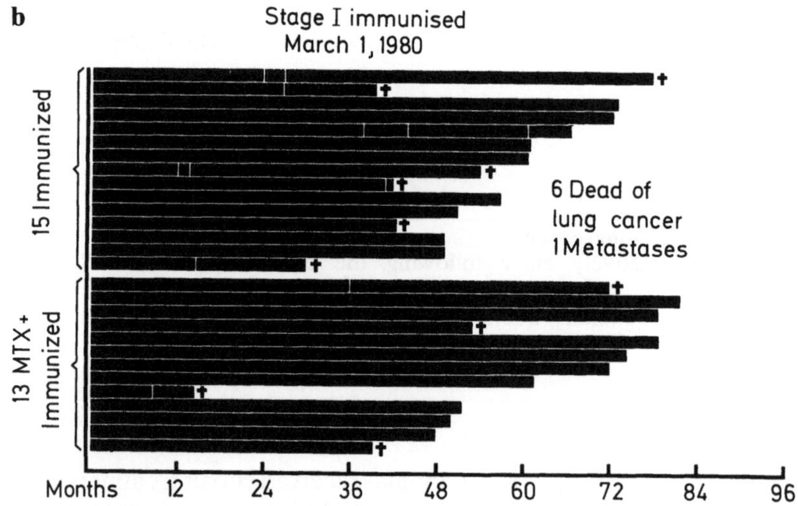

Fig. 1a, b. Status of patients with stage I lung cancer. **a** Of the 24 patients who were not immunized 12 have died of lung cancer; **b** of the 28 who were immunized six have died of lung cancer, four have died non-cancer deaths (see text) and one survives 2.5 years following inoperable intrathoracic recurrence

In Table 4, life-table survival is summarized as calculated by the method of Cutler and Ederer [3a]. Those patients who died a non-cancer death are shown as being lost to follow-up. Fig. 2 shows the survival curves for the control and treated groups, with one-sided 95% confidence limits for the control and treated group.
The survival experience of the treated group may be seen to diverge significantly from the control group beyond 24 months. While 96% of the immunized group reached a second anniversary, only 72% of the controls did so. The corresponding values for the

Table 4. The life-table survival experience is shown, with 95% confidence limits for the control and immunized groups

	MTX + controls		Immunotherapy + immunochemotherapy	
		95% One-sided-CL		95% One-sided-CL
P_6	1.00	1.00	1.00	–
P_{12}	0.91	1.00	1.00	–
P_{18}	0.86	0.97	0.96	0.89
P_{24}	0.72	0.82	0.96	0.89
P_{30}	0.63	0.76	0.92	0.84
P_{36}	0.54	0.69	0.92	0.84
P_{42}	0.54	0.69	0.85	0.74
P_{48}	0.50	0.65	0.80	0.67
P_{54}	0.50	0.65	0.76	0.61
P_{60}	0.50	0.65	0.76	0.61
P_{66}	0.44	0.67	0.76	0.61
P_{72}	–	–	0.66	0.46

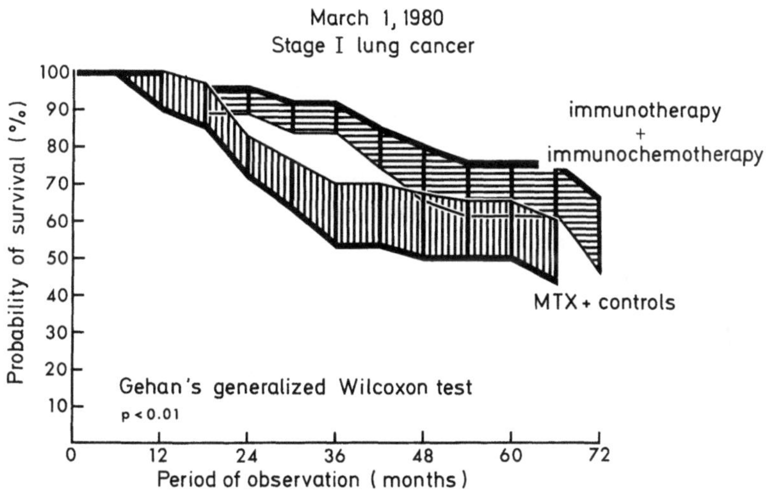

Fig. 2. This is a graphic representation of the data in Table 4. Note significant differences in survival experience after 2 years, until 4 years, and again at 5.5 years

fourth anniversary are 80% and 50% respectively. The overall comparison for the treated and control groups using Gehan's generalized Wilcoxon test [36] yielded a statistical significance of $P < 0.01$. In Fig. 3, survival of the immunized and immunochemotherapy groups is identical until 36 months following surgery. Thereafter the immunochemotherapy group perform better than the immunized group.

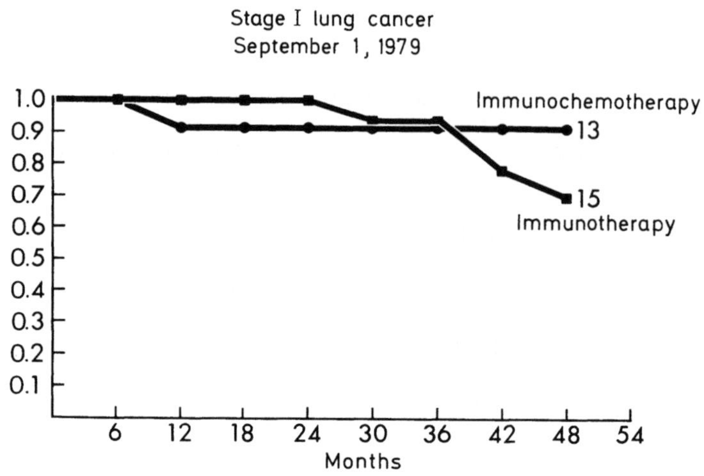

Fig. 3. Improved survival is seen after 3 years in favour of the group which received immunochemotherapy

Discussion

A clear correlation between resistance to tumour growth and a delayed hypersensitivity reaction to soluble tumour-associated antigens has been shown in experimental animal tumour systems [1–3, 9]. In general, such delayed hypersensitivity reactions last for 28–30 days. We believe that, in our patients, persistence of such hypersensitivity reactions to tumour antigens for 5 years or more is a sign of prolonged resistance to tumour growth. If this conclusion is valid, it becomes attractive to propose prophylactic immunization of healthy adults who are at very high risk of developing lung cancer, by virtue of heavy cigarette smoking and industrial exposure. A polyvalent vaccine can be made to contain soluble tumour-associated antigens derived from squamous cell carcinoma, adenocarcinoma and anaplastic large and small cell carcinoma. The inevitablle difficulties of launching a prophylactic approach for controlling lung cancer have recently been reviewed in depth [4]. We are optimistic that such an approach in humans would be effective, as in animal experiments [5].

References

1. Abe S, Yamazaki M, Mizuno D (1978) Antitumour immunity after surgical removal of 3-methylcholanthrene-induced murine tumours: Correlation between resistance and delayed hypersensitivity reaction. Gann 69: 323–329
2. Brannen GE, Santos GW (1975) Immune responses to soluble tumour antigen in various stages of tumour growth. Invest Urol 13: 79–84
3. Brannen GE, Adams JS, Santos GW (1974) Tumour specific immunity in 3-methylcholanthrene-induced murine fibrosarcomas. I. In vivo demonstration of immunity with three preparations of soluble antigens. J Natl Cancer Inst 53: 165–175
3a. Cutler SJ, Ederer F (1958) Maximum utilization of the life table method in analyzing survival. J Chronic Dis 8: 699–712
3b. Gehan EA (1965) Generalized two sample Wilcoxon test for doubly censored data. Biometrika 52: 650–653

4. Miller AB (1980) Methodological considerations for trials of lung cancer prophylaxis. Can Med Assoc J 122: 776
5. Prager MD, Gordon WC (1980) Specific immunoprophylaxis in experimental tumour-host systems. Can Med Assoc J 122: 780–784
6. Stewart THM, Hollinshead AC, Harris JE (1976) Immunochemotherapy of lung cancer. Ann NY Acad Sci 277: 436–466
7. Stewart THM, Hollinshead AC, Harris JE et al. (1977) Specific active immunochemotherapy in lung cancer: A survival study. Can J Surg 20: 370–377
8. Stewart THM, Hollinshead AC, Harris JE, Raman S (1978) Active immunochemotherapy in lung cancer: A survival study. Recent Results Cancer Res 68: 278–285
9. Vaage J, Jones RD, Brown BW (1972) Tumour specific resistance in mice detected by inhibition of macrophage inhibition. Cancer Res 32: 680–687

38. *Malnutrition in Lung Cancer: Incidence, Prognostic Implications, and Pathogenesis*

D. L. Kisner

National Cancer Institute, Division of Cancer Treatment,
Cancer Therapy Evaluation Program, Bethesda, MD 20205, USA

Summary

Malnutrition and weight loss are common in patients with lung cancer. Weight loss is an independent prognostic factor for survival in lung cancer treatment studies. Metabolic disturbances probably play a dominant role in weight loss in these patients rather than reduced food intake. The identification of the pertinent etiologic metabolic abnormalities and development of specific therapeutic intervention should be goals for future research.

Introduction

There has been an increasing awareness of malnutrition-related morbidity and mortality in patients with cancer. In one autopsy series [10] more than 22% of patients died without identifiable cause other than cachexia. There is little doubt that these patients die of their cancer, but they die of systemic effects of their tumor that produce the debilitating syndrome that is malignant cachexia, rather than from a tumor mass in an anatomically critical location.

The purpose of this paper is to assess the incidence of malnutrition in patients with unresectable lung cancer, and examine its impact on treatment results. Current thinking on the pathogenesis of malnutrition in lung cancer patients will also be reviewed briefly.

Frequency

Despite large-scale trials reporting surgical results in lung cancer, precise statistics relative to the incidence of weight loss on presentation for primary therapy are difficult to find. Because a relatively small proportion of patients are curatively resectable, the incidence of weight loss on entry into advanced disease studies may well be a fair approximation of the incidence at diagnosis.

Several pertinent small series have been reported. Issel et al. [5] reported that 22 of 49 (45%) patients with non-oat cell lung cancer had greater than 6% body weight loss on entry into a phase II chemotherapy trial. This same group reported that degree of

Recent Results in Cancer Research, Vol. 80

Table 1. Eastern Cooperation Oncology Group. Frequency of weight loss in lung cancer patients. Adapted from DeWys et al. [3]

Tumor type	No. patients	Weight loss in the 6 months prior to entry (%)			
		0	0–5	5–10	> 10
Small cell	436	43	23	20	14
Non-small cell	590	39	25	21	15

weight loss in 17 of 26 (65%) patients with epidermoid histology entering another trial [6]. Issel et al. [4] also reported a 30% incidence of more than 6% weight loss in patients with adenocarcinoma of the lung entering treatment.

In a larger series including all histologies Zelen [11] has reported 287 of 1,000 (28.7%) with greater than a 10 lb. (4.5 kg) weight loss at entry into several studies of the Veterans Administration Lung Study Group.

In a recent analysis of Eastern Cooperative Oncology Group advanced lung cancer trials DeWys et al. [3] reported weight loss data on a large group of both small cell and nonsmall cell lung cancer patients treated in Eastern Cooperative Oncology Group (ECOG) studies. Table 1 shows the frequency and severity of pretreatment weight loss in 1,026 cases. This study provides the most extensive detailed data currently available, and suggests that fully 60% of lung cancer patients have some appreciable weight loss by the time they enter advanced disease studies. This significant frequency of malnutrition in lung cancer patients demands consideration of its prognostic implications.

Prognostic Effects

There have been several studies reporting reduced survival time for patients having lost weight on entering therapeutic trials. Zelen [11] reported a 13.1-week median survival for patients having lost 10 lb. (4.5 kg) or more while patients without weight loss survived a median of 18.7 weeks. These data were calculated on a group of 1,000 patients with all histologies. It is not clear that weight loss is of prognostic importance independent of performance status in this series. It was stated that performance status was the most important single prognostic factor after stage of disease.

Issel et al. [4] has reported reduced chemotherapeutic response and survival in adenocarcinoma patients with greater than 6% weight loss. Weight loss seemed to correlate with performance status in this study, but no analysis of the independent role of weight loss was presented. In another report Issel et al. [5] demonstrated weight loss (more than 6%) to be more important than performance status as a prognostic factor in 49 nonsmall cell cancer patients treated with isophosphamide, adriamycin, and *C. parvum.*

In a thorough analysis of 316 patients Lanzotti et al. [8] examined several prognostic factors in patients with inoperable lung cancer of all histologies. In 129 patients with limited intrathoracic disease, pretreatment weight loss (more than 12%) was found to be the most important prognostic factor, with performance status being next in

Table 2. Eastern Cooperation Oncology Group. Effect of weight loss on survival. Adapted from DeWys et al. [3]

Tumor type	Median survival (weeks)		*P* value
	No weight loss	Weight loss	
Small cell anaplastic	34	27	< 0.05
Nonsmall cell	20	14	< 0.01

Table 3. Eastern Cooperation Oncology Group. Effect of weight loss subcategories on median survival in nonsmall cell lung cancer ($n = 590$). Adapted from DeWys et al. [3]

Weight loss (%)	Median survival (weeks)				*P* value
	None	0–5	5–10	> 10	
	20	17	13	11	< 0.01

Table 4. Eastern Cooperation Oncology Group. Relationship between weight loss, ECOG performance status (PS), and median survival. Adapted from DeWys et al. [3]

Tumor type	Median survival (weeks)					
	PS 0–1			PS 2–4		
	No weight loss	Weight loss	*P*	No weight loss	Weight loss	*P*
Small cell	39	29	< 0.01	19	25	NS
Nonsmall cell	28	18	0.01	14	10	< 0.05

importance. In 187 patients with extensive disease, weight loss was found to be of less prognostic importance than performance status and age.

More recently DeWys et al. [3] has reviewed the prognostic importance of pretreatment weight in 1,026 patients treated on ECOG protocols. Table 2 shows the relationship between pretreatment weight loss (any weight loss) and survival times. The existence of any pretreatment weight loss correlated significantly with shorter survival in both histologic groupings. In patients with nonsmall cell lung cancer, progressively more severe weight loss correlated with shorter survival (Table 3). While poor performance status correlated with a higher incidence of weight loss ($P < 0.01$ for both small cell and nonsmall cell histology), the negative prognostic effect of pretreatment weight loss was also found within most performance status groups (Table 4), with the exception of small cell patients with ECOG performance, status categories 2, 3, 4 pretreatment weight loss was found to be independent of performance status as a prognostic factor. Also of interest is that pretreatment weight loss did not correlate with tumor extent (as scored crudely by the number of metastatic sites involved at entry into study). Within the limitations of the methods used weight loss was not simply an indication of more advanced disease.

One possible mechanism by which weight loss might lead to reduced survival time might be by reducing the patients' likelihood of a good response to chemotherapy. Only in nonsmall cell lung cancer was a trend towards reduced response rates for the weight loss group noted, and it failed to reach statistical significance.

One must conclude from the studies available that pretreatment weight loss appears to be a significant prognostic factor for survival in advanced lung cancer patients, as important as and largely independent of performance status. With this established, the nature and pathogenesis of this weight loss and malnutrition becomes of interest as they may well have an impact on our choice of therapeutic options for these patients.

Pathogenesis of Malnutrition in Lung Cancer Patients

Malnutrition and weight loss in the cancer patient is a complex process that does not lend itself easily to study or analysis. In general, weight loss occurs whenever caloric (energy) intake (that is, calories ingested and absorbed) is exceeded by energy expenditure. The frequency of reduced food intake in patients with malignancy is high, but current information suggests that the loss of mass from the various body tissue compartments is probably the result of reduced food intake and increased energy expenditure [1]. One recent study by Warnold et al. [9] sheds considerable light on this subject. In a series of ten cancer patients, energy expenditure per 24 h was calculated from oxygen consumption and heart rate data. Energy intake was determined by records of food intake and standard food composition tables. The results were compared with similarly obtained data in a series of nine hospitalized control patients. Twenty-four-hour caloric intake for cancer patients and controls was 1,340 kcal and 1,470 kcal, respectively, while 24-h energy expenditures were 1,980 kcal and 1,420 kcal, respectively. This suggests both a decreased energy intake and increased energy expenditure in the cancer patients. Although this study included patients with several tumor types it is probably naive to assume that the relative roles of reduced food intake and increased energy expenditure do not vary with the type, bulk, and location of the tumor burden. For example, carcinoma of the esophagus is probably more likely to reduce food intake and cause weight loss early in the disease process than other tumors without specific gastrointestinal tract obstruction. For that reason, consideration of studies specifically dealing with lung cancer is necessary. One recent report by Costa et al. [2] examined spontaneous food intake and weight loss in 61 male patients with non resectable non small cell lung cancer compared to an age-matched group of 76 male controls. The cancer patients were divided into two groups: "weight losers", or those with more than 5% loss of body weight in the initial 60 days after diagnosis and "weight keepers", or those with less than 5% body weight loss in that same period. Food intake data for these three groups is presented in Table 5. The data demonstrate significantly reduced food intake for the lung cancer patients compared to normal controls. However, the food intake for the cancer patients losing weight was virtually identical to that of patients who were maintaining their weight. The conclusion is that anorexia and reduced food intake were clearly present, but that they are not capable of

Table 5. Relationship between food intake and weight loss in male lung cancer patients and male controls. Adapted from Costa et al. [2]

Group	N	Mean weight (% ideal)	Mean intake (kcal/24 h)
Controls	76	118	2,358
			$P < 0.005$ (controls vs. weight keepers)
Weight keepers	38	112	1,776
		$P < 0.005$ (weight keepers vs. weight losers)	
Weight losers	23	96	1,780

explaining the early weight loss seen in 38% of the patient population. The implication is that host metabolic disturbances must be playing some role in this weight loss. A survival analysis of this same group of patients indicated a significantly longer survival for patients maintaining weight compared to the weight-losing group (median 11 months versus 5 months, $P < 0.001$). This agrees well with data outlined above, suggesting a reduced survival for lung cancer patients with weight loss early in their course.

The precise metabolic disturbances that might be causing the excelerated energy expenditure in lung cancer patients are not yet delineated. In a recent review, Kisner and DeWys [7] considered metabolic alterations known to occur in the cancer-bearing patient in general. These include elevated energy expenditures and basal metabolic rates. Specific abnormalities of carbohydrate metabolism present in the weight-losing cancer patient include carbohydrate intolerance, systemic insulin resistance, reduced uptake of glucose into peripheral muscle, reduced glycogen storage, and accelerated (energy consuming) hepatic gluconeogenesis [7]. Aberrant protein metabolism has also been documented in cancer patients, including depressed albumin synthesis, increased hepatic glycoprotein synthesis, increased activities of proteolytic enzymes in peripheral muscles with accelerated protein degradation, and reduced protein synthesis [7]. All of these abnormalities may be present, in addition to an energy and nutrient drain by the tumor, in the form of energy required for transport of nutrients and ions as well as tumor protein synthesis during growth [7]. This superimposition of tumor metabolism upon the abnormal host metabolism may, in a general way, explain increased energy expenditures in cancer patients. The exact importance of these various factors in cancer of the lung specifically remains to be established.

Conclusions

Malnutrition is a frequent clinical feature in patients with carcinoma of the lung, occasionally being present early in the course of the disease before widespread bulk disease is present. This malnutrition has been demonstrated to be a negative prognostic factor in treatment studies as important as and independent of performance status. Future randomized clinical trials in lung cancer should probably be stratified for nutritional status or weight loss, in addition to other known prognostic factors.

Current data suggest that this malnutrition is not simply related to anorexia and reduced food intake, but rather has its origins in host metabolic disturbances caused by the presence of malignancy that increases host energy expenditure. Considerably more work is required to clarify the specific metabolic aberrations present so that specific therapeutic interventions can be developed.

References

1. Brennan M (1977) Uncomplicated starvation versus cancer cachexia. Cancer Res 37: 2359–2364
2. Costa G, Bewley P, Aragon M, Siebold J (to be published) Anorexia and weight loss in cancer patients. Cancer Treat Rep
3. DeWys W, Begg C, Lavin P, et al. (to be published) Prognostic effect of weight loss prior to chemotherapy in cancer patients. Am J Med
4. Issel B, Valdivieso M, Bodey G (1978) Chemotherapy for adenocarcinoma and large cell anaplastic carcinoma of the lung with ftorafur, adriamycin and cis-dichloro-diammineplatinum (II). Cancer Treat Rep 62: 1089–1091
5. Issel B, Valdivieso M, Hersch E, Richman S, Gutterman J, Bodey G (1978) Combination chemoimmunotherapy of extensive non-oat cell lung cancer. Cancer Treat Rep 62: 1059–1063
6. Issel B, Valdivieso M, Zaren H, Dudrick S, Freireich E, Copeland E, Bodey G (1978) Protection against chemotherapy toxicity by intravenous hyperalimentation. Cancer Treat Rep 62: 1139–1143
7. Kisner D, DeWys W (to be published) Anorexia and cachexia in malignancy. In: Newell G, Ellison N (eds) Cancer and nutrition. Raven Press, New York
8. Lanzotti V, Thomas D, Boyle L, Smith T, Gehan E, Samuels M (1977) Survival with inoperable lung cancer. Cancer 39: 303–313
9. Warnold I, Lundholm K, Schersten T (1978) Energy balance and body composition in cancer patients. Cancer Res 38: 1801–1807
10. Warren S (1932) The immediate causes of death in cancer. Am J Med Sci 184: 610–615
11. Zelen M (1973) Keynote address on biostatistics and data retrieval. Cancer Chemother Rep 4: 31–42

39. *Follow-Up of a Randomized Trial for Oat Cell Carcinoma Evaluating the Efficacy of Peripheral Intravenous Nutrition (PIVN) as Adjunct Treatment**

B. Serrou, D. Cupissol, R. Plagne, P. Boutin, P. Chollet, Y. Carcassonne, and F. B. Michel

Hôpital Saint-Eloi, Centre Paul Lamarque, Department of Immuno-Chemotherapy, F-34033 Montpellier Cedex, France

Summary

A randomized trial was initiated to compare the effects of peripheral i.v. nutrition (PIVN)-associated chemotherapy (adriamycin, vincristine, VP-16-213, and cyclophosphamide) versus a chemotherapy control group in patients with oat cell lung carcinoma. Thirty-nine evaluable patients were randomized. The test group included 19 patients, whereas 20 were followed in the control group. PIVN was scheduled each day the patient underwent chemotherapy. Each patient received 1,550 kcal day which included 10% glucose, 20% lipids, and amino acids which may or may not have been mixed in the same infusion bottle. The results show ten PIVN patients presently in complete remission at the end of three courses of treatment, compared to nine over the same time period in the chemotherapy control group. Thirty-three percent of patients are still alive after 15 months after the beginning of treatment. There was no significant difference in either general health or side effects, frequency or duration of complete remission, or survival time. After 1 year of treatment, 8 of 19 PIVN patients are still in complete remission, compared to 7 of 20 patients in the control group.

Introduction

Chemotherapy has begun to play an increasingly important role in cancer treatment, particularly for solid tumors. However, chemotherapy appears to be less effective in the immunodepressed subject [5, 14, 23]. In addition, nutrition status [21] can exert an influence on immunologic parameters as well as being implicated in patient response to chemotherapy [2, 4, 6, 7, 9, 13, 15, 16, 20, 24, 26]. The more a patient suffers from malnutrition, the less likely the possibility that adequate chemotherapy can be administered. Very briefly stated, a nutritional state which approaches cachexia may be responsible for cessation of chemotherapy. This has prompted a number of authors to employ parenteral hypernutrition to reestablish a normal nutritional state so that chemotherapy could be initiated. Several authors, including ourselves, have shown in nonrandomized trials that a patient under parenteral hypernutrition who is treated chemotherapeutically will present a significantly superior response to this treatment

* Done in the framework of the French-American agreement

Recent Results in Cancer Research, Vol. 80

compared to those patients not receiving parenteral hypernutrition [3, 13, 15, 23, 27–29].

Certain recent observations suggest that parenteral hypernutrition is not without risk and can, in certain circumstances, favor local relapse and the onset of metastases [1, 17, Kisner, personal communication]. This brings us to the framework of the French-American agreement, involving a randomized trial to evaluate the role of parenteral hypernutrition in anaplastic lung cancer patients treated by chemotherapy. We chose this tumor type because it evolves rapidly and major therapeutic advances have been made in the chemotherapeutic treatment of this type of cancer.

Patients and Methods

Patients

Our study is a randomized trial in which which has thus fan entered 39 patients. All patients were histologically diagnosed as anaplastic lung cancer. Following randomization, patients were either treated with chemotherapy (first group) or chemotherapy associated with parenteral i.v. nutrition (PIVN). All patients were evaluated both before and after each chemotherapeutic cycle. Evaluation was based on the following criteria: performance status; weight; blood count; inflammatory proteins; delayed hypersensitivity skin tests; and liver function. Before treatment and again after 3 months of therapy all patients underwent fiberscopy with histologic studies, examination of bone marrow and liver, and bone and cerebral scintigrams.

Parenteral i.v. Nutrition

This treatment was given over an 8-h period each day chemotherapy was administered. Each patient received 1,550 kcal per day which included 1,000 ml 10% glucose, 500 ml Protinutril, and 500 ml 20% Intra-lipids. This PIVN was introduced into a peripheral vein. On occasion we were forced to catheterize either the inferior or superior vena cava. PIVN was administered only during ECHO and ECHO prime chemotherapy.

Chemotherapy

Chemotherapeutic agents were introduced by the same peripheral access as PIVN. Patients were initially treated by intensive induction (ECHO program) chemotherapy using 50–70 mg/m^2 of adriamycin, 1.5 mg vincristine, and 0.75–1.2 g/m^2 cyclophosphamide on day 1. VP 16–213, 75–120 mg/m^2, was given on days 3, 4, 5, and 6. Treatment was completed on day 8 by 1.5 mg vincristine. If the patient entered remission, he was placed on a maintenance protocol (ECHO and ECHO prime) for 3 months during which he underwent three treatment cycles combining adriamycin (40 mg/m^2), cyclophosphamide (500 mg/m^2), and vincristine (1.5 mg) on day 1, followed by VP 16–213 (50 mg/m^2) on days 3, 4, and 5. Each cycle ended with vincristine (1.5 mg) on day 8. This is, therefore, the same as the ECHO treatment at lower doses. "PRIME" therapy was initiated if the patients continued in remission.

This protocol consisted of 100 mg/m² *pro*carbazine orally on days 1–10, 1,000 mg/m² *i*fosfamide on days 1–5, and 50 mg/m² i.v. *me*thotrexate on day 1.

Evaluation

Partial remission was defined as reduced tumor volume, equal or superior to 50% of the product resulting from multiplication of two perpendicular diameters, and when no new lesions occurred. Disease was considered to evolve if all lesions increased by 25% or more, or if new lesions were observed. Evaluation of nutritional state was based on weight and general appearance as judged by the Karnofsky scale.

Results

Disease-Free Survival

Patient characteristics are shown in Table 1. We have been unable to show any significant difference for survival time for patients up to this point in time (Fig. 1 and Table 2). Ten patients receiving chemotherapy and PIVN were in complete remission at the end of three courses of treatment. Two patients did not respond to treatment and died. Nine of 20 patients in the control group were in complete remission after three courses of treatment, while three others have died as a result of progressive disease. Results for the two groups are superimposable due to a comparable number of patients in each group; 33% of patients are still alive 15 months after the beginning of the treatment. After 1 year of treatment, 8 of 19 PIVN patients are still in complete remission compared to 7 of 20 patients in the control group.

Effects on Patient Weight

There was no significant difference in weight between the two groups (Table 3). It should be noted that those patients who did not respond to treatment lost at least 3 kg per therapeutic cycle. However, weight loss of partially responding patients was only

Table 1. Patient characteristics

	Parenteral nutrition	No parenteral nutrition
Sex: Female	1	0
Male	14	16
Age: Median	54	56
(years) Range	40–68	42–69
Performance status:		
Ambulatory	11	12
Non ambulatory	4	4

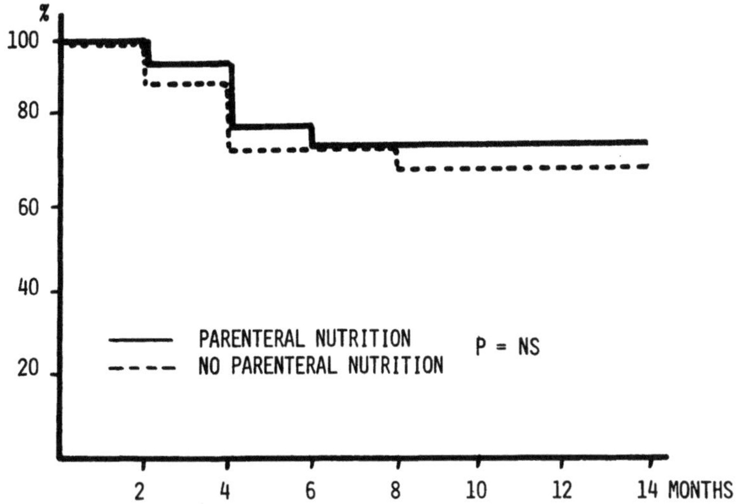

Fig. 1. Survival time for patients with oat cell lung carcinoma

Table 2. Clinical evaluation after 6 months of treatment

	Parenteral nutrition	No parenteral nutrition
Number of evaluable patients	15	16
Complete remission	7	6
Partial remission	3	3
No change	2	4
Progression	2	3
Relapse:		
Local	0	0
Metastatic	1	0

Table 3. Weight evaluation

	Parenteral[+] nutrition			No parenteral[+] nutrition		
	a	b	c	a	b	c
Weight gain (> 3 kg)	2	2		1	2	
No change (± 3 kg)	4	4		3	3	
Weight loss (> 3 kg)			3		3	4

a, Complete remission; b, Partial remission; c, No change and/or progressive disease
[+] Number of patients by groups

Table 4. Echo program: Effects of parenteral nutrition on chemotherapy induced myelosuppression

	Parenteral nutrition	No parenteral nutrition
No. patients/No. courses	15/42	16/45
Nadir median WBC/mm^3	700 ± 100	800 ± 170
Nadir median platelets × $10^3/mm^3$	80 ± 10	70 ± 20

p, Not significant

Table 5. Echo program: Median duration (days) of myelosuppression

	Parenteral nutrition	No parenteral nutrition
WBC ⩽ 1,000/mm^3	9 ± 2	10 ± 3
Platelets ⩽ 100,000/mm^3	8 ± 1	9 ± 2

p, Not significant

observed in the group not receiving PIVN. Patients who are presently in remission have not only avoided a weight loss, but have gained weight.

Toxicity

Concerning bone marrow toxicity, there was no significant difference in the nadirs of the two groups (Table 4). No significant difference was observed for the median duration of myelosuppression for the two groups (Table 5) or recuperation time for white cells and platelets. In the evaluation of toxicity to the digestive tract, no significant difference was noted between the two groups.

Complications

No major complication was associated with PIVN treatment. There were no incidences of sepsis, phlebitis, or complications linked to lipid administration.

Discussion

Results for survival time are still preliminary. However, the number of patients in the study is relatively high and an average of 12 months have passed since the study was begun. Results so far show that there is no significant difference between chemotherapy and chemotherapy-PIVN groups, thus, confirming our previous results

[30]. There was no significant difference between the complications for the two groups, particularly those associated with myelosuppression as a result of chemotherapy.

Our results suggest that our PIVN protocol was not quantitatively aggressive enough, since we employed only 1,550 kcal per day and only on days where chemotherapy was administered. It is also possible that PIVN does not remarkably ameliorate tumors particularly sensitive to chemotherapy. In fact, some results reported in the literature based on both experimental and clinical findings [1, 17; Kisner, personal communication] suggest that, under certain conditions, parenteral nutrition may facilitate tumor growth. This in turn could conceivably bring a greater number of cells into the cell cycle thereby augmenting the efficacy of a given chemotherapeutic agent. Perhaps parenteral nutrition would present a greater interest for tumors which are considerably chemoresistant or characterized by few cells in the cycle as opposed to those with many cells in the cycle and therefore particularly chemosensitive. These questions should be approached by randomized trials, particularly for digestive tract and epidermoid tumors. On the other hand, in vitro tests, such as clonogenic assay [10], may prove to be of considerable help in evaluating the role of nutrients in tumor cell growth, and potential in vitro response to different drugs.

These results suggest a very special role for randomized trials which have led us to entirely different results than those which we previously noted for various tumors in nonrandomized trials. This could also explain the different conclusions presented by certain research groups. At present, our results parallel those of Valdivieso et al. [17, 31] who employed a more aggressive parenteral nutrition (in terms of calories and increased frequency of administration) for the same type of patient using the same chemotherapeutic protocol.

In conclusion, it seems to us that simple and inexpensive parenteral nutrition can be administered through a peripheral vein during chemotherapy. This type of therapy can be given to the ambulatory patient, representing an undeniable advantage. Parenteral nutrition does not seem to ameliorate chemotherapeutic efficacy to particularly chemosensitive tumors. Our results and those in the literature suggest that cell cycle manipulation by parenteral nutrition be evaluated both in vitro and with well-executed randomized trials. The possibility that the cell cycle can be manipulated by parenteral nutrition should not be overlooked and the immunologic impact of this treatment should be kept in mind. Finanlly, it is clear that we should orient our approach toward qualitative rather than a quantitative nutrition. The role of each nutrient should be carefully examined to ascertain if it acts on the immune response or on the tumor cell cycle. It has already been shown that amino acids [16], lipids [11, 12, 24, 25], sugars and insulin [18, 32], vitamins [19], zinc [8, 22], as well as other nutrients can, under certain circumstances, act on a given function to yield results which can appear contradictory.

In our minds, it is not a question of whether parenteral nutrition represents a useful therapeutic tool, but rather a reorientation and expansion of complementary therapy which may play a major role in tumor pharmacology in the years to come.

References

1. Cameron IL, Pavlat WA (1976) Stimulation of growth of a transplantable hepatoma in rats by parenteral nutrition. J Natl Cancer Inst 56: 597–607

2. Ching N, Mills C, Grossi C (1978) The maintenance of optimal nutritional status in chemotherapy treatment. Proc Am Soc Clin Oncol 19: C-49
3. Copeland EM, Macfadyen BV, Lanzotti VJ, Dudrick SJ (1971) Intravenous hyperalimentation as an adjunct to cancer chemotherapy. Am J Surg 129: 167–173
4. Copeland EM, Macfadyen BV, Durdrick SJ (1976) Effect of intravenous hyperalimentation on established delayed hypersensibility in cancer patient. Ann Surg 184: 60–64
5. Cuttner J, Glidewell O, Holland J (to be published) A controlled trial of chemoimmunotherapy in acute myelocytic leukemia (AML). In: Terry WD (ed) Immunotherapy of cancer: Present status of trials in man. Elsevier North-Holland, New York Oxford
6. Daly JM, Copeland EM, Dudrick SJ (1978) Effects of intravenous nutrition on tumor growth and host immunocompetence in malnourished animals. Surgery 84: 655–658
7. Douglas SD, Schopfer K (1976) Analytical review: Host defense mechanisms in protein-energy malnutrition. Clin Immunol Immunopathol 5: 1–5
8. Fraker PJ, Depasquale-Jardieu P, Zwickl CM (1978) Regeneration of T cell helper function in zinc-deficient adult mice. Proc Natl Acad Sci 75: 5660–5664
9. Gertner MH, Mullen JL, Buzby GP (1978) Evaluation of nutrition and immunocompetence in cancer and noncancer patients. Proc Am Soc Clin Oncol 19: C-150
10. Hamburger AW, Salmon SE (1977) Primary bioassay of human tumor stem cells. Science 199: 461–471
11. Heiniger HJ, Brunner KT, Cerottini JC (1978) Cholesterol is a critical cellular component for T lymphocyte cytotoxicity. Proc Natl Acad Sci 75: 5683–5687
12. Humphries GMK, MacConnell HM (1979) Potent immunosuppression by oxidized cholesterol. J Immunol 122: 121–126
13. Issell BF, Valdivieso M, Zaren HA (1978) Protection against chemotherapy toxicity by IV hyperalimentation. Cancer Treat Rep 62: 1139–1143
14. Jones S, Salmon S, Haskins C (to be published) Chemoimmunotherapy of non-Hodgkin's lymphoma. In: Terry WD (ed) Immunotherapy of cancer: Present status of trials in man. Elsevier North-Holland, New York Oxford
15. Jordan WM, Valdivieso M, Freeman M (1979) Importance of nutritional assessment and pre-chemotherapy hyperalimentation in adenocarcinoma of the lung. Proc Am Soc Clin Oncol 20: C-497
16. Jose DG, Good RA (1973) Quantitative effects of nutritional essential amino acid deficiency upon immune response to tumors in mice. J Exp Med 137: 1–12
17. Kisner D (to be published) Nutrition and lung carcinoma. Recent Results Cancer Res
18. Kisner D, Hamosh M, Blecher M (1978) Malignant cachexia: Insulin resistance and insulin receptors. Proc Am Assoc Cancer Res 19: 796
19. Krishnan S, Bhuyan UN, Talwar GP (1975) Role of vitamin A and protein-calorie undernutrition in immunity and infection. In: Talwar GP (ed) Regulation of growth and differentiated function in eukaryote cells. Raven Press, New York, pp 283–286
20. Lanzotti VJ, Copeland EM, George SL, Dudrick SJ (1975) Cancer chemotherapeutic response and intravenous hyperalimentation. Cancer Chemother Rep 59: 437–439
21. Macdonald JS, Schein PS (1976) Mechanisms and management of malnutrition status in patients with cancer. Clin Gastroenterol 5: 809–826
22. MacMahon LJ, Montgomery DW, Guschewsky A (1976) In vitro effects of zinc chloride on spontaneous sheep red blood cell (E) rosette formation by lymphocytes from cancer patients and normal subjects. Immunol Commun 5: 53–67
23. Pouillart P, Palangic T, Huguenin P, Morin P, Gauthier H, Baron A, Mathe G, Ledendente A, Botto G (1978) Cancers épidermoides bronchiques inopérables. Etude de la signification pronostique de l'état immunitaire et résultats d'un essai d'immunorestauration par BCG. Nouv Presse Med 7: 265–267
24. Ryan JL, Shinitzly M (1979) Possible role for glycosphingolipids in the control of immune response. Eur J Immunol 3: 171–175

25. Schlager SI, Ohanian SM (1979) A role for fatty acid composition of complex cellular lipids in the susceptibility tumor cells to humoral immune killing. Proc Am Assoc Cancer Res 20: 311
26. Serrou B, Cupissol D (to be published) Nutritional support and the immune system in cancer management. A critical review. Cancer Treat Rep
27. Serrou B, Joyeux H, Dubois JB, Cupissol D, Solassol C (1979) Pilot study of peripheral intravenous nutrition in patients bearing solid tumors: A simple and valuable adjunct to chemotherapy. Proc Am Soc Clin Oncol 20: 48
28. Serrou B, Cupissol D, Favier C (1979) Phases 1 and 2 study of peripheral intravenous nutrition in patients bearing solid tumors. Med Oncol 2: 148
29. Serrou B, Cupissol D, Favier C (to be published) Peripheral intravenous nutrition as a potential adjunct to chemotherapy in patients bearing advanced solid tumors
30. Serrou B, Cupissol C, Plagne R, Boutin P, Chollet P, Carcassonne Y, Michel FB (to be published) Total parenteral nutrition as an adjunct to chemotherapy in small cell anaplastic lung carcinoma. Cancer Treat Rep
31. Valdivieso M (to be published) Evaluation of intensive chemotherapy and nutritional support in patients with small cell bronchogenic carcinoma. Cancer Treat Rep
32. Weiss J (1957) Experience with insulin and a low carbohydrate diet in incurable cancer patients. Med Klin 52: 1190–1191

VI. Melanoma

40. *Clinical Trials of Chemotherapy and Chemoimmunotherapy in Primary Malignant Melanoma*

C. Jacquillat, P. Banzet, and J. Maral*

Unité de Chimiothérapie, Institut de Recherches sur les Mélanomes Malins, Lariboisière Saint-Louis, 2 Place du Docteur Fournier, F-75475 Paris Cedex 10, France

Summary

We report here two randomized prospective clinical trials of adjuvant treatment in the management of primary malignant melanoma of Clark's level III, IV or V. All patients had curative resection of the primary tumor. In the first trial, 117 patients were randomized between control (surgery alone) systemic chemotherapy and intraarterial chemotherapy. Intraarterial chemotherapy consisted of DTIC 80 mg/m^2 + 8 days prior to surgery. Systemic chemotherapy consisted of courses of vinblastine (6 mg/m^2), thiotepa (6 mg/m^2), rufocromycine (60 µg/m^2), methotrexate (15 mg/m^2) on day 1, and procarbazine (30 mg/m^{12} × 7 days. Courses were repeated every 2 weeks × 6, then every 4 weeks × 15. Twenty-two of 55 patients relapsed in the control group versus 22 of 67 in the chemotherapy group (NS). For male patients, the difference in disease-free survival was significant ($P < 0.005$, log rank test), though not in women.
In the second trial, 352 patients were entered from July, 1976. Men were randomized between chemotherapy and chemoimmunotherapy. Women were randomized between surgery alone and chemoimmunotherapy. Chemotherapy was identical, except for the addition of DTIC (300 mg/m^2) for each course. Immunotherapy consisted of BCG every 4 weeks and *C. parvum* every week. Immunotherapy seemed to be of no additional benefit.

Introduction

The majority of patients with malignant melanoma die within 10 years from dissemination of the disease. The survival rate of patients with level II–V melanoma (Clark's classification) [2] is 70% to 25% at 5 years. In these patients, adjuvant

---

* For the Groupe de Recherches sur les Mélanomes Malins. Participating members: Aliaga, Boniche, Auclerc, Banzet, Banzet, Barrade, Biron, Belaich, Blanchet, Bonnet, Blanc, Brouaire, Cesarini, Chastang, Civatte, Cottenot, Cristo, Davan, Desprez, Curely, Dufourmentel, Edelstein, Fournier, Gauci, Goguel, Horay, Houdard, Izrael, Jacquillat, Jourdain, Lassau, Laurent, Lecam, Lepine, Maral, Najean, Noury, Duperrat, Palangier, Pecking, Picard, Pompidou, Reaux, Puissant, Real, Serrou, Texier, Trigalo, and Well

Recent Results in Cancer Research, Vol. 80

treatment, which could control subclinical metastases present at the time of primary treatment, may be expected to improve overall survival and lengthen the disease-free interval. We undertook two successive randomized trials on patients with localized primary malignant melanoma of level III, IV, or V. In the first trial, patients were treated by chemotherapy including currently available drugs of demonstrated activity against this type of malignancy [4], or a combination of vinblastine, thiotepa, methotrexate, rufocromycine and procarbazine [1]. When possible, DTIC was administered by intraarterial infusion [5].

In our second trial, chemotherapy was identical except for the addition of DTIC, which is now available in France. Immunotherapy by immunopotentiating agents, such as BCG and *C. parvum,* which may increase the immunocompetence and thereby improve progression, was used in half of the patients [3].

Patients and Methods

Patients with primary cutaneous malignant melanoma free of metastases of level III, IV, or V, either of the superficial spreading or the nodular type, were entered in the studies. Between April, 1973, and June, 1976, 117 patients were entered in our first trial (2-NK-73). They were stratified into two groups for randomization according to whether the site could or could not be treated by intraarterial infusion. These patients were randomized between control (surgery alone), systemic chemotherapy, and, eventually, intraarterial chemotherapy.

Between July, 1976, and December, 1979, 352 patients were entered into our second trial (4-NK-76). They were stratified according to histologic type, level, age, and site. Randomization depended on the sex of the patient: Men were randomized between chemotherapy and chemotherapy plus immunotherapy; women were randomized between control (surgery alone) and chemoimmunotherapy.

Intraarterial chemotherapy of 2-NK-73 patients consisted of infusion of vincristine (1 mg/m^2) as a synchronization agent on day 1, then, 2 days later, DTIC (80 mg/m^2 $\times$ 5 days) was given. This schedule was performed twice before surgery. All patients had a wide excision of the primary with split-thickness skin graft. Prophylactic lymph node dissections were not performed.

Systemic chemotherapy of 2-NK-73 patients was started 1 month after surgery and included IV vinblastine (60 mg/m^2), thiotepa (60 mg/m^2), rufocromycin (60 μg/m^2) and methotrexate (30 mg/m^2) on day 1 and procarbazine (30 mg/2/d $\times$ 7 days). These courses were repeated every 2 weeks for the first 3 months, then every 4 weeks for a total of 18 months.

Chemotherapy of 4-NK-76 patients was identical except for the addition of DTIC (300 mg/m^2 i.v.) on day 1 of each course.

Immunotherapy of 4-NK-76 patients coinsisted of 0.1 ml BCG (Institut Pasteur) intradermally on all four limbs every 4 weeks and 2 ml *C. parvum* (Institut Mérieux) s.c.

The major end-point of our trial was treatment failure, defined by local recurrence or metastatic disease.

Statistical computer analysis was performed by the actuarial life-table method, and the log rank test.

Results

2-NK-73

Trial 2-NK-73, was to study the effect of chemotherapy versus surgery alone, and the possible additional benefit of intraarterial chemotherapy in patients with limb melanoma. In these patients disease-free survival rate curves showed no difference between patients treated by intraarterial infusion (seven relapses in 23 patients) and those treated by systemic chemotherapy alone (four relapses in 15 patients). Therefore, in all the following results we combined the two chemotherapy groups with or without intraarterial infusion.

During follow-up, 22 of 55 patients in the control group and 22 of 62 patients in the chemotherapy group relapsed.

The difference between the disease-free survival rate curves is not significant (Fig. 1).

When we studied the prognosis factors and their incidence on the effect of therapy, we found that sex seemed an important factor. For men patients, there is a great difference between the disease-free survival rates of patients treated with chemotherapy (90% at 2 years) and surgery alone (60% at 2 years); however, this was not significant (the number of patients being too small) (Fig. 2). On the contrary, for women patients there is no difference (Fig. 3). This may be due to bias of skewed randomization (in our first trial the patients were not stratified according to prognosis factors). To eliminate this influence, we performed the log rank test in all patients, stratified according to prognostic factors (sex, histologic type, histologic level, and site), and found a significant difference in favor of chemotherapy ($\chi^2 = 4.12$, $P < 0.05$), especially for male patients ($\chi^2 = 4.2$, $P < 0.05$).

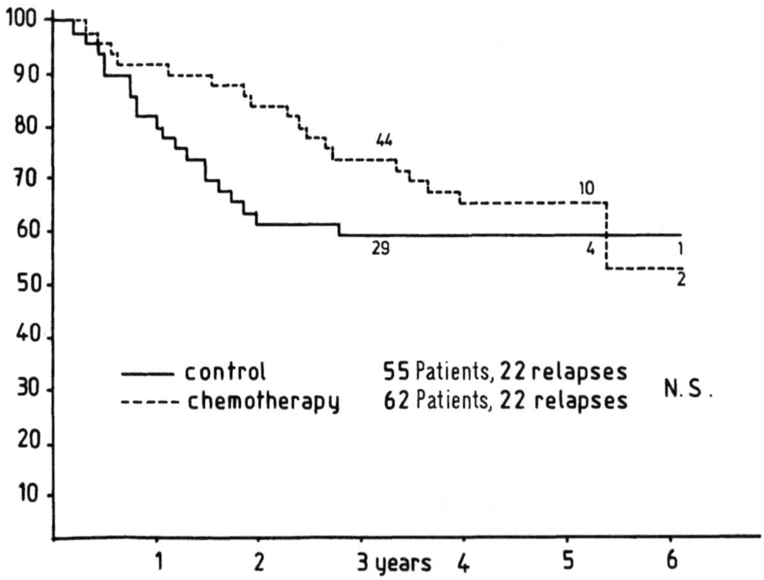

Fig. 1. 2 NK 73: Disease-free survival according to treatment

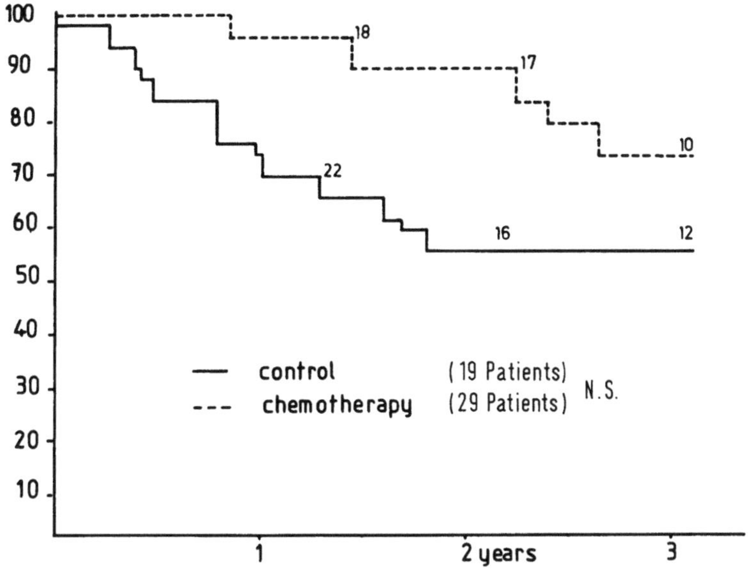

Fig. 2. 2 NK 73: Disease-free survival of men according to treatment

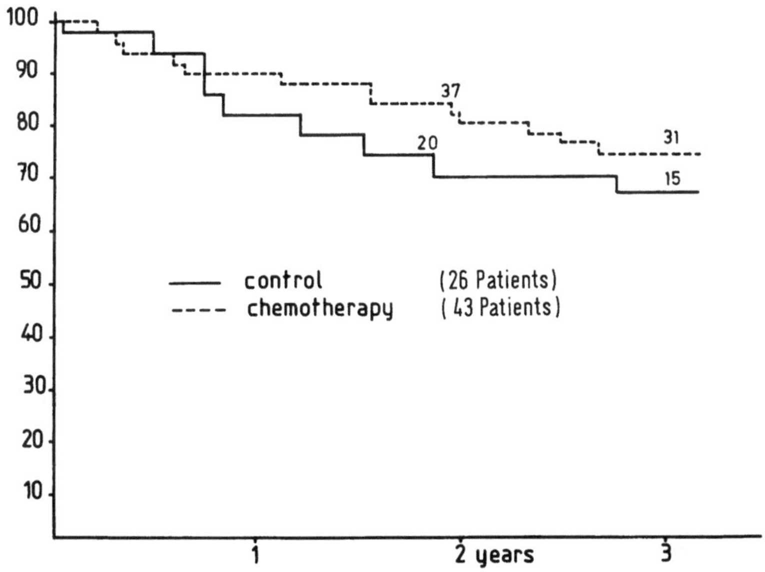

Fig. 3. 2 NK 73: Disease-free survival of women according to treatment

4-NK-76

In this study, 352 patients have been entered to date and, during the period of follow-up, 43 patients have had a recurrence. The overall disease-free period is 68% at 2 years, equivalent to that of 2-NK-73. All men were treated with adjuvant treatment, either chemotherapy (21 relapses in 78 patients) or chemoimmunotherapy (16 relapses in 79 patients).

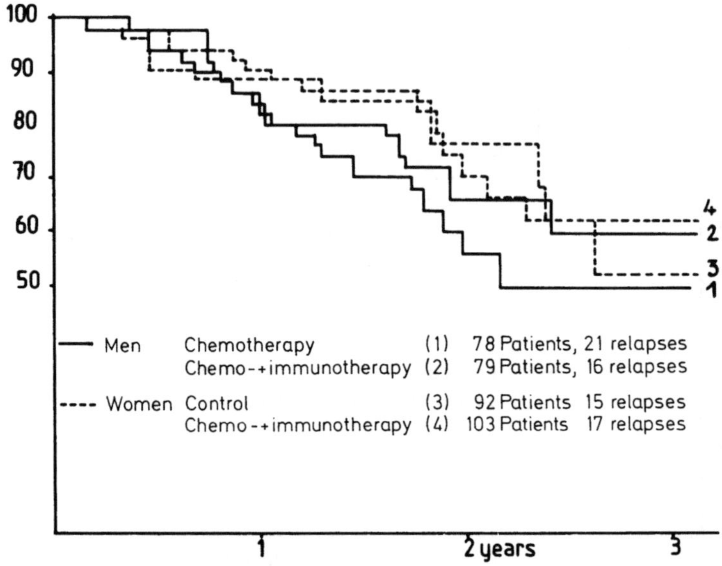

Fig. 4. 4 NK 76: Disease-free survival according to treatment

The disease-free rate curves showed no significant difference (at 2 years 60% and 68%, respectively).
For female patients, our previous trial did not show a significant benefit of chemotherapy and they were randomized between control (92 patients, 15 recurrences) and chemoimmunotherapy (103 patients, 17 relapses). The disease-free survival rate curves did not show a significant difference (at 2 years 70% and 75%, respectively) (Fig. 4).

Conclusion

Adjuvant treatment, as we performed it, may be of some benefit in lengthening the disease-free interval of patients with primary malignant melanoma. However, it seems to be only effective in male patients. Immunotherapy did not significantly improve the prognosis of malignant melanoma patients.

References

1. Banzet P, Jacquillat Cl, Civatte J (1978) Adjuvant chemotherapy in the management of primary malignant melanoma. Cancer 41: 1240–1248
2. Clark WH, From L, Bernardino EA, Mihm MC. The histogenic and biological behaviour of primary human malignant melanoma of the skin.
3. Gutterman JO, Mavligit G, Reed R, Richman S, Mc Bride CE, Hersh EM (1975) Immunology and immunotherapy of human malignant melanoma: historic review and perspective of the future. Sem Oncol 2: 155–174
4. Luce JK (1972) Chemotherapy of malignant melanoma. Cancer 30: 1604–1605
5. Stehlin JS, Chark RL, Vickers WE, Monges A (1963) Perfusion for malignant melanoma of the extremities. Am J Surg 105: 607–614

41. *Trial 6: Randomized Study of Prolonged Chemotherapy, Immunotherapy, and Chemoimmunotherapy as an Adjuvant to Surgery for Stage I and II Melanoma: A Progress Report**

G. Beretta**

Ospedale San Carlo, WHO Melanoma Group, Via Venezian 1, I-20133 Milan, Italy

Summary

WHO clinical trial 6 studies the effect of long-term adjuvant therapy (chemotherapy, immunotherapy, and chemoimmunotherapy) after radical surgery in malignant melanoma with high risk of recurrence. The randomized study has been running for 67 months with 845 patients. This intermediate report seems to indicate that, concerning the relapse-free period, adjuvant treatment appears superior to surgery alone. However, no significant difference in the duration of survival is evident among the four treatment groups.

Introduction

Due to the unsatisfactory prognosis of patients with malignant melanoma of the skin and/or locoregional node metastases (N+) after radical surgery (5-year survival rate of about 15–20%, and 80% relapse rate within 2 years), we the sixth WHO clinical trial. In 1974 the WHO Collaborating Centres for Evaluation of Methods of Diagnosis and Treatment of Melanoma began a controlled randomized study comparing three long-term medical treatments after radical surgery in malignant melanoma with high risk of recurrence (all stage II and stage I primary in the trunk with Clark's level 3–5) [7].

The adjuvant treatments dacarbazine (DTIC) and/or BCG were selected due to activity of both compounds against malignant melanoma in different clinical situations [3, 4].

Patients and Methods

According to the original protocol of trial 6 [7], adequate surgery is the basic requirement for patient entry: The primary melanoma must be removed with at least

* Supported by NIH-NCI, Bethesda (Contract N01-CM-43726)

** For Melanoma Group. Participating members: P. Rümke, R. Tomin, Z. Mechl, F. Lejeune, B. Kiss, A. Kulakowski, A. Cochran, R. McKie, J. Adamus, H. H. Peter, C. Aubert, E. Bajetta, G. Beretta, G. Bonadonna, N. Cascinelli, A. Morabito, U. Veronesi, J. Priario, J. Durand, J. De Marsillac, R. L. Ikonopoisov, and G. W. Milton

Recent Results in Cancer Research, Vol. 80

3 cm skin incision in healthy tissues, including the underlying muscular fascia; all the regional lymph nodes must be removed according the criteria of radical surgery. All patients with primary melanoma of the skin located in the head and neck, trunk, or extremities areas are eligible, provided that they present at nodal dissection lymph node metastases (N+, or stage II). Also cases showing N− (stage I) are included if the originate in the trunk and are histologically classified as 3−5 Clark's level.

Only patients geographically accessible and providing informed consent are included.

Subjects are not accepted if presenting any one of the following: fixed lymph nodes; in-transit metastases; previous cytotoxic chemotherapy treatments; being less than 15 or greater than 75 years of age; other concomitant tumors; major allergic or systemic (cardiovascular, hepatic, renal, pulmonary, or metabolic) diseases.

The patients are defined as untreated cases (including those having had an excisional biopsy within 6 weeks) and previously treated cases (radical surgery more than 6 weeks before randomization, or in whom a previous excision of primary melanoma has been followed by the appearance of regional lymph node metastases leading to further radical surgery).

At entry, the patients are stratified according to sex, site of primary melanoma, nodal involvement (N+ or N−), and whether then had prior surgery. Then the patients, all free of disease after radical surgery, are randomized into four groups to receive: no further treatment (controls); DTIC by i.v. bolus at daily dose of 200 mg/m^2 for 5 consecutive days every 4 weeks; BCG, by multipuncture Sterneedle (Heaf gun) technique (four shots 2 mm deep) into of one of the extremities in clockwise rotation, in two-vial doses (Pasteur, lyophilized vaccine) each containing $1.6 \pm 0.8 \times 10^8$ living bacterial units, weekly or monthly in the case of positive skin reaction; DTIC plus BCG in the same doses and modalities as above, with BCG given on the day 5 after starting DTIC.

Courses of adjuvant treatments had to be started 10−30 days after surgery, and repeated every 4 weeks for 2 years or until relapse is documented. A dose modification of DTIC in the presence of myelosuppression and of BCG in the case of excessive skin reaction was adopted as previously reported [1, 5, 7].

The follow-up is performed with the same modality in all four patient groups. It consists of physical examinations and blood counts (monthly), routine laboratory tests and chest X-rays (every 2−3 months), other special examinations, such as liver and brain scan or skeletal survey (whenever indicated by the clinical situation, and in all cases after 2 years of observation).

The end point of the study is considered at the first evidence of the treatment failure (locoregional or distantly recurrent disease). After recurrence, a detailed description of further treatments and responses and the time and cause of the eventual death are reported.

Results

Substantial data related to the patient accrual, the characteristics of the collected case material, and the toxicity can now be given, while only preliminary results concerning the clinical activity and the survival are available. From June 15, 1974, to January 15, 1980, 845 patients were randomized from 16 collaborating centers. The patient accrual per year is shown in Table 1.

Table 1. Patient accrual per year

Year	No. of cases
1974	43
1975	148
1976	181
1977	179
1978	160
1979	124
1980	10
Total	845

Table 2. Characteristics of 845 randomized patients according to stratification parameters

	Controls	DTIC	BCG	DTIC + BCG	Total
Total patients	193	226	206	220	845
Males	118	128	119	132	497
Females	75	98	87	88	348
Limbs, head, and neck	95	122	101	107	425
Trunk (N+)	65	70	70	80	285
Trunk (N−)	33	34	35	33	135
Untreated	103	118	101	109	431
Previous surgery	90	108	105	111	414

The Table 2 describes the collected case material according to the stratification parameters and treatments. The patient distribution among the treatment groups shows no significant difference at statistical analysis.

Of the randomized patients, 745 or 88.1% are considered evaluable for the present report.

The toxicity produced by the adjuvant treatments is limited and easily manageable (Table 3). After DTIC plus BCG, nausea and vomiting of short duration (1−2 days) are very commonly seen, while leukopenia is less than 10%, and thrombocytopenia is less than 5%. These side effects have not significantly modified the planned treatments in the majority of patients. Also the skin reactions to BCG administration have been well-tolerated and easily managed. No differences in toxicity, either additive or reductive, have been associated up to now with the use of combined DTIC-BCG, in comparison with the single-agent treatments.

The average follow-up is still 32 months and it will not substantially change due to the homogeneous patient accrual. The estimated time to recurrence and the mortality of the evaluable population in relation to different treatments is reported in Table 4.

The actuarial analysis indicates that, if we consider the time to recurrence in general, the disease-free interval from radical surgery to relapse is longer in the groups

Table 3. Side effects reported in the form according to treatments in 745 evaluable patients

	Controls (169)	DTIC (204)	BCG (182)	DTIC + BCG (190)
Myelosuppression				
Leukopenia	–	13	–	21
Thrombocytopenia	–	6	–	8
Gastrointestinal	–	62	4	56
Fever	–	2	6	7
Liver toxicity	–	1	2	3

Table 4. Time (days) to recurrence and mortality (actuarial analysis) according to treatments

	Controls	DTIC	BCG	DTIC + BCG
Cumulative proportion of relapsing patients				
25%	155	191	228	182
50%	355	730	620	483
75%	1,095	> 1,095	> 1,095	> 1,095
Rate of recurrence at 36 months	75%	58%	64%	72%
Cumulative proportion of dying patients				
25%	392	374	474	401
50%	730	> 1,022	1,022	912
75%	NR[a]	NR	NR	NR
Survival rate at 36 months	35%	53%	48%	49%

[a] Not reached

receiving the adjuvant treatments compared with the untreated controls. This difference is statistically significant only if we compare the adjuvant DTIC and the untreated controls.

Table 4 shows how the apparent favorable effect on the relapse-free period produced by the adjuvant therapy is presently not able to produce a difference in the survival of the four groups. This result does not change if we analyze separately the stage I or II patients.

Moreover, the evaluation of the patterns of relapse shows no differences in the four groups in relation to the sites of recurrences either local or distant as well as considering the brain metastases. After relapse, the response rate is very poor with any treatment, especially in the patients progressing after adjuvant DTIC plus BCG therapy.

Conclusion

Previous reports at meetings of the WHO Melanoma Group [8, 9] and a few open conferences [1, 2, 6, 10] have discussed the present status of clinical trial 6. It must be stressed that this study is still in a phase of active recruitment of case material, so the data reported should be considered as very preliminary and susceptible to changes. The clinical results have yet to be reassessed with a careful analysis of all entered cases, and with separate evaluation of the different patient subsets.

Also other parameters, such as the skin reaction to BCG and myelosuppression, versus the recurrences, and moreover other factors which are of possible importance, such as the number of involved nodes or the histologic characteristic of the primary or nodal tumors, have to be more deeply analyzed. To date, the number of entered patients appears nearly adequate for an initial, more consistent exploration of data can be forecast for early 1981.

References

1. Beretta G (1978) Controlled study for prolonged chemotherapy, immunotherapy, and chemotherapy plus immunotherapy as an adjuvant to surgery in stage I–II malignant melanoma: Preliminary report. In: Terry WD, Windhorst D (eds) Immunotherapy of cancer: Present status of trials in man. Progress in cancer research and therapy. Raven Press, New York, pp 65–72
2. Beretta G (1980) Randomized study of prolonged chemotherapy, immunotherapy and chemoimmunotherapy as an adjuvant to surgery for stage I and II malignant melanoma (trial 6). Second International Conference 'Immunotherapy of cancer: present status of trials in man', Bethesda, April 28–30, 1980, Abstract, p 8
3. Comis RL, Carter SK (1974) Integration of chemotherapy into combined modality therapy of solid tumors. IV. Malignant melanoma. Cancer Treat Rep 1: 285–304
4. Gutterman JU, Mavligit G, McBride C, Frei E III, Freireich EJ, Hersh EM (1973) Active immunotherapy with BCG for recurrent malignant melanoma. Lancet 1: 1208–1212
5. Veronesi U, Beretta G (1979) Controlled study for prolonged chemotherapy, immunotherapy, and chemotherapy plus immunotherapy as an adjuvant to surgery in malignant melanoma (trial 6): Preliminary report. In: Recent Results Cancer Res 68: 325–379
6. Veronesi U, Bajetta E, Cascinelli N, Clemente C, Rilke F (1978) New trends in the treatment of malignant melanoma. Int Adv Surg Oncol 1: 113–116
7. WHO Collaborating Centres for Evaluation of Methods of Diagnosis and Treatment of Melanoma (1974) Controlled study for prolonged chemotherapy, immunotherapy and chemotherapy plus immunotherapy as an adjuvant to surgery (trial 6). WHO, Geneva
8. WHO Collaborating Centres for Evaluation of Methods of Diagnosis and Treatment of Melanoma (1974–1979) Newsletters 2–7. WHO, Geneva
9. WHO Collaborating Centres for Evaluation of Methods of Diagnosis and Treatment of Melanoma (1974–1979) Progress reports of the review meetings. WHO, Geneva
10. WHO Group for the Study of Melanoma. Priario JC, Borges JF, D'Auria A, Mate M (1979) Adjuvants to surgery in the treatment of malignant melanoma. In: Kumar S (ed) Clinical cancer, principal sites 1, vol 10. Proceedings of of the 12th International Cancer Congress, Buenos Aires 1978, Pergamon, Oxford New York, pp 57–65 (Advances in medical oncology, research and education)

42. *Current Status of Melanoma Chemotherapy and Immunotherapy**

B. M. Czarnetzki, E. Macher, H. Behrendt, and F. Lejeune

Dermatologische Klinik, von Esmarchstraße 56, D-4400 Münster, Germany

Summary

In the search for an improved prognosis in malignant melanoma after radical surgery, randomized trials are being conducted examining the results of immunostimulation (BCG or levamisole) with chemotherapy dimethyl – triazeno – imidazole – carboxamide (DTIC) in stage I melanoma. So far, no significant differences between the groups are evident. In stage III melanoma, a series of new agents are being rapidly screened and some appear promising. A closer look at the basic immunopathologic process during the growth of melanomas is might lead to a more effective control of this malignancy.

Introduction

Malignancies of the human melanocyte system belong to the group of cancers that have proven to be most resistant to therapeutic measures. Until now, the most effective treatment is surgical excision with a wide margin as early as possible in the natural evolution of the tumor. The notoriously bad prognosis of malignant melanoma relates to its potential releases microemboli of tumor cell early in its evolution. Attempts to improve prognosis have therefore focused on eliminating these small groups of metastasized tumor cells through immunotherapy or chemotherapy, after the major tumor burden has been removed by surgery.

Therapy of Stage I Melanoma

During the period of enthusiasm for the concept that immunologic mechanisms play a primary role in the control of malignant growth of cells, numerous studies were started to prove the benefit of vaccination with BCG or similar agents in patients with deep primary or metastatic melanomas. Although an improved prognosis (~ 25%) was

* This work was made possible by the help of Deutsche Krebshilfe. The secretarial assistance of Ms. B. Kampmann is gratefully acknowledged

Recent Results in Cancer Research, Vol. 80

apparent in a number of these trials during the first few years of observation [4], the overall long-term prognosis was not altered [2, 6].
In 1974, the EORTC Malignant Melanoma Cooperative Group initiated a trial (18741) to test the benefit of a 2-year vaccination program with lyophilized Pasteur BCG in patients with surgically removed malignant melanoma of Clark grade III or greater. This trial was abandoned because, due to ethical considerations, there were no unvaccinated controls. At the dermatology clinic in Münster, we have nevertheless compared 37 vaccinated with 36 nonvaccinated, nonrandomized patients with stage I ($\geq$ 1.5 mm thickness) malignant melanoma. Fig. 1 shows that the two groups do not differ significantly after 5 years of observation and, although results of such a nonrandomized trial must be interpreted with caution, the data resemble closely those obtained with other trials [6].
Currently, the EORTC has initiated a randomized study (protocol 18781) comparing the effectiveness of vaccination of melanoma patients treated with two different BCG preparations (Pasteur Institute and Rijks Instituut voor de Volksgesondheid) with a control group receiving no adjuvant therapy. Vaccination is to be extended over 3 years to increase the benefit seen during the first 2 years of vaccination in other studies. Also, the trial hopes to solve some of the controversies about the benefit of one vaccine versus another in cancer therapy. This EORTC trial has been started only recently and even preliminary results are not yet available.
Another EORTC study (18761) compared a group of patients treated with the enthusiastically promoted adjuvant levamisole with a group receiving placebo tablets, and with a third group given six monthly cycles of injections with DTIC (250 mg/m^2) on 5 consecutive days. More than 200 stage I patients have been entered into this trial (as of spring, 1980), but no significant differences in survival or disease-free interval between the groups have been observed so far. There has been one sudden death due to hepatic failure in the DTIC group, which occurred during the second cycle of injections and was associated with massive hepatic vein thrombosis and a marked eosinophilia [3]. Several similar cases have since been reported or personally

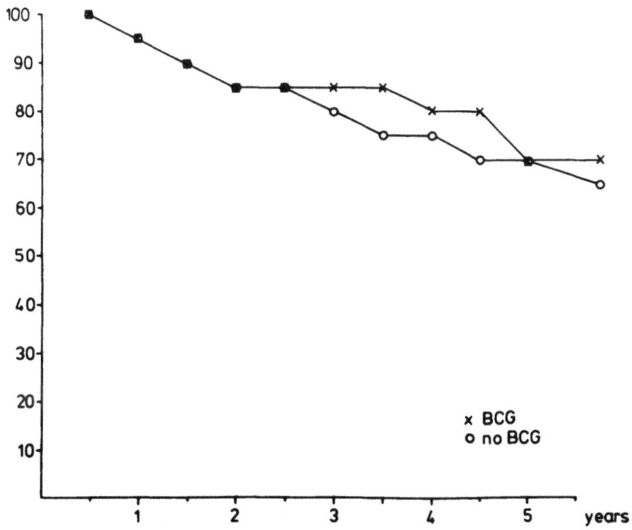

Fig. 1. Survival of stage I melanoma patients with $\geq$ 1.5 mm depth of invasion of the primary tumor. After surgery, 37 patients were vaccinated with BCG (———) and 36 patients served as controls (O———O)

communicated to us, and it is advised to carefully control peripheral eosinophil levels and liver enzymes to identify potential risk patients.

Therapy of Stage III Melanomas

While the therapy in patients with stage I melanoma is disappointing, the prognosis of these patients is still relatively good (Fig. 1) compared to the dismal prognosis of patients with metastatic melanoma. The best therapeutic results, apart from surgery, have been reported with the cytostatic agent dacarbazine (DTIC), with remission rates of about 25% [1]. All other more optimistic reports on trials with chemotherapeutic agents or with combinations of such agents have not withstood the test of extensive and prolonged investigations.

Realizing that the search for new and more effective chemotherapeutic agents is urgent, the EORTC melanoma group has decided to embark on a rapid screening program of new drugs in stage III melanoma patients. Vindesine (trial 18792) has been given to 23 patients, with only one questionable regression of measurable tumor mass, so that this trial has been discontinued. Twenty-four patients have been treated with N-phosphonoacetyl-L-aspartate (PALA), an inhibitor of aspartate transcarbamylase (trial 18793), four patients have so far been classified as responders. Side effects with this drug are mild and patient acceptance is high. More patients are being entered into this trial to see whether the early promising results can be maintained in a larger group. A trial testing a combination therapy of vindesine and cisplatinum (18802) has been started recently. Results are not yet available.

At the dermatology clinic in Münster, an extract of *Streptococcus pyogenes* with cytotoxic as well as adjuvant properties has been tested in eight patients with widespread metastases, with only one patient having entered complete remission. The extract is well-tolerated, but again, larger numbers of patients should be tested to see whether the drug offers any real advantage to the patients.

Alternative Approaches to Melanoma Therapy

The preceding discussion makes it very evident that, beyond surgical treatment, present therapy of malignant melanoma is unsatisfactory. Great hopes had been put into the search for specific immunologic alterations in melanoma patients to explain development and progression of the tumor, but these efforts have been disappointing. Current interest has reverted to nonspecific inflammatory events.

In the tissue surrounding malignant melanoma, a dense mononuclear infiltrate has been observed especially in areas of spontaneous regression. We have examined the cellular infiltrates of primary malignant melanomas by special staining methods and by electron microscopy and have noticed, besides macrophages, an unexpectedly high number of mast cells within the tumor and in the surrounding tissue. Fig. 2 shows a mast cell lying near a tumor cell, with many interlocking membranes allowing interaction between the cells. In one region, the mast cell is partly degranulated.

Mast cell granules have recently been shown to play a role in mediating tumor cell cytotoxicity via their peroxidases [5]. It remains to be seen whether this is indeed the role of these cells when in contact with tumor cells or whether they merely indicate an

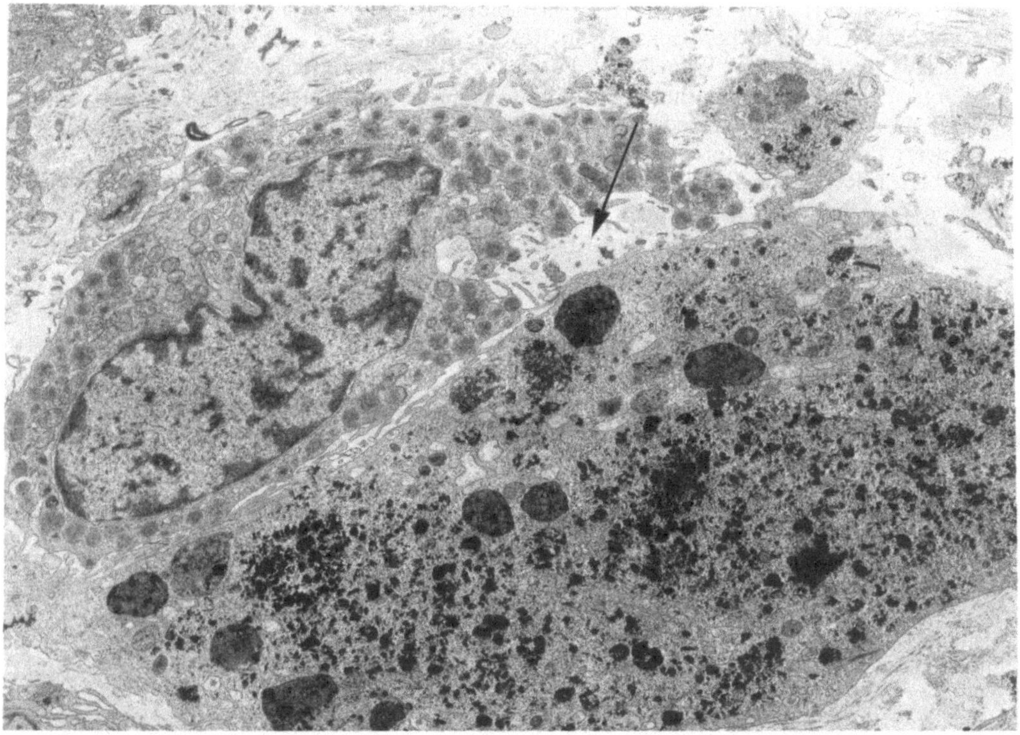

Fig. 2. Electron micrograph (× 10,500) showing a mast cell *(upper left)* closely attached to a tumor cell in a superficial spreading melanoma. Note the partial degranulation of the mast cell in the upper area of contact *(arrow)*

increased turnover of connective tissue in which mast cells are known to partake [7]. If indeed a beneficial role of mast cells could be demonstrated in the host's defense against the invading tumor, then an enhancement of this cell's activity might be a reasonable therapeutic goal.

Summing up, one must admit that the therapy, as well as the understanding of the biology of malignant melanoma is still at a very early stage, which is all the more a reason to investigate new pathways that may improve management of this tumor.

References

1. Carter SK (1976) Dacarbazine. Int J Dermatol 15: 59–63
2. Eilber FR, Morton DL, Holmes EC, Sparks FC, Ramming KP (1976) Adjuvant immunotherapy with BCG in treatment of regional lymph node metastases from malignant melanoma. N Engl J Med 294: 237–240
3. Frosch PF, Czarnetzki BM, Macher E, Grundmann E, Gottschalk I (1976) Hepatic failure in a patient treated with dacarbazine (DTIC) for malignant melanoma. J Cancer Res Clin Oncol 95: 281–286
4. Gutterman JU, McBride C, Freireich EJ, Mavligit G, Frei E, Hersh EM (1973) Active immunotheraply with BCG for recurrent malignant melanoma. Lancet 1: 1208–1212

5. Henderson WR, Jong EC, Chi EY, Klebanoff SJ (1980) Mast cell-mediated tumor cell cytotoxicity: Role of peroxidase. Clin Res 28:416
6. Pinsky CM, Hirshaut Y, Wanebo HJ, Fortner J, Mike V, Schottenfeld D, Oettgen HF (1978) Surgical adjuvant immunotherapy with BCG in patients with malignant melanoma. Results of a prospective randomized trial. In: Terry WD, Windhurs D (eds) Immunotherapy of cancer: Present status of trials in man. Raven Press, New York, p 27
7. Robinson RW, Likar IN, Likar LJ (1978) Mast cells in normal, aged and diseased arteries. Monogr Atheroscler 89:73–116

VII. Testicular Neoplasia

43. *Adjuvant Therapy of Testicular Carcinoma*

C. G. Schmidt

Innere Universitätsklinik und Poliklinik (Tumorforschung), Westdeutsches Tumorzentrum, Hufelandstrasse 55, D-4300 Essen, Germany

Introduction

Adjuvant chemotherapy could have a role in the management of stage I and II testicular tumors. The results presented in this paper deal with the treatment of stage II testicular tumors only.

The optimal management of patients with clinical stage II nonseminomatous testicular cancer has been a matter of controversy. Following orchiectomy most patients are subjected to bilateral lymphadenectomy. Unfortunately, this procedure is accompanied by considerable morbidity and serious side effects, such as ejaculatory disturbances.

The purpose of bilateral dissection of retroperitoneal lymph nodes is two-fold: It may be curative in early stage II disease and it serves to exactly define the extent of retroperitoneal lymph node involvement.

Patients and Methods

This report includes 140 patients with stage II, 68 with stage IIA, 40 with stage IIB, and 32 patients with stage IIC disease. All patients had histologic proof of testicular cancer after semicastration, and the histologic classification of Dixon and Moore [1] was used in most cases. The distribution of patients according to the extent of disease as defined by clinical and pathologic staging procedures is presented in Table 1. The clinical stage II (regional metastases) was subclassified as follows: biopsy-proven retroperitoneal metastases completely resectable at lymphadenectomy, with normal levels of (β-HCG, α-fetoprotein, and lactate dehydrogenase (LDH) 4 weeks after lymphadenectomy (stage IIA); minor residual disease (maximum diameter usually not exceeding 2–3 cm) after lymphadenectomy and/or positive markers 4 weeks after lymphadenectomy (stage IIB); and bulky residual abdominal disease, in most cases palpable, often with ureteral displacement (stage IIC).

It should be stated that although many authors are very precise with similar definitions of stage IIA–C disease, most of such classifications seem arbitrary. This also holds true for the separation of residual lymph node metastases with diameters below or above 2–3 cm, as necessary in the stage II subclassification used here. Some overlaps may occur between stages IIB and IIC. Stage IIA, however, should in all cases indicate

Recent Results in Cancer Research, Vol. 80

Table 1. Study criteria for the subclassification of stage II testicular carcinoma

Stage II Ragional lymphatic spread including tumor in the spermatic cord, iliac, inguinal, and/or periaortic nodes
Stage IIA Complete dissection of lymph nodes β-HCG, α-fetoprotein, and/or lactate dehydrogenase normal after lymphadenectomy
Stage IIB Minor irresectable abdominal disease (maximum diameter 2 cm) β-HCG, α-fetoprotein, or lactate dehydrogenase elevated after lymph node dissection
Stage IIC Advanced non-resectable abdominal disease (diameter > 2 cm) at laparotomy Palpable mass Ureteral displacement with or without obstructive uropathy Large abdominal mass, according to sonography after laparotomy

Table 2. Combination chemotherapy in stage III testicular cancer

Regimen A: Vinblastine (0.2 mg/kg i.v. daily × 2) plus bleomycin (30 units daily × 5, continuous infusion)

Regimen B: Adriamycin (60 mg/m^2 i.v.) plus DDP (20 mg/m^2 + 2,500 ml saline daily × 5)

Treatment (every 3–4 weeks)
Group I: A A B B A A B B A A B B
Group II: B B A A B B A A B B A A

	n	Complete remission	Partial remission	No change	Progressive disease
Group I	25	17 (68%)	6 (24%)	1 (4%)	1 (4%)
Group II	15	10 (67%)	2 (13%)	–	3 (20%)
Total	40	27 (68%)	8 (20%)	1 (2%)	4 (10%)

a clearly adjuvant clinical situation with no tumor present after lymphadenectomy (Table 1).

Thus far, adjuvant chemotherapy has only played a minor role in the treatment of stage II testicular cancer. However, this disease may be an ideal candidate for adjuvant chemotherapy because the disease tends to an early hematogenic spread and new effective chemotherapy has become available as shown by its efficacy in stage III disease.

The regimens currently used are mainly based on the synergistic combination of vinblastine and bleomycin, as originally reported by Samuels et al. [9], and on the additional effect of cis-dichlorodiammineplatinum (II) (DDP) [3]. At the West German Tumor Center (Essen) a sequential combination chemotherapy regimen including vinblastine, bleomycin, adriamycin (ADM), and DDP was studied [10], and was effective (Table 2).

The encouraging results of this sequential approach together with its low complication rate have been the rationale for its adjuvant application.

Table 3. Protocol for the treatment of stage II nonseminomatous testicular cancer every 4 weeks after laparotomy

Stage IIA	Stage IIB	Stage IIC
Two courses vinblastine/bleomycin (regimen A)		
Two courses adriamycin/DDP (regimen B)		
One course vinblastine/bleomycin (regimen A)		
One course adriamycin/DDP (regimen B)		
With or without irradiation to the bilateral paraaortic and homolateral ilioinguinal lymph nodes (3000–3600 rad)	Radiotherapy and/or second laparotomy only in individual cases Further chemotherapy for a minimum of another 6 months	

As outlined in Table 3, after laparotomy all patients were treated with chemotherapy for 6 months. In stage IIA, after complete transperitoneal lymph node dissection, this treatment was considered adequate with or without additional high-voltage irradiation to the bilateral paraaortic and homolateral ilioinguinal lymph nodes (3,000–3,600 rad). Stage IIB and IIC patients still showing disease after initial chemotherapy received radiotherapy (RT) or relaparotomy followed by further chemotherapy for a minimum of another 6 months. In stage IIB and IIC patients without evidence of disease, chemotherapy alone was continued up to a total of 12 months. After termination of chemotherapy all patients were followed-up at intervals of 6–8 weeks on an outpatient basis.

Out of a total of 68 stage IIA patients who all had initially received the sequence A-A-B-B-A-B chemotherapy at intervals of 4 weeks, 35 patients (nonrandomly assigned) were given additional RT to the bilateral paraaortic nodes and the homolateral iliac and inguinal lymph nodes (3,000–3,600 rad), starting 3 weeks after the last chemotherapy course.

As indicated in Table 3, all patients classified as stage IIB initially received the same chemotherapy sequence as described for stage IIA. Patients with persisting evidence of disease were then submitted to RT, and chemotherapy was continued at monthly intervals for a minimum of 6 months. During this period, chemotherapy had to be individualized in some patients, using dose reductions of the original regimens or a third combination (ifosfamide plus VP 16-213) depending on the individual toxicity.

Stage IIC patients were given sequential combination chemotherapy for at least 12 months. Bulky residual disease was resected in a second laparotomy whenever this was possible at the time of maximum chemotherapeutic response. Alternatively, some patients received local RT to bulky residual disease.

Results

The survival data of 68 patients with stage IIA, 40 patients with stage IIB, and 32 patients with stage IIC disease, who had all received sequential chemotherapy with vinblastine-bleomycin and ADM-cisplatin with or without RT as described are presented in Table 4 and Fig. 1. In addition, data on 34 patients surgically classified as stage I have been included. In this group, which has received no further treatment, the relapse-free survival time will be in the order of more than 90% after 4 years (median observation time is 24 months).

Stage IIA

The actuarial survival rate at 4 years after lymphadenectomy is 97% for the 35 patients who received both chemotherapy and RT and 87% in the group of 33 patients who received six sequential chemotherapy courses alone. These groups were not formed on a random basis and the differences are not statistically significant. No severe toxicity was encountered in these 68 patients. To this date, only three patients have relapsed, one in the combined modality and two in the chemotherapy-alone group. Interestingly, in both nonirradiated cases recurrent disease had involved both retroperitoneal nodes and visceral organs (Table 4) but it could not be decided which was the first site of relapse.

Table 4. Survival data for patients under chemotherapy with or without radiotherapy

Treated after OP and RND	Stage I No.	Stage IIA		Stage IIB	Stage IIC
		6 × Chemotherapy plus radiotherapy	6 × Chemotherapy	min. 12 × Chemotherapy ± radiotherapy	
Number of patients	34	35	33	40	32
Patients with ned	32/34 (94%)	34/35 (97%)	31/33 (94%)	34/40 (85%)	8/32 (25%)
Relapse					
Histology[a]					
II	1/10	1/14	0/13	3/14	13/17
III	0/12	0/4	0/6	1/7	6/6
IV	0/10	0/15	2/10	1/14	4/7
V	1/2	0/2	0/4	1/5	1/2
Site (S)					
Retrop. nodes	2	–	2	2	17
Mediastinum	–	–	–	1	1
Supraclav. nodes	–	–	–	1	1
Lung	–	1	1	3	9
Liver	–	–	1	–	2
Relapse-free at 48 months[b]	90 ± 7%	97 ± 3%	87 ± 8%	81 ± 7%	10 ± 6%
Alive at 48 months[b]	95 ± 5%	100%	80 ± 14%	92 ± 5%	12 ± 8%

[a] Dixon and Moore [1]
[b] Actuarial
OP, orchiectomy; RND, retroperitoneal lymph node dissection; NED, no evidence of disease; Retrop., Retroperitoneal; Supraclav., Supraclavicular

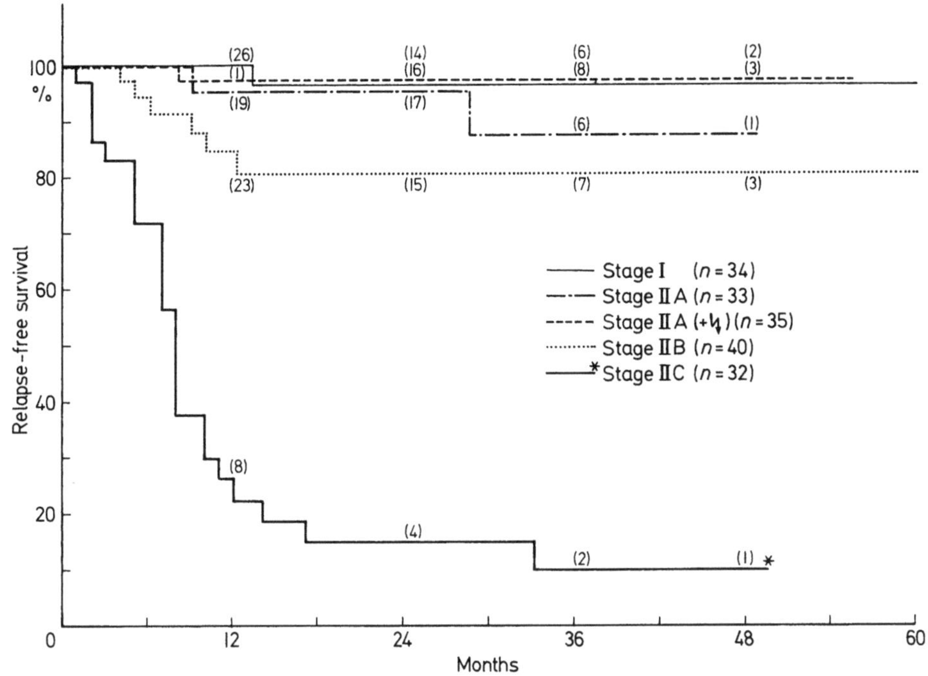

Fig. 1. Survival data for patients shown in Table 4, and including data on 34 patients surgically classified as stage I. ♂ + ϟ, plus radiotherapy

This 90% 4-year survival of 68 patients with pathologically staged IIA testicular teratomas compares favorably with survival data in stage II (43–81% at 3–5 years) obtained with lymphadenectomy plus RT [2, 5–7, 12, 16], and also to series using RT alone [7, 8, 14, 15]. However, the application of all three modalities in stage IIA, as done here, could imply overtreatment. Accordingly, the concept of delayed chemotherapy after complete lymph node dissection deserves further interest [4]. As an alternative line of development, modern combination chemotherapy and RT should be studied in early stage II testicular cancer staged either clinically (lymphogram, computerized tomogram, or sonogram) or by a nonradical surgical approach, which could avoid the serious side effects of lymphadenectomy. Very recently, a 100% disease-free survival at 36 months has been reported by Peckham et al. [8], using lymph node irradiation and delayed chemotherapy in 28 patients with stage I and IIA disease, though the stage I and IIA groups were not separated and the subgroup of stage II may have been very small. In spite of the encouraging data obtained thus far with the delayed chemotherapy concept [4], much more substantial data will be necessary to show its superiority to a program with adjuvant chemotherapy and RT which, at the risk of minor side effects, has produced a 3–4-year relapse-free survival rate of over 90%.

Stages IIB and IIC

In 40 patients with pathologic stage IIB, an actuarial survival of 92% at 48 months after lymphadenectomy (median observation 19 months) was obtained by sequential chemotherapy and RT (Table 4 and Fig. 1). This result is very encouraging, since all patients involved had, according to the definition, nonresectable abdominal disease, which meant that RT alone or delayed chemotherapy would not have been promising therapeutic alternatives. Again, with a low toxicity and without drug-related deaths, the sequential program used has shown its effectiveness in the prevention of visceral metastases and also its compatibility with RT for local tumor control. For this group of patients our future protocols will prefer a single efficient chemotherapy series for 4–12 months, followed by RT at the end of the program. It would be desirable to shorten the chemotherapy arm to a minimum without a loss in local and metastatic tumor control.

Patients with advanced irresectable retroperitoneal metastases (stage IIC, $n = 32$) still bear a fairly poor prognosis and only some 15% may expect long-term survival or cure (Fig. 1). Treatment should be largely individualized in this group. With aggressive chemotherapy, a significant tumor reduction should be possible in most cases and surgical and/or RT measures should follow at the time of maximum chemotherapeutic response. Data of other studies with a 40–50% long-term survival rate in this stage could have been derived from a more favorable patient selection (no pretreatment, lower perçentage of β-HCG positivity, etc.)

Discussion

A summary of previous results in the therapy of stage II testicular carcinoma is presented in Table 5 compared with our results. Most studies, unfortunately, have included only small numbers of patients. In addition, the evaluation of a number of reports is limited by the fact that subgroups according to the extent of retroperitoneal lymph node involvement have not always been defined. Overall 3–5-year survival rates of 70% and more achieved by lymphadenectomy alone seem to be closely related to highly sophisticated preparative work at lymph node dissection and are probably not realistic for all stage II patients. This view may be supported by the more recent results of combination of lymphadenectomy and RT with 3–5-year survival rates of 43–81%.

Thus far, controlled studies on adjuvant chemotherapy in stage II testicular cancer have not been reported. In the series of Skinner [11], stage I and early stage II patients were evaluated together. When stage II patients were separated from stage I, in this series the 5-year survival rate was 78%. It was, however, not specified which patients had lymphadenectomy alone and where chemotherapy or RT was added. It was further reported by Skinner that the survival rate of patients with stage A and B_1 (stage I and IIA and B) increased from 82–93% by the addition of adjuvant chemotherapy with actinomycin D. RT alone in stage II patients has resulted in 3–5-year survival rates of 46–82%. In this series stage II was defined by lymphography only. It cannot be concluded from the data in Table 5 that RT is less effective than lymphadenectomy in comparable stage II populations.

Although appropriate control groups have not been included in our series, the results in stage IIA and IIB patients appear promising and indicate that adjuvant chemotherapy may improve long-term survival in early stage II testicular cancer. Nevertheless, prospective randomized trials comparing lymphadenectomy alone, lymphadenectomy plus RT, and lymphadenectomy plus chemotherapy in well-defined early stage II testicular cancer are mandatory. If the benefit of adjuvant chemotherapy

Table 5. Three- to five-year survival rates of patients with stage II nonseminomatous testicular cancer

Lymphadenectomy			
Staubitz et al. [13]		15/20	(70%)
Walsh et al. [16]		3/4	(75%)
	Overall	18/24	(71%)
Lymphadenectomy and radiation therapy			
Slawson [12]		9/21	(43%)
Walsh et al. [16]		9/16	(56%)
Earle et al. [2]		13/20	(65%)
Hussey et al. [5]		17/25	(68%)
Lynch et al. [6]		10/14	(71%)
Maier and Mittemeyer [7]		26/32	(81%)
	Overall	84/128	(66%)
Lymphadenectomy with or without radiation therapy plus/minus chemotherapy			
Skinner [11]		28/36	(78%)
Lymphadenectomy plus chemotherapy and additive radiation therapy			
Schmidt [9a]	Stage IIA	34/35	(97%)
	Stage IIB	38/40	(85%)
	Stage IIC	8/32	(25%)
Radiation therapy			
Van der Werf-Messing [15]		16/35	(46%)
Tyrrell and Peckham [14]		14/29	(48%)
Maier and Mittemeyer [7]		9/11	(82%)
	Overall	39/75	(52%)

and RT can be demonstrated, a combination of chemotherapy and RT may be discussed for stage I and early stage II patients as defined by modern diagnostic procedures (sonography, lymphography, or computerized axial tomography) to possibly avoid the serious side effects of lymphadenectomy.

References

1. Dixon FJ, Moore RA (1953) Testicular tumors. A clinicopathological study. Cancer 6: 427–454
2. Earle JD, Bagshaw MA, Kaplan HS (1973) Supervoltage radiation therapy of testicular tumors. Am J Roentgenol 117: 653–661
3. Einhorn LH, Donohue J (1977) cis-Diamminedichloroplatinum, vinblastine, and bleomycin combination chemotherapy in disseminated testicular cancer. Ann Intern Med 87: 293–298
4. Einhorn LH, Donohue J (1979) Adjuvant chemotherapy for testicular cancer: Is it necessary? In: Jones SE, Salmon SE (eds) Adjuvant therapy of cancer II. Grune & Stratton, New York, pp 329–335
5. Hussey DH, Luk KH, Johnson DE (1977) The role of radiation therapy in the treatment of germinal cell tumors of the testis other than pure seminoma. Radiology 123: 175–180

6. Lynch DF Jr, McCord LP, Nicholson TC, Richie JP, Sargent CR (1978) Sandwich therapy in testis tumor: Current experience. J Urol 119: 612–613
7. Maier JG, Mittemeyer B (1977) Carcinoma of the testis. Cancer 39: 981–986
8. Peckham MJ, McElwain TJ, Barrett A, Hendry WF (1979) Combined management of malignant teratoma of the testis. Lancet 2: 267–270
9. Samuels ML, Johnson DE, Holoye PY (1975) Continuous intravenous bleomycin (NSC-125066) therapy with vinblastine (NSC-49842) in stage III testicular neoplasia. Cancer Chemother Rep 59: 563–570
9a. Schmidt CG (1980) Stellung der Chemotherapie in der Behandlung der teratoiden und embryonalen Hodentumoren. Urologe [B] 20: 119–128
10. Seeber S, Scheulen ME, Osieka R, Höffken K, Schmidt CG (1978) Development of chemotherapy programs containing vinblastine, bleomycin, adriamycin and cisplatin for testicular teratomas. In: Carter SK, Crooke ST, Umezawa H (eds) The bleomycins: Current status and new developments. Academic Press, New York, pp 215–226
11. Skinner DG (1976) Non-seminomatous testis tumors: A plan of management based on 96 patients to improve survival in all stages by combined therapeutic modalities. J Urol 115: 65–69
12. Slawson RG (1978) Radiation therapy for germinal tumors of the testis. Cancer 42: 2216–2223
13. Staubitz WJ, Early KS, Magoss IV, Murphy GP (1974) Surgical management of testis tumor. J Urol 111: 205–209
14. Tyrrell CJ, Peckham MJ (1976) The response of lymph node metastases of testicular teratoma to radiation therapy. Br J Urol 48: 363–370
15. Van der Werf-Messing B (1976) Radiotherapeutic treatment of testicular tumors. Int J Radiat Oncol Biol Phys 1: 235–248
16. Walsh PC, Kaufman JJ, Coulson WF, Goodwin WE (1971) Retroperitoneal lymphadenectomy for testicular tumors. JAMA 217: 309–312

VIII. Gastrointestinal Neoplasms

44. *Adjuvant 5-Fluorouracil and BCNU Chemotherapy in Gastric Cancer: 3-Year Results**

P. Schlag, W. Schreml, W. Gaus, C. Herfarth, M. M. Linder, W. Queisser, and M. Trede**

Universität Ulm, Abteilung für Allgemeine Chirurgie, D-7900 Ulm-Safranberg, Germany

Summary

One hundred-three patients with a potentially curative operation of a histologically proven gastric cancer were randomly assigned to a control and chemotherapy group after stratification according to tumor stage II and III. Chemotherapy courses with 5-fluorouracil (10 mg/kg/day) and BCNU (40 mg/m^2/day) for 5 days were administered eight times in 6–8 week intervals. Age, sex, and tumor location were matched in the chemotherapy and control groups. Five patients declined treatment after randomization. Three years after initiating the study, the tumor has recurred in 38 of the 103 patients. There were 21 recurrences of 54 controls and 14 recurrences of 44 patients who received chemotherapy, and 17 and ten deaths, respectively, due to tumor relapse. The results of our study to data show a high degree of statistical probability that adjuvant chemotherapy with the regime used has no influence on the recurrence-free interval and survival time in gastric cancer.

Introduction

For gastric cancer, except in the early stages, results of treatment are singularly disappointing. Only about 60% of those patients with gastric cancer are eligible for potentially curative resection, and of those patients only about 20% survive for 5 or more years [7, 10]. Despite an extended and standardized surgical procedure, stage-dependent survival time has not been significantly influenced over the last 20 years [5, 9]. Considering this situation, no further improvement of the prognosis can be expected from exclusively surgical measures. Therefore, the concept of adjuvant systemic therapy appears attractive [14]. However, most of the trials concerning adjuvant chemotherapy in gastric cancer had negative or highly equivocal results [1, 2, 14]. Positive studies have been reported only from Japan [4, 12]. In these trials, long-term treatment and the use of mitomycin-C (MMC) relatively effective in gastric cancer, may have been the decisive factors. However, these data from Japan cannot be

* Joint Studies of the Tumor Centers Mannheim and Ulm, Germany

** We thank Mrs. B. Rappenecker for statistical evaluation and Mrs. H. Mayr for preparation of the manuscript

applied to other situations without critical reevaluation. Furthermore, due to the considerable side effects, adjuvant chemotherapy poses may problems, in particular when MMC is used. A less toxic treatment of equal effectiveness should therefore be given preference.

Some progress achieved with combination chemotherapy of gastric cancer in the disseminated tumor stage stimulated new interest in adjuvant trials [1, 14]. In comparison with response rates of 20% usually obtained with monotherapy, remissions of up to 40% could be achieved in metastasizing gastric cancer with a combination chemotherapy of 5-fluorouracil (5-FU) and nitrosoureas [8a, 11]. At the same time, the survival rate of responding patients could be prolonged. Since the side effects of the treatment were also tolerable, it appeared justified to examine the effectiveness of a combination chemotherapy with 5-FU and BCNU under adjuvant conditions. In the following, we will report on the 3-year results of a study jointly conducted by the tumor centers in Mannheim and Ulm.

Patients and Methods

All patients entered in the study had received a potentially curative operation of a histologically proven gastric cancer in the tumor stage II or III, according to the UICC

Table 1. Design of the adjuvant chemotherapy trial

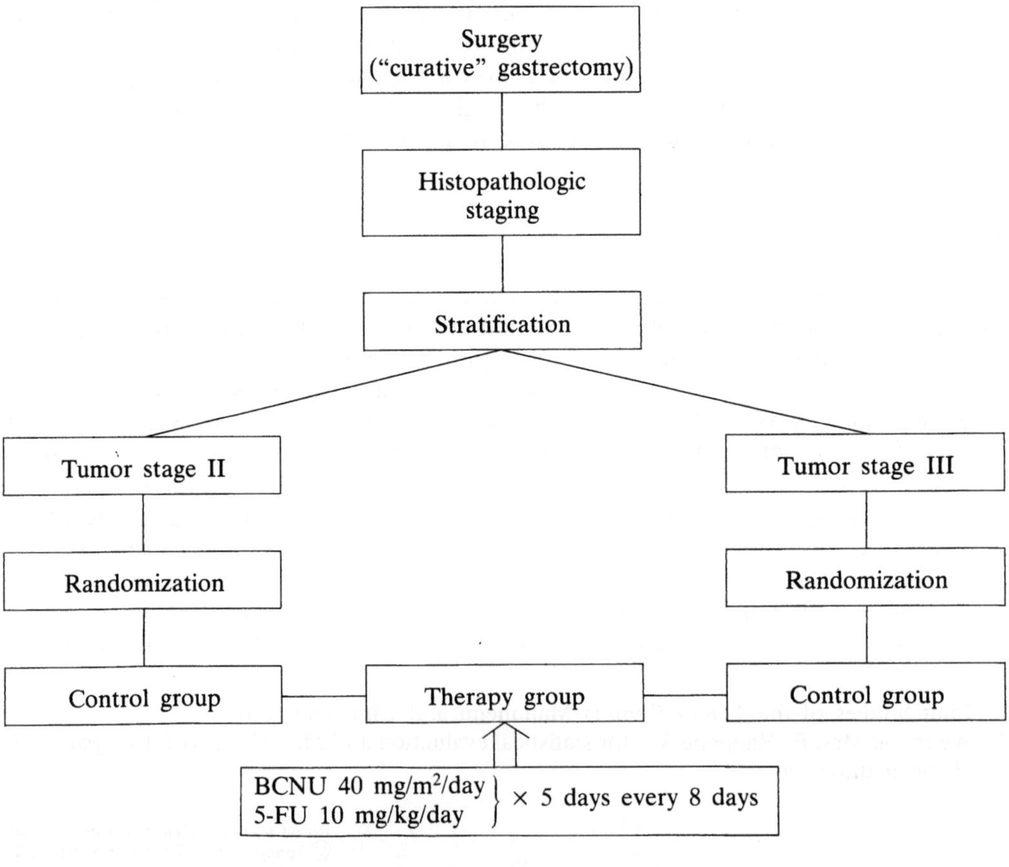

classification of malignant tumors. The stage classification was based on the operative findings as well as the histomorphologic evaluation of the surgical specimen. Criteria excluding a patient from this study were: (1) age over 68 years; (2) histology other than a primary adenocarcinoma of the stomach; (3) presence of a second tumor; (4) clinically demonstrable or suspected metastases; (5) a clinical condition leading to an unjustifiably high risk of side effects; (6) previous therapy with cytostatics; or (7) refusal of the patient.

Following the stratification of the patients according to tumor stage, they were randomly assigned to a control or chemotherapy group. Chemotherapy courses of 5 days were administered eight times in 6–8-week intervals. 5-FU was given i.v. in a dosage of 10 mg/kg/day and BCNU was given in a dosage of 40 mg/m^2/day (Table 1). The first course was administered between days 42–46 postoperatively. Both groups were reexamined with clinical and laboratory techniques every 2 months in the beginning and every 3 months after a 1.5-year postoperative period. X-Ray examination of the lung, an abdominal sonograph, and an upper-intestinal endoscopic examination were performed every 6 months.

The time of relapse and the survival time were considered as criteria for the effectiveness of therapy. The probability of the disease-free interval (DFI) or the survival of the patients were determined per month according to the life-table method. The statistical evaluation was done with the log rank test described by Peto [13]. The present data were evaluated 40 months after the beginning of the study in November, 1976.

Results

One hundred-three patients have been included in this study to date. The last patient was randomized 3 months before the study was evaluated. Fifty-four patients were in the control group and 49 patients were randomized in the chemotherapy group. Five patients of the chemotherapy group declined treatment after randomization. The age and sex of the patients were matched in the chemotherapy and control group. The frequency of various tumor locations in the upper, middle, and lower part of the stomach was also quite identical for both groups (Table 2). The tumor has recurred in 38 of the 103 patients to date. There were 21 recurrences of 54 controls and 14 recurrences of 44 patients in the chemotherapy group, and there were 17 and 10 deaths, respectively, due to tumor relapse. In two-thirds of the patients, the recurrence was found to be primarily locoregional. In one-third, the first sign of a relapse was detected in the form of metastases in the liver, lung, or bone marrow. The type of localization of the recurrence was largely identical for the control and the chemotherapy groups, except for a slight predominance of distant metastases in the therapy group (Table 3).

After an observation period of about 3 years, a comparison of DFI shows no statistical difference between groups of treated and untreated patients. Also the probability for survival for the two groups is nearly identical. There exists no statistically proven benefit for the treatment group. Probability for survival was 52% in both groups for a 36-month postoperative interval (Fig. 1).

Consideration of the stratified prognostic subgroups of tumor stages II and III also shows no trend. The treatment performed shows no gain at all with regard to DFI or survival rate compared with the untreated control group (Figs. 2 and 3). Furthermore, the side effects which occurred in part of the chemotherapy patients have yet to be mentioned. Half of this patient group complained of relatively severe gastrointestinal distress, such as nausea, vomiting, and diarrhea, in connection with the therapy performed. Four patients discontinued treatment due to these symptoms and the psychological strain. Chemotherapy had to be discontinued in a further four patients

Table 2. Distribution of age, sex, and tumor location in control versus chemotherapy group

	Chemotherapy group $n = 49$	Control group $n = 54$
Age (years)	59.8	57.6
Sex (male/female)	30/19	33/21
Upper part	14	13
Middle part	14	15
Lower part	21	26

Table 3. Number and distribution of recurrences in control versus chemotherapy group

	Chemotherapy group $n = 49$	Control group $n = 54$
Anastomosis	2	2
Locoregional	6	14
Distant metastases	7	5
Uncertain location	2	–
Total	17	21

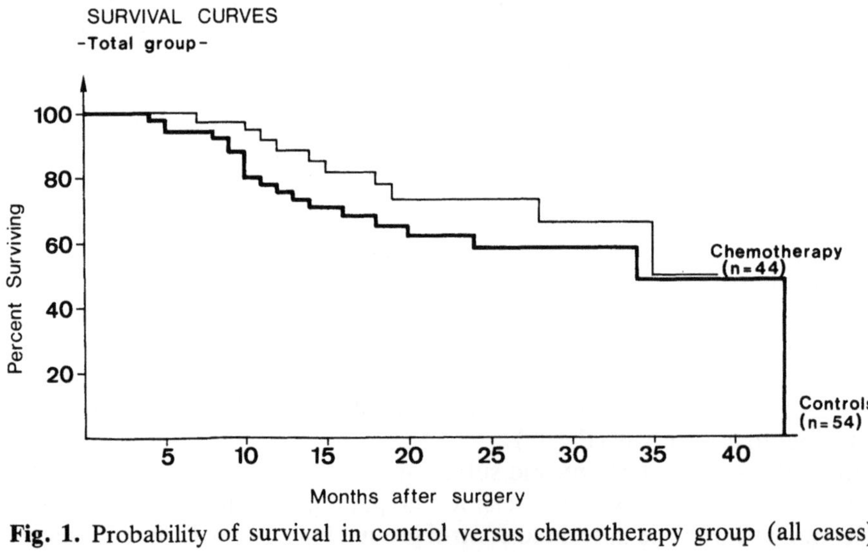

Fig. 1. Probability of survival in control versus chemotherapy group (all cases)

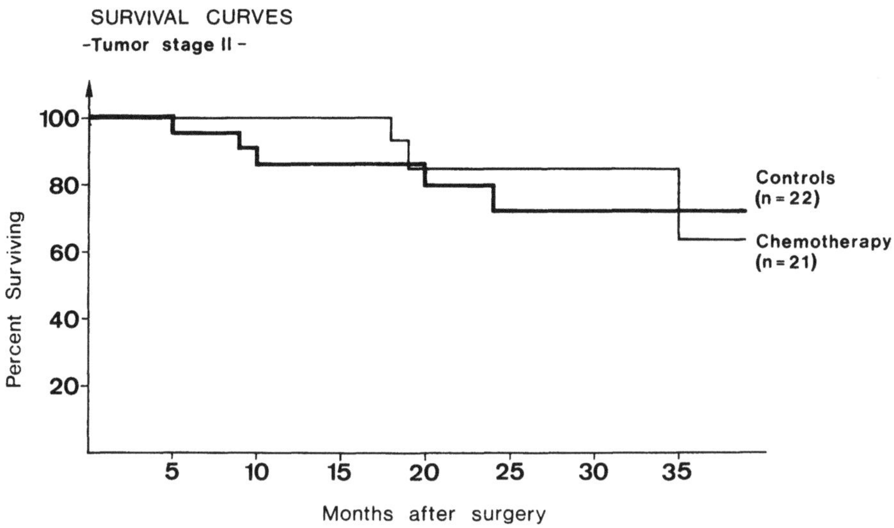

Fig. 2. Probability of survival in control versus chemotherapy group (stage II)

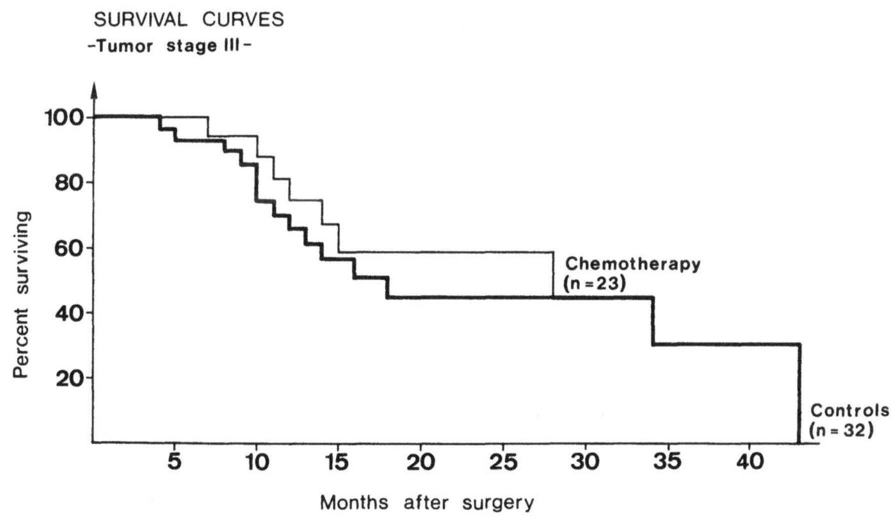

Fig. 3. Probability of survival in control versus chemotherapy group (stage III)

because of persisting hematologic side effects (thrombocytopenia and granulocytopenia).

A comparison of the recurrence-free interval within the chemotherapy group with regard to complete or interrupted treatment also shows no significant difference between the two groups. Patients refusing treatment appear to have a higher frequency of recurrences, though this difference is not statistically significant (Fig. 4).

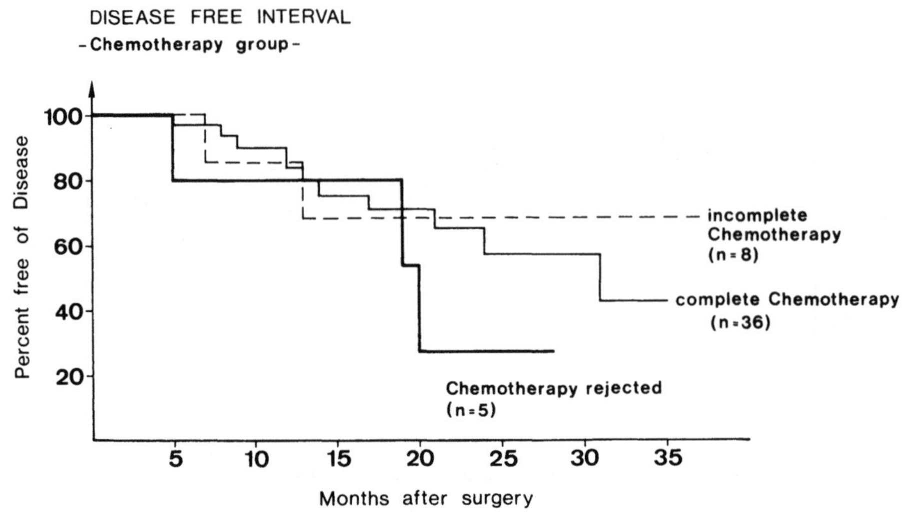

Fig. 4. Disease-free interval by treatment

Discussion

The current results of our study show, with a high degree of statistical probability, that 5-FU and BCNU in the doses and schedule used, have no influence on DFI and survival time when used as adjuvants in patients who have been surgically treated for gastric cancer. It becomes even more evident that no therapeutic benefit for gastric cancer patients resulted from this adjuvant therapy when patients of the therapy group who declined treatment after randomization are included in the evaluation.

The results add to the negative experiences obtained in previous studies with adjuvant monotherapy [1, 2] and are in accordance with preliminary results of other trials with adjuvant polychemotherapy in gastric cancer [3]. Preliminary data of 5-FU chemotherapy in combination with radiotherapy have also shown no benefit as adjuvants in gastric cancer [6]. So, the results of combination chemotherapy do not seem superior to monotherapy under adjuvant conditions in the modalities tested. This is at variance only with the Japanese treatment results [4, 12, 15]. It remains to be seen whether the failure of adjuvant therapy in most of the trials is founded in the lack of sufficiently effective cytostatic modalities [8], or whether a different biology of gastric cancer requires concepts beyond an exclusively systemic chemotherapy. The conspicuous frequency of locoregional recurrences, which may indicate a reduced accessibility in systemic chemotherapy, supports these thoughts.

References

1. Carter SK, Comis RL (1977) Gastric cancer: Current status of treatment. J Natl Cancer Inst 58: 567–578
2. Dixon WJ, Longmire WP, Holden WD (1971) Use of triethylenethiophosphoramide as an adjuvant to the surgical treatment of gastric and colorectal cancer: Ten-year follow-up. Ann Surg 173: 26–39

3. Engström P (to be published) Adjuvant therapy of gastric carcinoma: ECOG protocol comparing 5-FU plus MeCCNU versus untreated control. EORTC Symposium on Progress and Perspectives in the Treatment of Gastrointestinal Tumors, Brussels. Eur J Cancer
4. Fujimoto S, Akao T, Itoh B, Koshizuka I, Koyano K, Kitsukawa Y, Takahashi M, Minami T, Ishigami H, Miyazaki M, Amamiya K, Ohyama Y, Ono K, Kure M, Itoh K, Hikosaka T (1977) Protracted oral chemotherapy with fluorinated pyrimidines as an adjuvant to surgical treatment for stomach cancer. Ann Surg 185: 462–466
5. Gilbertsen VA (1969) Results of treatment of stomach cancer. An appraisal of efforts for more extensive surgery and a report of 1,983 cases. Cancer 23: 1305–1308
6. Goffin IC (to be published) Controlled clinical trial for the treatment of patients with gastric cancer using surgery, radiotherapy and chemotherapy. Preliminary results. EORTC Symposium on Progress and Perspectives in the Treatment of Gastrointestinal Tumors, Brussels. Eur J Cancer
7. Herfarth C, Schlag P (eds) (1979) Gastric cancer. Springer, Berlin Heidelberg New York
8. Karrar K (1972) Importance of dose schedules in adjuvant chemotherapy. Cancer Chemother Rep 56: 35–45
8a. Kovach JS, Moertel CG, Schutt AJ, Hahn RG, Reitemeier RJ (1974) A controlled study of combined 1,3-bis-(2-chlorethyl)-1-nitrosurea and 5-fluorouracil therapy for advanced gastric and pancreatic cancer. Cancer 33: 563–567
9. Longmire WP (1977) Gewandelte Aspekte des Magenkarzinoms. Münch Med Wochenschr 119: 613–616
10. Merkle P, Schlag P, Herfarth C (1979) Aktuelle Aspekte bei der Therapie des Magenkarzinoms. Zentralbl Chir 104: 1111–1116
11. Moertel CG (1978) Chemotherapy of gastrointestinal cancer. N Engl J Med 299: 1049–1052
12. Nakazato H, Imanaga H (1979) Results of surgery for gastric cancer and effect of adjuvant chemotherapy. In: Herfarth C, Schlag P (eds) Gastric cancer. Springer, Berlin Heidelberg New York, pp 344–356
13. Peto R, Pike MC, Armitage P, Breslow NE, Cox DR, Howard SV, Mante N, McPherson K, Peto J, Smith PG (1977) Design and analysis of randomized clinical trilas requiring prolonged observation of each patient. Br J Cancer 35: 1–39
14. Schlag P, Merkle P, Herfarth C (1979) Neue Aspekte in der Konzeption adjuvanter und nachsorgender Therapie des Magencarcinoms? Chirurg 50: 432–435
15. Taguchi T, Hattori T, Inoue K, Kondo T, Ichiji I, Kikuchi K, Sugie S, Inokuchi K (1979) Multihospital randomized study on adjuvant chemotherapy with mitomycin + Futraful for gastric cancer. In: Jones SE, Salmon SE (eds) Adjuvant therapy of cancer II. Grune & Stratton, New York London Toronto Sydney San Francisco, pp 581–586

45. *Adjuvant Chemotherapy in Colon and Gastric Cancer*

J. S. Macdonald, D. G. Haller, and D. L. Kisner

National Cancer Institute, Division of Cancer Treatment,
Cancer Therapy Evaluation Program,
Bethesda, MD 20205, USA

Summary

The adjuvant chemotherapy of colorectal and gastric cancer is being actively investigated. Studies of both single antineoplastic agents and combinations of several drugs have been used. In colorectal cancer, single-agent therapy has not resulted in improved survival. Combination chemotherapy studies are at too early a stage to be evaluated. In gastric cancer, single-agent chemotherapy has not been effective as adjunctive treatment to surgery. Combinations of active agents in gastric cancer hold promise as effective surgical adjuvant therapy.

Introduction

Both colorectal cancer and gastric cancer are major causes of cancer-related death in the United States [19]. There are 100,000 new cases of cancer of the colon and rectum in America, and 50,000 cancer deaths each year are directly attributable to this disease. Gastric cancer is not as great a problem numerically as colon cancer, but is still significant. There are 22,000 cases of adenocarcinoma of the stomach each year in the United States [19] and 15,000 deaths from this disease. Stomach cancer is the sixth most common cause of cancer-related mortality in America. On an international level, gastric cancer is of extreme importance [15] and represents the major cause of cancer-associated mortality in Japan and China.

Colorectal cancer and gastric cancer may be cured only by surgical resection. However, in both diseases, resection is frequently not curative even though all visible disease is surgically excised. It can be assumed that 40–50% of patients with colon cancer [13] and 50–70% of patients with gastric cancer [8] will develop recurrent disease after surgical resection. Patients who develop recurrent cancer after resection will, with very rare exception, die of cancer. Therefore, it is clear that if an effective adjunctive treatment to surgery could be developed for patients with colorectal and gastric carcinoma, the benefits in improved survival time and decreased patient morbidity would be highly significant. This paper will review the current status of adjuvant therapy in these diseases.

Recent Results in Cancer Research, Vol. 80

Colon Cancer

Although chemotherapy appears to be of limited value in advanced colorectal cancer, many efforts to apply this treatment as an adjuvant to surgery have been carried out. Selection of cases for adjuvant chemotherapy depend upon the determination of the probability of relapse in patients undergoing surgical therapy for primary colon cancer. Pathologic evaluation of the primary tumor is used to assess the probability of recurrence. Dukes' classification, which correlates the degree of penetration of the colonic wall and involvement of lymph nodes with probability of relapse, has been widely used. The derivation and value of Dukes' classification has been extensively reviewed [13]. It is sufficient to note here that patients with tumor that has invaded through the muscularis and serosa (Dukes' B_2) or that has spread to lymph nodes (Dukes' C) have a greater than 40% probability of relapse after resection with curative intent. These patients are candidates for postoperative adjuvant chemotherapy trials.

Since the early 1960's, extensive studies on surgical adjuvant chemotherapy of colon cancer have been performed. Most studies have been of single agents and the Veterans' Administration Surgical Oncology Group (VASOG) has been a leader in these investigations.

VASOG first tested thiotepa [3] and subsequently floxuridine (FUDR) [4] administered at the time of operation and in the immediate postoperative period. In these prospectively randomized trials, neither drug improved 5-year survival rates. The next drug investigated was 5-fluorouracil (5-FU). Five- and seven-year survival data are now available on the VASOG 5-FU trials [8]. In the initial 5-FU study, patients were stratified into three subgroups, group A (curative resection), group B (palliative resection with histologic evidence of residual disease), and group C (clinically palliative resection with no histologic proof of residual tumor). Within these groups, patients were randomized to receive drug or no treatment. 5-FU was given (12 mg/kg body weight i.v.) daily for 5 days. Curative resection patients and clinically palliative resection patients were given a second course in 7 weeks, while pathologically proven palliatively resected patients received 5-FU courses at 6–8-week intervals until their disease progressed.

The results of this trial demonstrated evidence of minimal benefit from 5-FU treatment. Although, within the curative resection group, the 5-year survival rate was 58% among 142 patients receiving 5-FU versus 49% for 146 control patients, these differences were not statistically significant. The trend toward better survival times with 5-FU therapy was seen in the clinically and histologically proven palliative resection groups, although statistical significance was not attained.

VASOG [8] subsequently evaluated prolonged intermittent 5-FU therapy in poor-prognosis patients with colorectal cancer. The unfavorable prognostic signs qualifying patients for inclusion in this study included presence of positive lymph nodes, serosal involvement, and invasion of a resected organ other than the colon. Patients were stratified for curative resection or palliative resection with proved residual disease. Randomization was between 5-FU treatment after surgery and surgery alone. Treatment consisted of 5-FU (12 mg/kg i.v.) daily for 5 days. The courses were repeated at 6–8 week intervals. The curative resection group was treated for 18 months (about 12 drug courses). The palliatively resected patients were maintained on repeated courses of 5-FU until disease progression or death. Follow-up has exceeded 4 years (46 patients) and actuarial survival at 7 years shows some benefit for the treated group. Thirty-three percent [8] of patients receiving 5-FU and 26% of control patients are alive at 7 years. These differences are not statistically significant. For those patients undergoing palliative resection, the 18-month survival rate is 38% for 5-FU-treated cases versus 26% for controls. These results are also not significantly different.

A possible explanation of the failure of the various VASOG 5-FU studies to show benefit as adjuvant treatment in colon cancer is lack of intensity of therapy. The 5-FU preparation can be given in a more intensive manner, and, in fact, only 30% of the VASOG patients evidenced symptoms of drug toxicity [8]. With this in mind, the Central Oncology Group [6] has examined the effect of 5-FU on disease-free interval (DFI) and survival times in 210 patients who had curative resections for colorectal cancer. In this randomized study, patients receiving 5-FU were treated with an

Table 1. Controlled trials of systemically administered fluorinated pyrimidines as adjuvant therapy to surgery in colorectal cancer

Drug	Number of patients	Statistical survival benefit with treatment
FUDR [3, 4]	548	None
5-FU [8]	308	None
5-FU [8]	522	None
5-FU [6]	210	None

Table 2. Adjuvant combination chemotherapy in colon cancer

Group	Regimen	Duration of therapy	Untreated control	Patients eligible
ECOG	5-FU vs. 5-FU + methyl-CCNU	18 months	No	Dukes' B + C
VASOG	5-FU + methyl-CCNU vs. surgery-only control	12 months	Yes	Dukes' B + C
GITSG	5-FU + methyl-CCNU vs. MER vs. 5-FU + methyl-CCNU + MER vs. surgery-only control	12 months	Yes	Dukes' B + C
SWOG	5-FU + methyl-CCNU vs. 5-FU + methyl-CCNU + oral BCG	12 months	No[a]	Dukes' B + C
NSABP	5-FU + methyl-CCNU vs. BCG vs. surgery-only control	12 months	Yes	Dukes' B + C
NCCTG	Levamisole vs. levamisole + 5-FU vs. surgery-only control	12 months	Yes	Dukes' B + C

[a] Untreated control arm added after trial initiated

aggressive-loading dose schedule of drug in the postoperative period followed by 1 year of i.v. 5-FU weekly (12 mg/kg). There were 113 patients in the control arm and 97 patients in the treatment arm of this trial. Fifty-seven of 113 controls (50%) and 54 of 97 (56%) treated patients are surviving free of disease. These results are not significantly different. However, in the patients with Dukes' C lesions, there was statistically significant ($P = 0.04$) prolongation of DFI in the patients receiving 5-FU therapy. In a group of 29 patients with rectal cancer, 5-FU therapy was associated with significant prolongation in survival ($P = 0.011$).

One study of 5-FU utilizing an innovative method of drug delivery has shown early positive results and deserves confirmation. This is the study of Taylor et al. [19] in which patients with resected colon cancer were randomized to either 7 days of postoperative 5-FU via continuous infusion into the portal vein or no adjunctive treatment. Taylor et al. have performed a randomized trial [19] in which 24 patients received 5-FU by portal vein infusion and 26 were treated with surgery alone. Eight of the 26 patients in the surgery-only group had developed metastases after 15 months of follow-up. There were six patients with liver metastases and two with local recurrence. None of the 24 patients treated with 5-FU developed metastases. The Gastrointestinal Tumor Study Group (GITSG) in the United States will attempt to confirm this study.

Table 1 summarizes the results obtained with controlled trials of adjuvant therapy with systemically administered fluorinated pyrimidines. When overall survival of all patients in any one trial is examined, there is no evidence of statistical benefit in survival from fluorinated pyrimidine therapy. It should be noted that these trials all show some small benefit from 5-FU therapy. However, the maximum 5-year survival benefit that can be demonstrated in controlled trials is only 5–10% above controls. Such results are of marginal biologic or clinical significance.

Adjuvant therapy studies in colon cancer have been initiated with combination chemotherapy and immunotherapy treatment protocols. Published results from these studies are not currently available as they are of recent origin. The design of currently active studies are illustrated in Table 2. The total number of patients to be evaluated in these trials will be in excess of 2,000 and the majority are designed with a prospectively randomized surgery-only control arm. This study design should allow for clear definition of the role of 5-FU plus methyl-CCNU and nonspecific immunostimulants in the surgical adjuvant therapy of colorectal cancer.

The status of adjunctive therapy in colon cancer can be summarized. There are no prospectively randomized controlled trials of systemically administered single-agent chemotherapy showing clear benefit in overall or disease-free survival for patients receiving the adjunctive chemotherapy. Combination chemotherapy trials are still at too early a stage for analysis, although one would predict that these studies will show no dramatic benefits since combination treatment is not superior to single-agent therapy in advanced colon cancer. The situation in adjuvant chemotherapy of colon cancer will only improve through the development of more active single agents and combinations, and the innovative use of currently available drugs, as illustrated by the study of 5-FU by portal vein reported by Taylor et al. [19].

Gastric Cancer

As is the case with colon cancer, there are also clinicalpathologic risk factors in gastric cancer which predict for a high likelihood of relapse after surgical resection. VASOG has examined prognostic factors in 503 patients undergoing gastrectomy for stomach cancer [7, 17]. Performance status before operation is of significant importance [7, 17], since patients with weight loss, anorexia, and weakness have a higher likelihood of dying of recurrent cancer after operation than patients without these factors. Similarly to the situation in colon cancer, patients with locally advanced stomach carcinoma [7, 17], as evidenced by tumor invasion through the gastric serosa, into blood vessels, or lymphatics or involvement of perigastric lymph nodes, have a poor prognosis. Patients with any of these indications of local invasion have less than 20% probability of being cured by gastric resection [7]. Proximal position of the primary tumor in the stomach necessitating a total gastrectomy is an adverse prognostic factor. In the VASOG studies [7], only 15% of patients requiring proximal or total gastrectomies for resectable gastric cancer survived 5 years as opposed to 27% survival rate for those having distal gastrectomies. The pathologic characteristics of the primary tumor constitute very important information in predicting survival. Of patients with linitis plastica [7], only 2% survived 5 years after resection.

The adjuvant chemotherapy of gastric cancer has depended upon the availability of active single agents and combinations of drugs in advanced disease. Fluorinated pyrimidines [1], mitomycin-C [5], nitrosoureas [9], and anthracyclines [13] have all been demonstrated to produce objective regression in 15–30% of patients with advanced gastric cancer. In contradistinction to the findings in colon cancer, combination chemotherapy produces better response rates than single agents in stomach cancer [9, 11, 14]. Thus, the use of combinations of cytotoxic agents might be the most reasonable approach in gastric cancer adjuvant therapy.

VASOG has actively pursued the surgical adjuvant therapy of gastric cancer in the United States. The data derived from this group have shown that single-agent chemotherapy with thiotepa [2] or fluorodeoxyuridine [16] failed to influence disease-free survival at 5 years after resection. In the thiotepa study, treatment with chemotherapy adversely influenced survival [2]; however, this difference is not significant. This negativity of the VASOG studies has not, unfortunately, been an isolated phenomenon since the vast majority of well-designed adjuvant chemotherapy studies reported have failed to show significant benefit for treatment with chemotherapy. Table 3 describes a series of studies in which more than 2,500 patients were evaluated. It is clear that in an adjuvant therapy study it is exceedingly important that a prospectively randomized design be utilized. Only in this way can one be assured of balancing prognostic factors between treated and control groups. All of the studies detailed in Table 3 were prospectively randomized controlled trials of chemotherapy versus treatment with surgery alone.

Because of the very high incidence of gastric cancer in Japan, there has been great interest in the surgical adjuvant therapy of gastric cancer in that country. Table 3 describes the combined results of a series of six randomized controlled trials including over 1,950 patients. Drugs tested included 5-FU, mitomycin-C, cyclophosphamide, and chromomycin-A_3. In no instance was chemotherapeutic treatment superior to surgery alone.

The majority of patients in these studies (Table 3) were treated with single-agent chemotherapy and, as previously described, there is now clear evidence that combination chemotherapy is superior to single-agent treatment in advanced gastric cancer. It is presumed that the combinations would also be more active in the surgical adjuvant situation and several such studies are underway. Adjuvant chemotherapy studies using the moderately active 5-FU plus methyl-CCNU [14] and the highly active

Table 3. Randomized controlled trials of adjuvant chemotherapy in stomach cancer

Group	No. patients	Design	Survival benefits for treated patients	Reference
VASOG	194	Thiotepa vs. control	None	[2]
VASOG	276	FUDR vs. control	None	[16]
VASOG	110	5-FU + methyl-CCNU vs. control	In progress	–
ECOG	144	5-FU + methyl-CCNU vs. control	In progress	–
GITSG	123	5-FU + methyl-CCNU vs. control	In progress	–
SWOG	24	FAM vs. control	In progress	–
CALGB	10	FAM vs. control	In progress	–
Stomach cancer study group (Japan)	1,967	Six studies including mitomycin-C, thiotepa, cyclophosphamide, 5-FU, and chromomycin-A_3 vs. control	None	[10]

5-FU, adriamycin, mitomycin-C (FAM) [11] regimen are now being pursued in well-designed trials by VASOG, GITSG, SWOG, ECOG, and CALGB (Table 3). These studies are still too early for analysis, but their results will have major impact on the appropriate postoperative management of patients undergoing gastric resection for cancer.

Conclusion

Both colon and gastric cancer should serve as challenges to the oncologist interested in clinical trials. In both diseases the "standard" form of therapy, surgical resection, has realized its maximal potential and still fails in at least 50% of patients with resectable disease. It is clear that such a situation must challenge the medical oncologists to establish effective surgical adjuvant therapy. This brief review has pointed out that currently we are at an early stage in the development of adjuvant chemotherapy in gastric and colon cancer. We are plagued by relatively inactive drugs in colon cancer, but it may be possible to alleviate this disadvantage by innovative use of the available agents. In gastric cancer, trials with active combination chemotherapy regimens are still at an early stage, but have the potential to clearly answer the question of the value of postoperative chemotherapy in this disease.

Of most importance is the necessity for clinical investigators to carefully design and evaluate clinical trials so that the questions posed can be clearly answered. At present, a well-designed clinical trial of adjuvant therapy in gastrointestinal cancer requires a prospectively randomized control arm and stratification for known prognostic factors. It is only through the use of such rigorously structured protocols that answers to the major challenges posed by the adjuvant therapy of colon and gastric cancer will be found.

References

1. Comis RL, Carter SK (1974) Integration of chemotherapy into combined modality treatment of solid tumors. III. Cancer Treat Rep 63: 1863–1868
2. Dixon WJ, Longmire P, Holden WD (1971) Use of triethylene-thiophosphoramide as an adjuvant to the surgical treatment of gastric and colorectal cancer. Ten-year follow-up. Ann Surg 173: 16–34
3. Dwight RW, Higgins GA, Keehn RJ (1973) Factors influencing survival after resection in cancer of the colon and rectum. Am J Surg Oncol 5: 243–254
4. Dwight RW, Humphrey EW, Higgins GA (1973) FUDR as an adjuvant to surgery in cancer of the large bowel. J Surg Oncol 5: 243–249
5. Frank W, Osterberg AE (1960) Mitomycin-C (NSC 26989). An evaluation of the Japanese reports. Cancer Chemother Rep 9: 114–120
6. Grage TB, Hill GJ, Cornell GN, Frelick RW, Moss SE (1979) Adjuvant chemotherapy in large bowel cancer: Updated analysis of single-agent chemotherapy. In: Jones SE, Salmon SG (eds) Adjuvant therapy of cancer II. Grune & Stratton, New York, pp 587–594
7. Higgins GA, Serlin O, Amadeo JH, McElhinney J, Keehn J (1976) Gastric cancer factors in survival. Gastroenterol Surg 10: 393–399
8. Higgins GA, Lee LE, Dwight RW, Keehn RJ (1978) The case for adjuvant 5-fluorouracil in colorectal cancer. Cancer Clin Trials 1: 35–41
9. Kovach JS, Moertel CG, Schutt AJ (1974) A controlled study of combined 1,3-bis(2-chloroethyl)-1-nitrosourea and 5-fluorouracil therapy for advanced gastric and pancreatic cancer. Cancer 33: 563–569
10. Koyama Y, Kimura T (1978) Preventive chemotherapy after radical operations in stomach cancer. In: Thatcher N (ed) Digestive cancer. Pergamon Press, Oxford (Advances in medical oncology. Research and education, vol IX, pp 255–268)
11. Macdonald JS, Schein P, Ueno W, Woolley P (1979) 5-Fluorouracil, mitomycin-C and adriamycin (FAM): A new combination chemotherapy program for advanced gastric carcinoma. Cancer 44: 42–47
12. Moertel CG (1973) Large bowel. In: Holland JF, Frei E III (eds) Cancer medicine. Lea & Febiger, Philadelphia, pp 1597–1627
13. Moertel CG, Lavin PT (1979) Phase II–III chemotherapy studies in advanced gastric cancer. Cancer Treat Rep 63: 1863–1868
14. Moertel CG, Mittelman JA, Bakermeier RF, Engstrom P, Hanely J (1976) Sequential and combination chemotherapy of advanced gastric cancer. Cancer 38: 678–684
15. Piper DW (1978) Stomach cancer. UICC Tech Rep Ser 34: 3–26
16. Serlin O, Wolkoff JS, Amadeo JM, Keehn RJ (1969) Use of 5-fluorodeoxyuridine (FUDR) as an adjuvant to the surgical management of carcinoma of the stomach. Cancer 24: 223–230
17. Serlin O, Keehn RJ, Higgins GA, Harrower HW, Mendeloff GL (1977) Factors related to survival following resection for gastric carcinoma. Cancer 40: 1318–1326
18. Silverberg E (1980) Cancer statistics 1980. CA 30: 23–38
19. Taylor I, Brooman P, Rowling JT (1977) Adjuvant liver perfusion in colorectal cancer: Initial results of a clinical trial. Br Med J 2: 1320–1322

46. *Chemotherapy of Metastatic Gastrointestinal Cancers: Prospects for Future Adjuvant Systemic Therapies*

D. L. Kisner and J. S. Macdonald

National Cancer Institute, Division of Cancer Treatment,
Cancer Therapy Evaluation Program,
Bethesda, MD 20205, USA

Summary

Overall survival enhancement for patients with gastrointestinal malignancies is most likely to come from the integration of active systemic drug therapies into combined modality programs, applied in the surgical adjuvant or locoregional disease setting. Recent results of chemotherapy trials in advanced disease are discussed with emphasis placed on regimens that appear to be likely candidates for future early-stage disease studies. The ultimate success of this overall strategy depends heavily on identification of new active chemotherapeutic agents. Meticulous disease-oriented phase II testing of all new agents in gastrointestinal cancers is critical to this effort.

Introduction

Gastrointestinal (GI) tract cancer is the leading cause of cancer mortality in the United States, causing more than 100,000 deaths a year. Approximately 99,000 new cases and 49,000 deaths occur annually from large bowel cancers alone [12]. These figures are virtually unchanged in the last three decades. Carcinoma of the pancreas is increasing in incidence in the United States and is currently the fourth most common cause of cancer death. More than 21,000 cases occur annually with virtually all patients eventually dying of their disease [12]. Carcinoma of the stomach has progressively decreased in incidence in the United States over the past four decades, but still accounts for more than 14,000 deaths annually [12]. Because of the high rate of primary nonresectability and recurrence after resection, most patients at some time become candidates for therapy directed at locoregional or metastatic disease. Recent clinical research has aimed at identifying and confirming the activity of new drugs or drug combinations in metastatic disease with an eye towards their application in the locoregional or surgical adjuvant setting. The purpose of this report is to highlight the pertinent recent data in chemotherapy trials in advanced GI cancer.

Gastric Cancer

Recent work in advanced gastric carcinoma has concentrated heavily on adriamycin combination therapies in light of two recent reports demonstrating a greater than 20%

Recent Results in Cancer Research, Vol. 80

response rate for that drug as a single agent [4, 8]. The combination of 5-fluorouracil (5-FU) (600 mg/m^2 i.v. on days 1, 8, 29, and 36), adriamycin (ADM) (30 mg/m^2 i.v. on days 1 and 29), and mitomycin C (MMC) (10 mg/m^2 i.v. on day 1) (FAM) was initially reported by Macdonald et al. [7] to produce responses of 18 of 36 (50%) patients with a median response duration of 9.5 months. Overall patient survival was 5.5 months. FAM activity has now been confirmed by the Southwest Oncology Group (SWOG) [11], where it has produced a 44% partial response rate with an overall survival of 25 weeks for all patients treated.

The Gastrointestinal Tumor Study Group (GITSG) has reported results with a second ADM combination consisting of 5-FU (350 mg/m^2 i.v. on days 1–5), ADM (40 mg/m^2 i.v. for 4 weeks), and methyl CCNU (150 mg/m^2 orally on day 1) (FAMe) [4]. Forty-seven percent of previously untreated patients responded objectively to FAMe chemotherapy with an overall median survival of 24 weeks. In a second study [10] the GITSG has demonstrated that both FAM and FAMe are superior to combinations consisting of methyl CCNU plus 5-FU and 5-FU plus ICRF-159 plus methyl CCNU with regard to survival. This suggests that ADM and 5-FU may well be the two important agents in FAM and FAMe. The GITSG is now randomly comparing ADM plus 5-FU with the other two ADM-containing regimens. The superior activity of these regimens suggests that their use in the surgical adjuvant setting or in locally residual disease might have a significant survival impact. With this as the goal, SWOG and the Cancer and Leukemia Group B (CALGB) are currently evaluating FAM as a surgical adjuvant therapy compared to surgery alone. Both of these trials are still in the early stages.

Pancreatic Cancer

Chemotherapy of pancreatic carcinoma remains a frustrating problem for both clinical researchers and practitioners. Although several active agents have been identified, it is safe to say that single-agent therapy has produced no significant benefit to the patient with metastatic disease.

Results with combination chemotherapy have been only slightly more encouraging. Wiggans et al. [14] reported 10 of 23 (43%) responses to a combination of 5-FU (600 mg/m^2 i.v. in weeks 1, 2, 5, and 6), streptozotocin (1.0 g/m^2 i.v. in weeks 1, 2, 5, and 6), and MMC (10 mg/m^2 i.v. in week 1) (FMS). Responders survived a median of 10 months, with overall survival for all patients treated a median of 6 months. One patient in that trial is alive and disease-free more than 5 years after biopsy-proven diagnosis of metastatic disease.

A second drug combination reported by the same group is FAM, developed initially for gastric cancer and described above [13]. FAM chemotherapy produced 10 of 25 (37%) objective responses. The median duration of survival for responders is 1 year. Activity for FAM in pancreatic cancer has been confirmed by Bitran et al. [1] in a report of one complete response (CR) and five partial response (PR) in 15 patients treated with the regimen (CR plus PR, 40%). Median survival for responders was in excess of 13 months compared to 3.5 months for nonresponders.

FMS and FAM chemotherapies are currently being randomly compared by the GITSG. One or both of these regimens may well be in the next generation of early disease studies in pancreatic cancer.

A very recent report of a new active drug combination has come from Brown et al. [2]. The regimen consisted of combined 5-FU (30 mg/kg/day i.v. × 5 days by constant infusion), MMC (10 mg/m^2 i.v. on day 1), and hexamethylmelamine (150 mg/m^2 orally on days 2–15) every 5 weeks (hex-MF). Hex-MF chemotherapy was given to 21 ambulatory, adequately nourished patients with biopsy-proven pancreatic adenocarcinoma. Six of 15 (40%) evaluable patients responded objectively, with disease stabilization seen in an additional six patients. Median survival for all patients is 42+ weeks suggesting hex-MF to be roughly comparable to FMS and FAM. Evaluation of hex-MF in larger series of patients with comparison to the other active combinations is desirable to validate its usefulness in advanced disease and potential use in early-stage disease.

Colorectal Cancer

The chemotherapy situation in advanced colorectal cancer is similar to that in pancreatic cancer. Single agents have been extensively studied, but do not provide overall survival benefit to the patient population as a whole. Emphasis in recent years has, therefore, been on testing agents with known activity in various combinations. For this reason and the lack of new agents active in this disease this section will concentrate on combination chemotherapy.

In 1975, Moertel et al. [9] reported the results of a randomized trial comparing combined 5-FU (10 mg/kg/day i.v. × 5 days), vincristine (1.0 mg/m^2 i.v. on day 1), and methyl CCNU (125 mg/m^2 orally on day 1) (FMV) versus 5-FU alone in 80 advanced colorectal cancer patients. They reported a partial response rate of 43% for the combination compared to 19.5% for 5-FU alone ($P < 0.05$). Many attempts have been made to confirm activity for this combination, but the most recent was reported by the Eastern Cooperative Oncology Group (ECOG) [3]. Table 1 shows the results of five drug combinations in a randomized study containing 396 evaluable patients. The FMV combination achieved a dismal 12% partial response rate with a median survival of 33 weeks, firmly indicating no superiority to 5-FU alone.

Of interest, however, in this same ECOG study is that the two regimens with the longest median survival times both contained DTIC (dimethyl triazeno imidazole carboxamide). This is of even more interest considering the recent report of Haegele et al. [5], presenting results with a combination of DTIC (300 mg/m^2/day i.v. × 5 days)

Table 1. Eastern Cooperative Oncology Group: Advanced colon cancer trial. Adapted from Engstrom et al. [3]

Treatment	Responses	(%)	Median survival (weeks)
5-FU + MeCCNU + VCR	10/81	(12)	33
5-FU + MeCCNU	9/88	(10)	26
5-FU + Hydroxyurea	15/73	(21)	33
5-FU + MeCCNU + DTIC	14/83	(14)	41
5-FU + MeCCNU + DTIC + VCR	11/71	(15)	40
Historical 5-FU data		(16)	31

and MMC (50 μg/kg/day × 5 days) repeated every 3 weeks. Twenty-six patients with measurable abdominal or hepatic (17 cases) metastases were entered in the trial. All patients had progressed on previous combination chemotherapy consisting of 5-FU plus hydroxyurea or 5-FU plus nitrosourea. Five complete responses and eight partial responses were seen in the 26 patients (PR and CR, 50%). Median survival times were 10 months for responders and 3 months for nonresponders, with an overall median survival of 8 months. These results are particularly impressive in light of the prior treatment of the patient population, and suggest that further studies using DTIC in combinations are required and the routine inclusion of 5-FU in any new drug combination is probably not justified. The combination of MMC and DTIC is currently being evaluated in previously untreated patients in a group-wide study by the ECOG.

One ray of hope for 5-FU plus nitrosourea combinations comes in a recent report from Memorial Sloan Kettering by Kemeny et al. [6]. They report results of a randomized comparison of combined methyl CCNU (35 mg/m^2 orally daily × 5), 5-FU (350 mg/m^2 i.v. daily × 5), and vincristine (1 mg i.v. on day 1) (MOF) versus combined methyl CCNU (30 mg/m^2 orally daily × 5), 5-FU (300 mg/m^2 i.v. daily × 5), vincristine (1.0 mg i.v. on day 1), and streptozotocin (500 mg/m^2 i.v. weekly) (MOF-strep). The complete plus partial response rates for MOF and MOF-strep were 7% and 36%, respectively, ($P = 0.011$) with superior survival times as well for MOF-strep. Thus the addition of a second nonmyelosuppressive nitrosourea to the MOF regimen appears to enhance activity. Both the MOF-strep and MMC-DTIC combinations require further evaluation, but represent reasonable candidates for systemic therapies to be included in future surgical adjuvant therapy programs.

Conclusion

Slow progress has been made with combinations of established drugs in advanced GI cancers which may be useful in the next generation of early-stage disease protocols. Despite this, future advances depend heavily upon the development of new chemotherapy agents, and their meticulous testing in disease-oriented phase II studies. Careful consideration must be given to phase II study design and known prognostic factors so as to avoid inappropriate rejection of a potentially useful agent.

Integration of active systemic therapies into combined modality programs in the locoregional or surgical adjuvant setting remains the most likely approach to enhance overall survival of these malignancies.

References

1. Bitran J, Desser R, Kozloff M, Billings A (1979) Treatment of metastatic pancreatic and gastric adenocarcinoma with 5-fluorouracil, adriamycin and mitomycin-C (FAM). Cancer Treat Rep 63: 2049–2051
2. Brown JC, Bruckner HW, Storch J, Chamberlin K, Pressman PI (1980) Combination chemotherapy for pancreatic cancer. Proc Am Assoc Cancer Res Am Soc Clin Oncol 21: 420

3. Engstrom P, MacIntyre J, Douglass H, Carbone P (1978) Combination chemotherapy of advanced bowel cancer. Proc Am Assoc Cancer Res Am Soc Clin Oncol 19: 384
4. Gastrointestinal Tumor Study Group (1979) Phase II–III studies in advanced gastric cancer. Cancer Treat Rep 63: 1871–1876
5. Haegele LA, Conroy JF, Brodsky I, Kahn SB (1979) Dimethyl triazene imidazole carboxamide (DTIC) and mitomycin-C in the treatment of advanced colon carcinoma. Proc Am Assoc Cancer Res Am Soc Clin Oncol 20: 342
6. Kemeny N, Yagoda A, Golbey R (1980) A prospective randomized study of methyl-CCNU, 5-fluorouracil and vincristine (MOF) vs MOF plus streptozotocin (MOF-Strep) in patients with metastatic colorectal carcinoma. Proc Am Assoc Cancer Res Am Soc Clin Oncol 21: 417
7. Macdonald JS, Schein P, Ueno W, Woolley PV (1979) 5-Fluorouracil, mitomycin-C and adriamycin (FAM): A new combination chemotherapy program for advanced gastric carcinoma. Cancer 44: 42–47
8. Moertel CG, Lavin P (1979) Phase II–III chemotherapy studies in advanced gastric cancer. Cancer Treat Rep 63: 1863–1869
9. Moertel CG, Schutt AJ, Hahn RG, Reitemeier RJ (1975) Therapy of advanced gastrointestinal cancer with a combination of 5-FU, methyl-CCNU and vincristine. J Natl Cancer Inst 54: 69–71
10. O'Connell M, O'Fallon J, Lavin P, Moertel C, Bruckner H, Douglass H, Livestone E, Lokich J, Mitchell M, for the Gastrointestinal Tumor Study Group (1980) A comparative assessment of combination chemotherapy in advanced gastric carcinoma. Proc Am Assoc Cancer Res Am Soc Clin Oncol 21: 420
11. Panettiere F, Heilbrun L (1979) Comparison of two different combinations of adriamycin, mitomycin-C and 5-FU in the management of gastric carcinoma: A SWOG study. Proc Am Assoc Cancer Res Am Soc Clin Oncol 20: 315
12. Silverberg E (1980) Cancer statistics 1980. CA 30: 39
13. Smith FP, Macdonald JS, Woolley PV, Hoth DF, Smythe TA, Lichtenfeld L, Levin B, Schein P (1979) Phase II evaluation of FAM in advanced pancreatic cancer. Proc Am Assoc Cancer Res Am Soc Clin Oncol 20: 415
14. Wiggans G, Woolley PV, Macdonald JS et al. (1978) Phase II trial of streptozotocin, mitomycin-C and 5-fluorouracil (SMF) in the treatment of advanced pancreatic cancer. Cancer 41: 387–391

47. *Chemotherapy of Carcinomas of the Digestive Tract**

C. Gisselbrecht, D. Belpomme, L. Mignot, M. Marty, G. Mathé, and M. Boiron

Unité d'oncologie Clinique, Hôpital Saint-Louis, 2 Place du Docteur Fournier, F-75475 Paris Cedex, France

Summary

Adjuvant chemotherapy trials in gastric and colorectal carcinomas are reviewed and no clear benefit from such treatment could be observed. To improve existing chemotherapy regimens, several pilot studies were performed in 95 gastric cancer and 85 colorectal carcinomas patients. Response rate for gastric carcinomas using the mitomycin C plus adriamycin plus 5-fluorouracil (5-FU) (FAM) regimen was 40% and was not improved by the addition of nitrosoureas. In colorectal carcinomas none of the combinations used gave better results than 5-FU alone. Fourteen patients with esophageal carcinoma were treated with combination CDDP and the response rate was as high as 50%.

Introduction

Despite high incidence and the recent advances in chemotherapy, tumors of the digestive tract still have a poor prognosis. Advanced carcinomas remain insensitive to chemotherapy combinations [9]. However, from both theoretical and animal data, it has been suggested that even less effective antineoplastic drugs could have positive effects in treating residual tumor cells after surgery [14].
From the adjuvant chemotherapy studies performed, (4-5-11-9) no clear positive effect could be noted either in gastric or colorectal carcinomas. One reason for this could be the lack of an effective chemotherapy regimen available for treatment of gastrointestinal carcinomas. At the present time, one of the main tasks for oncologists interested in tumors of the digestive tract should be to find new treatment approaches. New drugs or new chemotherapy combinations can be, at best, tested in advanced carcinomas.
In this paper, we report some of the most significant ajuvant trials in gastrointestinal carcinomas, and present a series of recent pilot studies conducted in gastric, colorectal, and esophagal carcinomas.

* This work was supported in part by the NCI French-American Cancer Research Agreement

Table 1. Adjuvant chemotherapy for gastric carcinoma

Author	Regimen	Comparative survival
Blixenkrone-Moller (1967)	Cyclophosphamide	No significant difference
Karrer et al. (1968)	Cyclophosphamide	No significant difference
VASAG (1965)	Thio tepa	No significant difference
Dixon et al. (1971)	Thio tepa	No significant difference
Serlin et al. (1969)	FUDR	No significant difference
Fujimoto et al. (1977)	5-FU	Significant improvement
Nakazato et al. (1979)	Mitomycin C	Significant improvement
Mayer et al. (1979)	5-FU BNCU	No significant improvement
VASOG (1979)	5-FU Methyl CCNU	No significant improvement
GITSG (1980)	5-FU Methyl CCNU	No significant improvement

Adjuvant Chemotherapy for Gastric Carcinomas

Adjuvant chemotherapy trials with curative-operated stomach cancer are summarized in Table 1.

For some years, it has been hoped that the combination of chemotherapy and radical gastric resection would improve the curability of gastric cancer. Studies with fluorodeoxyuridine, thiotepa, or cyclophosphamide as adjuvant treatment had no positive effect on survival. However, chemotherapy used in earlier studies was usually of short duration and of moderate intensity with a single agent [5].

Other studies, using more intensive and prolonged treatment either with mitomycin C, 5-fluorouracil (5-FU), or with a combination of 5-FU and nitrosoureas showed a slight increase in disease-free interval (DFI) although without significantly increasing long-term survival, except in some Japanese studies. Nakazato [11] reported that mitomycin C twice weekly for 5 weeks increased the overall survival by 13.5% and produced a highly significant 36.6% increase in 5-year survival times in patients with stage II cancer. Mitomycin C was particularly effective in preventing hematogenous metastases to the liver in patients who did not have serosal invasion, but it was not effective when the cancer invaded the serosa. Well-differentiated carcinomas did benefit from adjuvant chemotherapy compared to poorly differentiated carcinomas.

However, all the published data have used combination regimens without adriamycin (ADM) or combination 5-FU-ADM, since this represents the backbone of the most active chemotherapy treatment for advanced gastric carcinomas. Several controlled studies are now using, after curative resection, and adjuvant chemotherapy composed of 5-FU, ADM, and mitomycin C, but are at a stage too early to be evaluated.

Adjuvant Chemotherapy for Colorectal Cancer

In spite of a few isolated, uncontrolled series that have suggested benefit with postoperative 5-FU, the consistent conclusion reached by the prospective randomized trials (Table 2) make it painfully clear that 5-FU as a single-agent adjuvant therapy in

Table 2. Randomized trials of adjuvant chemotherapy for colorectal cancer from Carter [4]

Author	Regimen	Comparative survival
Higgins et al. (1971)	5-FU IV 2 weeks and 8–10 weeks postoperatively	No significant difference
Higgins et al. (1976)	5-FU IV every 6 weeks for 1.5 years	No significant difference
Dwight et al. (1973)	FUDR IV and orally	No significant difference
Lawrence et al. (1975, 1978)	5-FU intraluminal + every 2 months orally for 1 year	No significant difference
Grage et al. (1977)	5-FU IV weekly for 1 year	No significant difference
Grossi et al. (1977)	5-FU intraluminal	No significant difference

colorectal cancer is doomed to failure [4]. Despite the large number of patients with various modalities of treatment with 5-FU, only in the trial conducted by the Central Oncology Group [6] did the DFI for Dukes' C curative resection cases approach statistical significance, with a median of 24 months for the chemotherapy group versus 16 months for control. However, this did not extend to increased survival for the treated group.

Lately, some new approaches are being tested by the Gastrointestinal Tumor Study Group. Patients with Dukes' B2 and C colon cancer who have undergone surgical resection are being randomized to chemotherapy with 5-FU plus methyl CCNU, immunotherapy, chemoimmunotherapy, or no treatment (controls). As far as preliminary results are concerned, no increase in survival can be observed with such treatment, even though treated patients did better than nontreated ones [7].

Adjuvant Immunotherapy in Colorectal Carcinomas

Past and current attempts at controlling the growth of colon cancer by immunologic means have been dominated by the use of nonspecific immunomodulators, which have been used as components of adjuvant therapy after surgery [12]. The same disappointing results were observed as when immunotherapy was utilized alone or associated to chemotherapy. In the studies (Table 3) with levamisole no benefit could be seen, except in one study where an increased DFI could be observed. As yet, there is little evidence that BCG, MER, or *C. parvum* are effective in this context [10].

Chemotherapy experience with the less common gastrointestinal carcinomas has, in the main, been too fragmentary to allow any evaluation. In 1980, it must be concluded that there is no clear adjuvant chemotherapy approach to gastrointestinal carcinoma. However, by no means should this conclusion imply that efforts should be abandoned.

Table 3. Randomized trials of adjuvant immunotherapy in colorectal carcinoma from Second International Conference Immunotherapy of cancer: Present status of trials in man. Bethesda (1980)

Author		Comparative disease free
Verhaegen et al. (1980)	Levamisole	Significant Improvement
Borden et al. (1980)	Levamisole + 5-FU	No significant difference
EORTC (1980)	Levamisole	No significant difference

Table 4. Chemotherapy in advanced gastric carcinoma

Regimen	Patients	Response rate
Vm FM-CCNU (1978) [2]	20	32%
FAM (1979) [8]	61	43%
FAM Chloro (1980) [a]	10	40%
FAM-RFCNU (1980)[a]	14	28%

[a] Unpublished datas

One reason which could explain the failure of such an adjuvant program, might be the rather poor efficacy of combination chemotherapy in tumors of the digestive tract.

Response rate in advanced gastrointestinal carcinomas are characterized by the variability of response rate from study to study, the fairly low rate of partial response (40%) and the almost inexistent complete response rate, and the short duration of response.

In other words, chemotherapy seems unable to eradicate completely all tumor cells in advanced carcinomas. Resistant clones of cells allow gastrointestinal cancer to recover. Although no strong correlation should be drawn between chemotherapy activity in advanced cancer with bulky disease and activity in residual tumor cells, these points should be kept in mind when designing new therapeutic approaches. From the results obtained in previous studies, one recommendation for the future is that new drugs or new combination chemotherapies should be tested in both phase II and pilot studies [3].

Chemotherapy for Advanced Gastric Carcinomas

In the past 3 years some significant progress has been made in treating advanced gastric carcinomas.

Mcdonald et al. [8] treated 61 patients with a combination of 5-FU (600 mg/m^2 on days 1 and 8), ADM (30 mg/m^2 on day 1), and mitomycin C (10 mg/m^2 on day 1 every two cycles) (FAM). A 43% partial response rate was observed with a median remission of 9 months. The median survival for responders was 14 months and the median survival time for nonresponding patients was 3 months. The survival for responding patients was significantly better. The FAM combination represents the most popular drug therapy for advanced gastric cancer. To improve this regimen, we ran two studies adding to the FAM protocol chlorozotocin or chloroethyl-ribofuranosyl nitrosourea (RFCNU), two nonmyelotoxic nitrosoureas. As seen in Table 4, the response rate was 40% in a group of ten patients treated with FAM-chlorozotocin and 28% in 14 patients who had received FAM-RFCNU. The addition of nitrosoureas did not seem to improve the overall results of the FAM combination.

In another study [2] 20 patients were treated with a cyclic sequential combination of drugs consisting of VM 26 (60 mg/m² on day 1), mitomycin C (12 mg/m² on day 2), CCNU (60 mg/m² on days 3 and 4), and 5-FU (400 mg/m² on days 2–5). The response rate was 32% with a median survival for responders of 7.8 months.

Considering these results, it seems likely that chemotherapy can achieve partial remission with an improvement of survival in about one-third to one-half of the patients. The synergistic association of 5-FU and ADM accounts for this improvement. All these results are far from impressive but further progress could be made by using new associations with new drugs such as *cis*-platinum compounds.

Chemotherapy in Advanced Colorectal Cancer

In colorectal carcinoma, despite the large number of drugs tested, no major advance has been made since the use of 5-FU (Table 5).

In the first study using the same combination of VM 26, mitomycin C, CCNU, and 5-FU, 40 patients with advanced colorectal carcinomas were treated. The partial response rate was 25%, while the median survival time was 4.7 months for nonresponders and 8.5. months for responder patients [2].

A great hope has been put in new nitrosoureas derivatives, such as chlorozotocin (chloro) and RFCNU, because of their less myelotoxic action which allows greater flexibility in combination chemotherapy. Twenty-seven patients were treated with a combination of 5-FU (300 mg/m² for 5 days) and chlorozotocin (80 mg/m² on day 1). The partial response rate was only 18%. Eighteen additional patients with advanced colorectal carcinomas were treated with RFCNU (300 mg/m² every 5 weeks), 5-FU (600 mg/m² in weeks 1, 2, 5, 6, and 9), cyclophosphamide (600 mg/m² in weeks 1, 5, and 9), and mitomycin C (6 mg/m² in weeks 1 and 9). The response rate was 16%.

With the evident inadequacy of fluorinated pyrimidine therapy, there is no doubt that colorectal carcinoma represents one of major fields were new drugs should be tested in phase II programs.

Table 5. Chemotherapy in advanced colorectal carcinoma

Regimen	Patients	Response rate
Vm FM-CCNU (1980) [2]	40	25%
FEM-RFCNU (1979)[a]	18	16%
5-FU Chloro (1980)[a]	27	18%

[a] Unpublished datas

Chemotherapy for Advanced Esophageal Cancer

The overall results of carcinoma of the esophagus treatment are not encouraging. Less than 5% of patients who develop it will indeed be cured of disease and alive 5 years after first diagnosed [1]. Moreover, it seems to be very resistant to chemotherapy. However, with the use of *cis*-diammine-dichloride-platinum (CDDP), important progress has been made in chemotherapy management of epidermoid carcinoma [13].

In a preliminary study, we treated eight patients with esophagus carcinoma with a combination of 5-FU, ADM, and CDDP, and six patients with CDDP-bleomycin-vinblastine. Dramatic tumor regression was observed in seven patients and in three patients the remission was complete. Our study compared very favorably with the 40% response rate reported with CDDP alone [13].

More patients are needed to confirm these results but we can be more optimistic about this difficult field of chemotherapy of digestive tract carcinomas.

References

1. Beatty JD, deBoer G, Rider WD (1979) Carcinoma of the esophagus. Cancer 43: 2254–2267
2. Belpomme D, Bohu A, Musset M (1979) Controlled ECR 1 and ECR 2 trials of chemotherapy and chemoimmunotherapy in advanced gastric and colorectal carcinoma: Value of a cyclic sequential combination using VM 26, 5 fluorouracil, mitomycin C, CCNU and BCG. Eur J Cancer 15: 189–196
3. Belpomme D, Bohu A, Gisselbrecht C, Marty M (1979) Nécessité d'essais coopérateurs contrôlés de chimiothérapie et d'immunothérapie pour le traitement des tumeurs digestives. In: Mathé G, Hoerni B (eds) Actualités cancérologiques 1979. Expension Scientifique Française, Paris, pp 31–41
4. Carter SK (1979) 5-Fluorouracil as adjuvant chemotherapy for large bowel cancer: Is it appropriate for routine community use? Cancer Chemother Pharmacol 2: 81–84
5. Comis RL, Carter SK (1974) Integration of chemotherapy into combined modality treatment of solid tumors. Cancer Treat Rev 1: 221–238
6. Grage TB, Metter GE, Cornell JG, Strawitz JG, Hill GJ, Frelich RW, Moss SE (1977) Adjuvant chemotherapy with 5-fluorouracil after surgical resection of colorectal carcinoma (COG protocol 7041): A preliminary report. Am J Surg 133: 59–66
7. Lokich JJ (1979) Adjuvant therapy for surgically curable colon cancer: A controlled study of chemo- and immunotherapy. Proc Am Assoc Cancer Res Am Soc Clin Oncol 20: 423
8. MacDonald JS, Schein PS, Woolley PV et al. (1979) 5-Fluorouracil (5-FU), mitomycin-C (MMC) and adriamycin (ADR) FAM combination chemotherapy results in 61 patients with advanced gastric cancer. Proc Am Assoc Cancer Res Am Soc Clin Oncol 20: 396
9. Moertel CG (1978) Current concepts in cancer. Chemotherapy of gastrointestinal cancer. N Engl J Med 299: 19, 1049–1052
10. Moertel CG, O'Connel MJ, Ritts RE, Schutt AJ, Reitemeier RJ, Huhn RG, Frytak SK, Rubin J (1978) A controlled evaluation of combined immunotherapy (MER-BCG) and chemotherapy for advanced colorectal cancer. In: Terry WD, Windhorst D (eds) Immunotherapy of cancer: Present status of trials in man, vol 6. Raven Press, New York, pp 573–586

11. Nakazato H, Imanaga H (1979) Results of surgery for gastric cancer and effect of adjuvant chemotherapy. In: Herfarth C, Schlag P (eds) Gastric cancer. Springer, Berlin Heidelberg New York, pp 344–356
12. Oettgen HF, Old LJ (1980) Immunotherapy of colon cancer: Prospects for developing immunogenic vaccines based on autologus serological typing. Cancer 45: 1218–1222
13. Ravry MJR, Moore M (1980) A phase II study of *cis*-platinum (II) (DDP) in advanced squamous cell esophageal cancer (SCE). Proc Am Assoc Cancer Res Am Soc Clin Oncol 21: 353
14. Schabel FM (1977) Rational adjuvant chemotherapy. Cancer 39: 2875–2882

IX. Conclusions and Prospects

48. *Clinical Trials on Adjuvant Therapies in Cancer: Short-Term and Long-Term Results**

P. Valagussa and G. Bonadonna

Istituto Nazionale Tumori, Division Medical Oncology, Via Venezian 1, I-20133 Milano, Italy

Summary

Short-term results of adjuvant treatments of cancer have been reported all over the world with the specific aim of reducing the period required to determine the cure rate of a potentially curative treatment. While this motivation is important, short-term analyses are not totally unbiased and they require careful evaluation. The most peculiar aspect is that short-term results should properly predict long-term results. Therefore, a complete knowledge of the natural history of the disease under evaluation, an adequate number of patients, adequate follow-up of these patients, as well as a proper statistical analysis are essential to derive useful information from intermediate analysis. This paper attempts to point out these aspects and summarizes the experience of the Istituto Nazionale Tumori of Milan in two different adjuvant studies (breast cancer and non-Hodgkin's lymphomas).

Introduction

In the vast majority of advanced neoplastic diseases and with the available therapies, even the best treatment modality is only able to palliate and not cure. Therefore, in the past few years, innumerable attempts have been made to combine different therapeutic modalities and to apply them in the early stages of disease to patients with unfavorable prognostic characteristics. These treatments, called adjuvant therapies, are specifically aimed at improving the cure rate at least in a fraction of patients [4].

A suggested definition for cure of a neoplastic disease is that "we can speak of cure when in time, probably a decade or so after treatment, there remains a group of disease-free survivors whose progressive death rate from all causes is similar to that of a normal population of the same age and sex constitution" [5]. While this definition is acceptable, The major limitation is that the period required to determine the cure rate of a potentially curative treatment is very long [6]. The rapid progress in therapeutic research has focused upon the need for determining the probability of cure as early as

* Supported in part by contract N01-CM-33714 with DCT, NCI, NIH, Bethesda, MD (USA)

possible. In an attempt to determine the presence and degree of curative treatment within a shorter period of time, the relapse-free survival (i.e., the time from start of treatment to the first evidence of new disease manifestation) has been studied and has shown to be a reliable index measure. However, even if relapse-free survival requires a shorter period of observation, a few years should elapse to properly evaluate the effect of a certain treatment.

About a decade ago, preliminary favorable results on adjuvant treatments were accepted with great enthusiasm by some oncologists, while more skeptical investigators were waiting for long-term results. A few years later, the enthusiasm was tempered by less brilliant results reported in subsequent analyses. These findings stimulated discussion and controversies about the reliability of short-term results to predict long-term results. There is no doubt that the evaluation of results in cancer clinical trials poses a number of problems that are usually not encountered in other areas of medicine. Up to now, only the very first studies on adjuvant treatments have reached the ideal long-term results (i.e., 10-year results). Therefore, 5-year results will be presented, assuming that this is a sufficiently long observation time.

Motivation and Biases of Short-Term Results

Table 1 attempts to summarize the different steps in the analysis of clinical trials. The first two points are general descriptions of the status of a trial, and are related to the feasibility of a proposed protocol. As the study progresses in time, interim analyses on short-term results of treatments are usually performed. They are described in steps 3 and 4. These reports still need a proper statistical evaluation.

There is no doubt that the most important aspect of a clinical trial is the final result, and that the essence of a successful trial is a sufficient number of patients [11]. The usual question concerns how many patients are needed to yield a result which is statistically significant at the 1% level. If is beyond the scope of this paper to describe mathematical models and calculations. Suffice it to say that to, properly answer this question in an adjuvant trial, we need to assume that a certain number of events (failures or death) have taken place within a certain number of years. If a few years have elapsed and demonstrated that a difference is statistically significant, why report short-term results?

The most important reason to report short-term results is that it is almost impossible to supervise a clinical trial for months or years without ever looking to see which way the

Table 1. Steps in analysis of clinical trials

1. Accrual rate, compliance to protocol eligibility, monitoring of data submitted for completeness, and consistency
2. Rate of adverse reactions and acute toxicity, and compliance to treatment program
3. Rate of tumor regression, early recurrences, and deaths
4. Intermediate results on total series and prognostic subgroups, and preliminary ancillary studies
5. Final analysis reporting positive and negative results, and answers to the objective(s) of the trial

results are drifting. In addition, we might expect great enthusiasm from the trial originators, while other participants may be less motivated. However, over time, the interest tends to progressively decrease and it is always difficult to maintain the initial motivation. Therefore, trial participants should be kept informed on the status of the study and rough comparison with results of other trials can be made, keeping in mind that patient populations may be not totally comparable. Another factor is that, at the end of the accrual period, a decision must be made about the treatment of incoming patients and we must rely on past experience.

Obviously, short-term analyses are not totally unbiased. The most important bias is that repeated testing on accumulating data implies a greater risk of error than the risk for each single test. To overcome this problem, no easy universal solution exists, and this aspect deserves a proper full explanation [1, 9]. Furthermore, when reporting short-term results, we must be aware of two other aspects: 1) Interesting, but not statistically significant differences usually produce unconvincing results and many clinical trials are abandoned prior to reaching valid conclusions; and (2) improvement in short-term results may be associated to a decline in long-term analysis.

Reliability and Aims of Short-Term Results

The experience of the Istituto Nazionale Tumori of Milan on two different types of neoplasia will be briefly described. In June, 1973, patients with operable breast cancer and positive axillary nodes were entered into a prospective randomized study and were allocated to receive no further treatment after radical mastectomy of 12 cycles of a combination chemotherapy known as CMF (cyclophosphamide, methotrexate, and

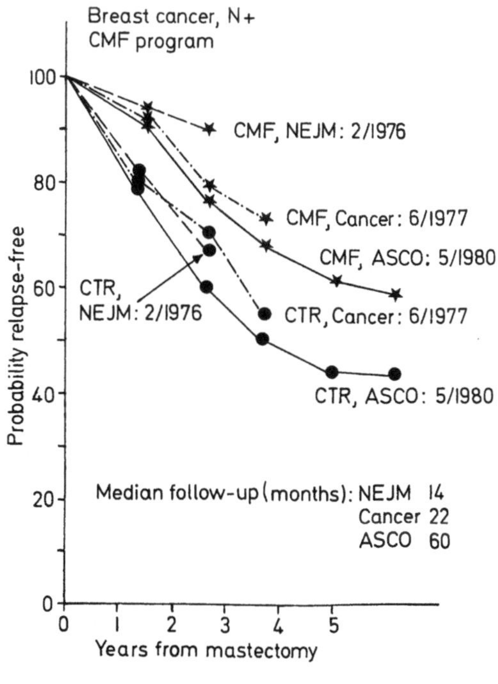

Fig. 1. Results of analysis as reported at three time intervals

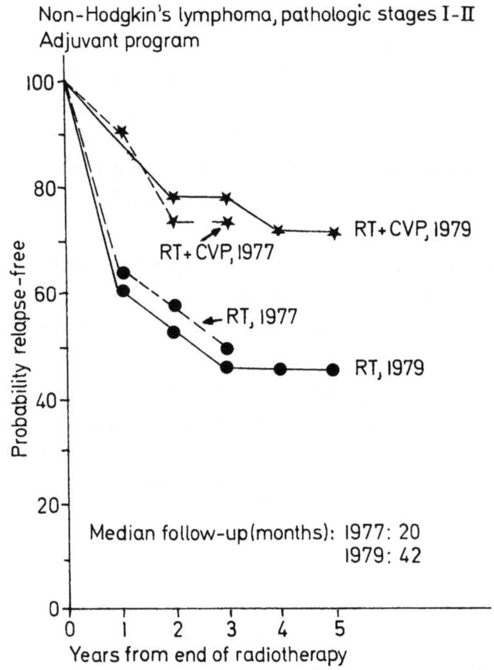

Fig. 2. Results at 3 and 5 years (actuarial analysis)

fluorouracil). Details of selection of patients, treatment program, and follow-up have been previously reported [2, 3].

Fig. 1 shows results of analysis as reported at three different time intervals. The early results of the first CMF program were reported on February, 1976 [2], and all patients were entered into the study and had a median follow-up of 14 months. Analyses of the status of the trial were performed previously but, in spite of good results, they did not influence the decision to stop patient entry prior to reaching the sample size required in the protocol. Early findings favored the treated group compared to later results reported at 3 [3] and 5 years [13]. It must be reemphasized that we concluded our first report by interpreting our preliminary results with a cautious attitude [2]. In fact, the natural history of operable breast cancer with positive axillary nodes shows that about 50% of patients relapsed within 3 years after locoregional modality alone. By approaching this crucial time, more sound data was derived and many other additional findings were reported. They could explain, in part, the differences in the various analyses.

In an other clinical trial, patients with nonHodgkin's lymphoma (pathologic stages I and II), after radiation therapy (RT), were randomly allocated to receive no further treatment or adjuvant CVP (cyclophosphamide, vincristine, and prednisone) for six cycles. Fig. 2 illustrates the results presented through actuarial analysis at 3 years [7] and then at 5 years [10]. No important fluctuations took place between the two different analyses. In fact, according to the natural history of this disease, very few relapses were expected after 2–3 years from RT. Therefore, the 3-year results were sufficiently predictive for the long-term results.

What type of information can be derived from short-term results? First of all, we need to distinguish between very preliminary results and intermediate results. Preliminary analyses aim at informing other investigators that certain hypotheses are being tested. Scientific motivations, reasons for choosing a certain type of treatment, details on plan of treatments, selection of patients, and criteria for evaluation should be reported, and data on feasibility of treatments, hematologic toxicities, and possible adverse reactions should be fully discussed. In an adjuvant setting, very preliminary statistical analyses are not mandatory especially when only very few patients have a sufficiently long follow-up.

In reporting short-term results, a sufficient number of patients should be followed-up and some dozens of events should be accumulated. Detailed plans of treatment and detailed plans of statistical analysis must be clearly reported. It must be emphasized that a *proper* and clear statistical analysis, reporting results derived from life tables and by using tests which take into account exactly the extent of risk of exposure, must be performed [8, 12].

Short-term results must be carefully interpreted. In doing so, knowledge of the natural history of the disease under treatment is essential. In fact, in almost all neoplastic diseases, there is an initial constant rate of failure followed by a decreasing rate. Therefore, we must know where the "break" could be to derive sound information. Short-term results should also indicate whether the working hypothesis is valid and whether subsequent refinements of the treatment applied could be worthy of subsequent studies to achieve even better results. In fact, adjuvant treatments should be sufficiently aggressive to be effective in the presence of large as well as small residual tumor burdens after locoregional modality [14]. Failure to show early effects is almost invariably associated with failure to show any effect, and while short-term results should not allow for definite conclusions, they should properly predict long-term results. Last, but not least, short-term results are more valid when derived from randomized studies with a concomitant control group [15]. In fact, we must realize that there could have been improvements in diagnostic procedures, as well as a discovery of new important prognostic variables or improvements in supportive care. Furthermore, as a consequence of successful educational programs, paients come in for diagnosis and treatment earlier than in the past. Therefore, we must be sure that the "improvement" we claim to have achieved through a given therapy is *entirely* due to the new treatment applied.

In conclusion, the conservative approach is to follow-up all patients for their total life span prior to making judgements. Ten years observation might be considered reasonably conservative, while 5 years observation is much less conservative. Looking for trends at a lesser period, with full knowledge that additional events may be expected, is *not* desirably conservative. However, we need to learn how to interpret short-term results so as to derive useful information to properly treat our cancer patients. Failure to do this will result in failure to achieve any progress in therapeutic research within a reasonable period of time and, what is more important, in failure to save the lives of thousands of patients.

References

1. Armitage P (1975) Sequential medical trials, 2nd edn. Blackwell, Oxford
2. Bonadonna G, Brusamolino E, Valagussa P, Rossi A, Brugnatelli L, Brambilla C, de Lena M, Tancini G, Bajetta E, Musumeci R, Veronesi U (1976) Combination chemotherapy as an adjuvant treatment in operable breast cancer. N Engl J Med 294: 405–410

3. Bonadonna G, Rossi A, Valagussa P, Banfi A, Veronesi U (1977) The CMF program for operable breast cancer with positive axillary nodes: Updated analysis on the disease-free interval, site of relapse and drug tolerance. Cancer 39: 2904–2915
4. Bonadonna G, Gasparini M, Rossi A (to be published) Adjuvant therapies of post-surgical minimal residual disease. Recent Results Cancer Res
5. Easson EC, Russel MH (1963) The cure of Hodgkin's disease. Br Med J 1: 1704–1707
6. Frei E III, Gehan EA (1971) Definition of cure for Hodgkin's disease. Cancer Res 31: 1828–1833
7. Lattuada A, Bonadonna G, Milani F, Banfi A, Valagussa P, de Lena M, Monfardini S (1977) Adjuvant chemotherapy with CVP after radiotherapy (RT) in stage I–II non-Hodgkin's lymphomas. In: Salmon SE, Jones SE (eds) Adjuvant therapy of cancer. Elsevier North-Holland Biomedical Press, Amsterdam, pp 537–544
8. Mantel N (1966) Evaluation of survival data and two new rank order statistics arising in its consideration. Cancer Chemother Rep 50: 163–170
9. McPherson K (1974) Statistics: The problem of examining accumulating data more than once. N Engl J Med 290: 501–504
10. Monfardini S, Banfi A, Bonadonna G, Rilke F, Milani F, Valagussa P, Lattuada A (1980) Improved five-year survival after combined radiotherapy-chemotherapy for stage I–II non-Hodgkin's lymphomas. Int J Radiat Oncol Biol Phys 6: 125–134
11. Peto R, Pike MC, Armitage P, Breslow NE, Cox DR, Howard SV, Mantel N, McPherson K, Peto J, Smith PG (1976) Design and analysis of randomized clinical trials requiring prolonged observation of each patient. I. Introduction and design. Br J Cancer 34: 585–612
12. Peto R, Pike MC, Armitage P, Breslow NE, Cox DR, Howard SV, Mantel N, McPherson K, Peto J, Smith PG (1977) Design and analysis of randomized clinical trials requiring prolonged observation of each patient. II. Analysis and examples. Br J Cancer 35: 1–39
13. Rossi A, Bonadonna G, Valagussa P, Banfi A, Veronesi U (1980) CMF adjuvant program for breast cancer: Five-year results. Proc Am Soc Clin Oncol 21: 404
14. Schabel FM Jr, Griswold DP Jr, Corbett TH, Laster WR Jr, Dykes DJ, Rose WC (1979) Recent studies with surgical adjuvant chemotherapy or immunotherapy of metastatic solid tumors of mice. In: Salmon SE, Jones SE (eds) Adjuvant therapy of cancer II. Grune & Stratton, New York, pp 3–17
15. Schneiderman MA (1975) How do you know you've done any better? Cancer 35: 64–69

49. *Long-Term Costs of Adjuvant Radiotherapy*

F. Volterrani and D. Sigurtà

Istituto Nazionale Tumori, Division Medical Oncology, Via Venezian 1,
I-20133 Milano, Italy

Introduction

Before discussing long-term costs it is worthwhile to define adjuvant radiotherapy. We cannot surely define as adjuvant the irradiation that follows a nonradical operation, because such treatment is compulsory and long-term costs are the price of recovery. We cannot talk about adjuvant treatment also after radical but limited surgery, such as a partial resection of the larynx or of the breast. In these cases the eventual long-term costs must also be seen from the esthetic and functional points of view and the value of this combined conservative approach must be proved with respect to the conventional treatment. We are in a different situation when we have to irradiate a patient after a radical and conventional operation, such as a radical mastectomy. In this case, the irradiation follows a treatment which is definitive in itself and this is exactly what we mean by adjuvant radiotherapy.

The aim of adjuvant radiotherapy is to control the residual disease in the locoregional area, that does not clinically appear, but that we can assume by histologic examination or natural history studies. Long-term costs must be strictly considered because patients with long life expectancy are involved. The usefulness of this kind of treatment is much debated due to the vast clinical data which varies in opinion.

Let's have a look now at the most important field of adjuvant radiotherapy.

Head and Neck Tumors

The incidence of serious and disabling lesions is hard determine since it is seldom clearly reported. In our experience of more than 1,200 patients with head and neck tumors treated from January 1959 to December 1970 long-term costs occurred in 10% of cases. The most frequent complications are xerostomia and subsequent dental pathology and the most dangerous are carotid necrosis and permanent myelitis. These are critical factors concerning permanent myelitis which depend on the treatment, such as fields overlap, short-term treatment, and length of the medulla involved, but patient-dependent factors, like previous or concomitant vertebral-medullar pathology and extreme ages, should not be forgotten. To minimize such risks, irradiation should be accurately planned and carried out, the dose limit respected (35–45 Gy), and the treatment prolonged.

Recent Results in Cancer Research, Vol. 80

Breast Cancer

Horrendous anecdotal incidents are certainly a consequence of radiotherapeutic malpractice. Generally severe injuries occur only in 3% of cases [2]. Concerning arm edema, surgery is the most important factor. In fact, this complication is twice as frequent after radical mastectomy alone than after simple mastectomy plus adjuvant radiotherapy. While we can find posttreatment studies reporting higher incidences of, for example, pulmonary fibrosis in 18% [7] or atrophic changes of bone and related sequelae in 12% [4], such numbers are likely derived from atypical treatments. In our series of cases, lesions of the brachial plexus occur only in 3.3% [1], while they reached 34.6% with nonconventional treatments [10].

Colorectal and Uterine Tumors

Intestinal injuries require a minimum dose of 40–50 Gy. Obstruction, hemorrhage, and fistula formation are dangerous complications. The rate of such lesions in postoperative radiotherapy for colorectal carcinoma is 14% [9], while in uterine tumors it depends on the extent of surgery. After conventional surgery these injuries occurred in 4.9% [11], but they reached higher incidences (25–48%) [3, 8] after extensive surgery (pelvic and paraaortic lymphadenectomy).

Soft Tissue Sarcomas

High radiotherapy doses are required and most patients exhibit some degree of clinically detectable fibrosis in the irradiated area. Soft tissue necrosis, edema, significant fibrosis, and bone necrosis were the main sequelae and occurred in 27.4% of cases treated for localizations in the upper or lower extremities. Besides, amputation may become necessary in 6.4% of these patients. In the head-neck and trunk localizations, significant complications are virtually nonexistent [5, 6] because doses are lower.

Secondary Tumors and Radiation-Related Leukemias

Many clinical observations are reported but definitive data of incidence are not available. According to studies of the ICRP, the expected risk of mortality from secondary tumors or radiation-related leukemias is 10^{-2} when a dose of 1 Gy is given to the whole body. When only a portion of the body is irradiated, this number is related to the fraction of the irradiated volume. Under standard conditions, this risk is 10^{-3}–10^{-2}.

Host-Defense Depression

This problem has often been acknowledged and many times denied by clinical observations. The role of adjuvant radiotherapy is hard to estimate and is not yet defined. However, it is a precocious effect that quickly returns to normal.

Conclusions

There are few data about long-term costs of adjuvant radiotherapy, but all published research should report this information. The seriousness of complications depends on the technique of irradiation. In adjuvant radiotherapy, atypical splitting-up techniques should be banished, given doses strictly valued, and healthy tissues saved. The problem of secondary tumors exists and their incidence mathematically depends not only on the given dose but on the irradiated volume.

References

1. Basso Ricci S, Della Costa C, Viganotti G, Ventafridda V, Zanolla R (1980) Report on 42 cases of post irradiation lesions of the brachial plexus and their treatment. Tumori 66: 117–122
2. Bruce J (1975) The treatment of early cancer of the breast: Some personal reflections. JR Coll Surg Edinb 20: 287–303
3. Delgado G, Caglar H, Walker P (1980) Survival and complications in cervical cancer treated by pelvic and extended-field irradiation after paraaortic lymphadenectomy. AJR 130: 141–143
4. Howland WJ, Kennet Loeffler R, Starchman DE, Johnson RG (1975) Post-irradiation atrophic changes of bone and related complications. Radiology 117: 677–685
5. Lindberg RD, Martin RG, Romsdahl MM (1975) Surgery and post-operative radiotherapy in the treatment of soft tissue sarcomas in adults. AJR 123: 123–129
6. Lindberg RD, Fletcher GH, Martin RG (1975) The management of soft tissue sarcomas in adults. J Radiol Electrol Med Nucl 56: 761–767
7. Oppedal T, Kolbensstvedt A (1976) Pulmonary contraction following ^{60}Co irradiation of mammary carcinoma. Acta Radiol Ther Phys Biol 15: 329–336
8. Piver MS, Vongtama V, Barlow JJ (1975) Paraaortic lymph node irradiation for carcinoma of the uterine cervix using split cause technique. Gynecol Oncol 3: 168–175
9. Romsdahl MM, Withers HR (1978) Radiotherapy combined with curative surgery. Arch Surg 113: 446–453
10. Svensson H, Westling P, Larsson LG (1975) Radiation-induced lesions of the brachial plexus correlated to the dose-time-fraction schedule. Acta Radiol [Diagn] (Stockh) 14: 228–238
11. Volterrani F, Prosperini G, Sigurtà D, Vona S, Musumeci R, Milano A, Luciani L (1979) Present status of treatment for invasive cervical carcinoma. Tumori 65: 611–624
12. Weishselbaum RR, Merk A, Hellman S (1976) The role of post-operative irradiation in carcinoma of the breast. Cancer 37: 2682–2690

50. *Long-Term Cost of Combined Radiotherapy and Chemotherapy**

M. Weil, C. Jacquillat, G. Auclerc, P. F. Unger, and J. Bernard

Unité de Chimiothérapie, Institut de Recherches sur les Maladies du Sang, Hôpital Saint-Louis, 2 Place du Docteur Fournier, F-75475 Paris Cedex 10, France

Summary

Complications after treatment of Hodgkin's disease are a good model to evaluate the long-term cost of combined chemo- and radiotherapy. Secondary malignancies and mainly acute myelocytic leukemias are the main complications. The 35 of 1,889 cases reported represent increased risk by factor 129. Often preceded by a leukemic phase, they are of poor prognosis. Solid tumors are increased by factor 2.8. They may occur in patients treated by prolonged chemotherapy with alkylating agent without radiotherapy. In seven of 31 patients, solid tumors appeared in the irradiated area. Sterility in young males was present during the first year, though some recuperation was observed thereafter. Better adjustment of treatment to individual risk, to drug sensitivity, and active combinations devoid of alkylating agents are required to reduce the rate of these complications.

Introduction

Adjuvant treatment is a relatively recent strategy in the field of solid tumors and the long-term cost may not be fully appreciated yet. Therefore, the main part of this presentation will be devoted to our personal experience of the long-term cost of treatment of Hodgkin's disease, a good model for conjecture. The two main late iatrogenic complications of Hodgkin's disease are secondary malignancies, especially leukemias, and gonadal alteration, especially sterility in young men.

Secondary Complications After Hodgkin's Disease Therapy

Risk of Acute Leukemias

Out of 1,889 patients with Hodgkin's disease treated at Hôpital Saint-Louis during 1957–1976, we have observed 35 cases of acute leukemias (AL). Most were acute

* This research was carried out with the aid of Contrat INSERM, Commission 8, Subvention du Comité Franco-Américain de Recherche sur le Cancer (INSERM), USPHS Research Grant, CA 13 239-05 du National Cancer Institute, Caisse Régionale d'Assurances Maladies de Paris, Formation de Recherche Associée n° 42 INSERM

Recent Results in Cancer Research, Vol. 80

myeloblastic leukemia, which does not fit well into any category of the FAB classification.

They are atypical and preceded by a preleukemic phase (median duration 3 months). This preleukemic phase consists of monocytopenia bi- or tricytopenia with maturation disorders. When AL was discovered, 11 patients were in their initial remission, 13 in their first relapse, and 11 had more than one relapse. On the whole, 23 patients were in complete remission (CR), two were in partial remission, and eight were in an relapsing stage of their Hodgkin's disease when AL occurred.

If we consider the 11 patients whose leukemia occurred during initial Hodgkin's disease remission, we can distinguish two categories: localized (I or II) stage patients who were treated with short-term combination chemotherapy (3 courses of MOPP in three stage I patients or 6 course of MOPP in three stage II patients followed by mantle radiotherapy; and stage III and IV patients who were treated by prolonged polychemotherapy (6 months of MOPP and MOPP every 3 months thereafter) (Table 1). Short-term remission of leukemia was more frequent in the first category. The relationship between treatment and leukemia is relevant in two patients because of the unusual cytologic type of secondary leukemia (M_3 and M_5) and because of the short interval between the two diseases.

In 18 patients AL occurred after one relapse: ten of them had received MOPP, four of them had received mantle radiotherapy, and four others total nodal radiotherapy. Only one patient did not receive any alkylating agent in addition to radiotherapy.

The 11 patients who had AL after more than one relapse were heavily treated patients who had received several courses of radiotherapy and of polychemotherapy.

Finally, the risk of AL is about 2% at 5 years. This risk is probably increased by MOPP, but we must not forget that the rate of cures is increased by MOPP in a much larger proportion (Table 2).

Table 1. Relationship between anatomic stage and first treatment of Hodgkin's (H) disease and time of occurrence of leukemia (AL) during first remission

	No. patients	Poly-chemo-therapy duration	Radio-therapy + VLB	Radiotherapy + poly-chemotherapy (years)	H–AL interval	Treat-ment results of AL
Stage I A	3		1	2	6-2[a]-2.5[b]	2 CR 1 F
Stage II B	3			3	4-5-5	2 CR 1 F
Stage III B	4	4	–	–	-4-6-6-8	1 CR 4 F
Stage IV B	1	1	–	–	4	

[a] A.U.L.

[b] M3

Abbreviations: 1 F, 1 failure; 4 F, 4 failures; AUL, acute undifferentiated leukemia; M3, acute promyelocytic leukemia; VLB, vinblastine

Table 2. Risk for AL according to time and to treatment of Hodgkin's disease

	Patients at risk	3 Years	5 Years	10 Years
Conventional Rx + chlor.	886	0.3%	0.6%	1.9%
E.F. Rx + VLB	208	0.6%	0.6%	1.6%
E.F. Rx + MOPP	260	2.4%	8.1%	
E.F. Rx + MOPP + VLB	329	0.3%	1.8%	3%
MOPP + VLB	173		4.9%	10.4%
VTRP[a]	33		4.7%	16.2%
Total	1,889	9/1044 (0.6%)	16/756 (2.1%)	10/293 (4.1%)

[a] Velbe-Thioripe-Mafochromycine-Predonizome (monthly)
Abbreviations: VLB, Vinblastine; E.F. Rx, extended field radiotherapy

Table 3. Incidence of solid tumors according to time and treatment of Hodgkin's disease

	No. of patients	Observed tumors/patients at risk between brackets actuarial incidences		
		At 3 years	At 5 years	At 10 years
Radiotherapy + Vinblastine	208	0/139 (0%)	1/119 (0.8%)	3/75 (3.8%)
MOPP + Vinblastine, H4, H6	206	4/112 (2.5%)	4/89 (6.3%)	3/31 (10.9%)
MOPP + radiotherapy + Vinblastine	589	7/335 (1.4%)	5/276 (2.8%)	3/43 (4.6%)
Monochemotherapy	91	0/67 (0%)	1/43 (1.8%)	0/17 (1.8%)
Total	1,094	11/753 (1.2%)	11/527 (2.9%)	9/166 (5.4%)

Calculated by patients per year, the number of leukemias expected in this population was 0.27. We observed 35 cases, thus, the risk for AL was multiplied by 129 in patients treated for Hodgkin's disease, that is, patients treated for Hodgkin's disease are 129 times more likely to contract AL.

The prognosis for these leukemias, where cytogenetic abnormalities are an almost constant finding, is poor. Even when CR seems to be achieved, it is of short duration (maximum 10 months).

Risk of Solid Tumors

We have observed, in a population of 1,094 patients, 36 solid tumors. In five cases, Hodgkin's disease had not been treated (four cases of simultaneous discovery). Thus, 32 solid tumors occurred in 31 patients who had previous treatment. Table 3 shows the incidence of solid tumors according to time and treatment. Twelve patients were treated by chemotherapy alone and 19 patients by combined radiotherapy and chemotherapy. The sites of the tumors are shown on Table 4. In seven patients, this site was located in a previously irradiated area. In this population, according to

Table 4. Sites of 33 solid tumors observed in 31 patients treated for Hodgkin's disease

All cases (31) (19 irradiated and 12 nonirradiated)

Esophagus	3	Cavum	1	Melanoma	2[a]	
Stomach	3	Tongue	1[a]	Basoc	3	
Colon	2	Tonsils	2[a]	Kaposi	1	
Rectum	2	Larynx	1[a]	Thyroid	2	
Hepatoma	1			Lung	3[a]	
Pancreas	1			Breast	2[a]	
				Cervix	1	
				Kidney	1	
				Brain	1	(oligodendroglioma)

[a] Patient previously irradiated

Table 5. Number of leukemias in patients with other malignant disease

	Chemo θ	Chemo θ + drug treatment	References
Ovarian cancers	9	12	[12]
Myeloma	28	19	[11]
Breast cancers (70 patients)	15	11	[13]

patients per year, the expected number of solid tumors was 12.9. Thus, the observed number of 32 in 31 patients represents an increase of 2.4.

Gonadal Alteration

Another serious drawback of Hodgkin's disease treatment, especially in young men, is the development of sterility. A recent study at Hôpital Saint-Louis dealing with serial spermograms of ten patients confirms that azoospermia is constant during the first year and very frequent thereafter. In women older than 35 years of age, early menopause is frequent and may require substitutive hormonal therapy.

Thus, the long-term cost of combined treatment in Hodgkin's disease is mainly the risk of AL and, to a lesser degree, by the increased risk of solid tumors. After 12 months, azoospermia is no more constant but still frequent. We must confirm whether combinations with intercalating agents, as suggested by Valagussa and Bonadonna data [14] and by theoretical models, are less leukemic than combinations with alkylating agents.

Long-Term Cost of Adjuvant Treatment of Solid Tumors

Several papers report leukemias in ovarian cancers, in myeloma, and in breast cancers and this list is not extensive. However, it must be emphasized that, besides treatment, there is an increased frequency of AL in myelomas and in breast cancers. As others, we have observed leukemias in such patients and, for instance, four patients included in the study of Rosner and the CALGB (Table 5). More recently, Pedersen reported eight cases of AML among 553 women treated with treosulfan for ovarian cancer. Although, the probability for leukemia was 7.6% at 5 years, the survival curve of these patients was only slightly affected by leukemic deaths.

Conclusion

The main long-term cost of adjuvant treatment is the development of secondary malignancies. The registration of all these cases is most important. They may be related to three factors; host, disease, and treatment. But, at the present time, the only factor that we can influence is the latter. We must adjust the treatment to the individual risk of each patient and to the sensitivity to therapy. We must design active combinations avoiding alkylating drugs. Antipromoters appear as an attractive but remote possibility.

References

1. Arsenau JC, Sponzo RW, Levin DL et al. (1972) Non-lymphomatous malignant tumours complicating Hodgkin's disease: Possible association with intensive therapy. N Engl J Med 287: 1119
2. Arsenau G, Canellos GP, Johnson RE, de Vita VT (1977) Risk of new-cancer patients with Hodgkin's disease. Cancer 40: 1912
3. Auclerc G, Jacquillat C, Auclerc MF et al. (1979) Post-therapeutic acute leukemia. Cancer 44: 2017
4. Berg JW (1967) The incidence of multiple primary cancers. Development of further cancers in patients with lymphoma, leukemia and myeloma. J Natl Cancer Inst 38: 741
5. Canellos GP, De Vita VT, Arseneau JC et al. (1974) Carcinogenesis by cancer chemotherapeutic agents: Second malignancies complicating Hodgkin's disease in remission. Recent Results Cancer Res 49: 108
6. Carey RW, Holland JF, Shege PR et al. (1967) Association of cancer of breast and acute myelocytic leukemia. Cancer 20: 1988
7. Crosby WH (1969) Acute granulocyticleukemia: A complication of therapy in Hodgkin's disease. Clin Res 17: 463
8. Jacquillat C, Weil M, Auclerc G, Teillet F, Weisgerber C, Tanzer J, Boiron M, Bernard J (1973) Les néoplasies simultanées et successives. A propos de 18 observations d'affections malignes compliquant l'évolution de la maladies de Hodgkin. Nouv Presse Med 2: 3039
9. Jacquillat C, Auclerc G, Weil M, Boiron M, Bernard J (1976) Acute leukemia, Kaposi sarcoma, epitheliomas, complicating 30 observations of Hodgkin. Proc Am Soc Clin Oncol 17: 247
10. Neufeld H, Weinermann BH, Kemel S (1978) Secondary malignant neoplasms in patients with Hodgkin's disease. JAMA 239: 2470
11. Kyle RA, Pierre PV, Bayrd ED (1975) Multiple myeloma and acute leukemia associated with alkylating agents. ARCM Intern Med 135: 185
12. Reimer RR, Hoover R, Fraumeni JF (1977) Acute leukemia after alkylating agent theory of ovarian cancer. N Engl J Med 297: 177
13. Rosner F, Carey RW, Zarrabi MH (1978) Breast cancer and acute leukemia. Report of 24 cases and review of the literature. Am J Hematol 4: 151
14. Valagussa P, Santoro R, Kenda R (1980) Second malignancies in Hodgkin's disease: A complication of certain forms of treatment. Br Med J 280: 216

51. *Studies of Clonogenic Human Tumor Stem Cells*

S. E. Salmon*

University of Arizona, Health Sciences Center, Hematology/Oncology Section,
Department of Internal Medicine and the Cancer Center, Tucson, AZ 85724, USA

Summary

In vitro tissue culture methods for cloning human tumor cells from fresh biopsy samples appear to provide a simple yet quantitative approach to study the biology and chemosensitivity of neoplastic cells which are likely to be responsible for micrometastasis and tumor progression in vivo. Use of this assay technique may provide a useful empirical approach to improve adjuvant therapy of cancer.

Introduction

During the past 5 years, a concerted effort has been made to develop simple quantitative in vitro techniques to study the biology, proliferative kinetics, and drug sensitivity of clonogenic human tumor cells from fresh biopsy samples [1, 3–5, 7, 12, 14]. These efforts have recently been summarized [11]. The impetus for these investigations was the recognition that clonogenic tumor stem cells are the key cells in a cancer in vivo [3]. They are the seeds of metastasis which circulate through the bloodstream and lymphatics and implant in "fertile soil" to form secondary colonies or micrometastases [10]. Prior studies with animal tumor systems in vivo [2] and in vitro [8] had indicated the behavior of clonogenic tumor stem cells, and their chemosensitivity was predictive of the biology and clinical sensitivity or resistance of the neoplasm [8]. Quite recently, techniques have been developed to perform in vitro colony culture on human tumor cells [1, 3–5, 7, 10, 11, 12, 14]. These efforts have been increasingly successful, with a wide variety of neoplasms. While the initial developmental work with these assay techniques for human tumors was carried out with grossly metastatic neoplasms, recent efforts have had greater focus on assessment of primary tumor biopsies from common invasive malignant neoplasms. Lines of

* I thank my current and former faculty colleagues, D. Alberts, R. Buick, B. Durie, A. Hamburger, S. Jones, F. Meyskens, T. Moon, T. Stanisic, E. Surwit, J. Trent, and technical staff including D. Curtis, S. Fry, M. Kim, D. Listowski, B. Soehnlen, and L. Young, for their efforts. This work was supported by grants CA 17094, CA 21839, and CA 23074 from the National Cancer Institute, DHEW, Washington, DC (USA)

Table 1. Identifiable features of human tumor colony-forming units (TCFU) which are consistent with in situ tumor stem cell origin

1. Expression of reproducible markers of clonality by tumor colonies

    Histology (e.g., melanin or mucin production, characteristic electron microscopic features)

    Cytogenetics (marker chromosomes, aneuploidy, and other characteristic chromosomal abnormalities)

    Production of tumor-associated biomarkers (e.g., monoclonal immunoglobulin, carcinoembryonic antigen, hormones)

2. Uniformity of cell type in developing colonies (colonies composed of neoplastic cell types and not mixed with normal cells)
3. TCFU are physically separable from non-neoplastic elements in the biopsy (centrifugal gradients or elutriation, "staput" analysis, phagocytic or rosette depletion, surface adherence, etc.)
4. TCFU manifest self-renewal properties (growth of secondary colonies after plucking, dispersing, and replacing primary colonies in vitro or in vivo in immune-deprived mice)
5. TCFU reflect in vivo tumor behavior (serial increase in relative cloning efficiency are associated with increasing malignancy in vivo, and a strong correlation between in vitro drug sensitivity or resistance and clinical response)

evidence that are required to demonstrate that in vitro tumor colony-forming units (TCFU) grown from biopsy samples are related to clonogenic tumor stem cells in situ are summarized in in Table 1.

Of all of the characteristics of tumor stem cells, their defining property can be considered to be the ability to undergo self-renewal. This can best be demonstrated by plucking colonies from the agar, dispersing them, and replating in semisolid medium followed by demonstration of growth of secondary colonies. Alternatively, cells dispersed from colonies can be implanted into immune-deprived mice and the growth of tumor gross nodules can be taken as evidence of the ability of human tumor stem cells to repopulate in situ. Preliminary evidence in breast cancer, colon cancer, ovarian cancer, melanoma, myeloma, and leukemia does, in fact, suggest that some TCFU have self-renewal properties as well as morphologic [12] and cytogenetic features [11, 18] of the tumor of origin. Clonal heterogeneity has often been apparent in these studies; for example, variable melanin content in different melanoma colonies [12], multiple clones on cytogenetic banding analysis [11, 18], and a mixture of sensitive, and resistant TCFU's as determined with cycle-nonspecific anticancer drugs [11, 14].

Chemosensitivity Studies

Perhaps the most important practical application of the in vitro clonogenic assay has been for studies of drug sensitivity of patient's tumor colony-forming cells [11, 14, 19]. Evidence which has accumulated at several centers has involved measurements carried out on patient biopsy samples in the human tumor stem cell assay. These studies

Table 2. Correlations of in vitro and in vivo resistance (R) and sensitivity (S) with the human tumor stem cell assay[a]: cumulative experience at two institutions. Reproduced from Salmon [11] with permission of the publisher

Investigative group	No. patients	No. clinical trials	Tumor-sensitive both in vitro and in vivo (S/S)	Tumor-sensitive in vitro and resistant in vivo (S/R)	Tumor-resistant in vitro and sensitive in vivo (R/S)	Tumor-resistant both in vitro and in vivo (R/R)
Tucson	96	193	34	22	5	132
San Antonio	101	123	15	6	2	100
Total	197	316	49	28	7	232

True positive rate (S/S)/(S/S + S/R) × 100 = 64%
True negative rate (R/R)/(R/R + R/S) × 100 = 97%

appear to be predictive of the patient's clinical response to cancer chemotherapy with specific agents. Both our group [11, 14] and Von Hoff's [19] have observed predictive correlation frequencies of 60–65% for drug sensitivity and more than 95% for drug resistance when in vitro and in vivo response data were compared ($P < 0.0001$).

A summary of the clinical correlations of in vitro sensitivity for metastatic neoplasms appears in Table 2. Results to date are reminiscent of those initially obtained with the estrogen receptor and prediction of response to hormonal therapy in breast cancer. Based on these promising initial correlations, a number of investigative groups are now exploring applications of the in vitro assay for biologic studies and for prospective correlative clinical trials of standard and new anticancer drugs, as well as for new drug screening. In fact, the NCI recently announced a new contract program to test the in vitro human tumor stem cell assay systematically as an alternative to the mouse models for new drug screening [9]. This same approach also appears to be a useful alternative or addition to clinical trial for assessing phase II activity of new anticancer drugs [13, 15–17].

Relevance of the Clonogenic Assay to Adjuvant Therapy of Cancer

As techniques for mechanical and enzymatic disaggregation of primary human cancers improve, in vitro assay gains relevance to the study of chemosensitivity of primary tumors from original surgical resections. Table 3 lists some of the high-risk human tumor types which have been successfully grown from primary tumor specimens and would have relevance to future predictive clinical trials of adjuvant therapy of cancer.

For each of these tumor types, occult micrometastases commonly result in locoregional and/or distant recurrences, leading to an increasing emphasis on the development of effective systemic adjuvant therapy. At present, overall sufficient growth (more than 30 colonies per plate) to conduct drug sensitivity assays is obtained in approximately 40% of primary biopsy specimens. Therefore, improvement of in

Table 3. Human cancers with a known high risk of recurrence which have been grown in soft agar from primary tumors

Bladder carcinoma	Pancreatic carcinoma
Breast carcinoma	Prostatic carcinoma
Colon carcinoma	Ovarian carcinoma
Lung carcinoma	Endometrial carcinoma
Stomach carcinoma	Thyroid carcinoma
Renal carcinoma	Various sarcomas

Table 4. Proposed study design for decision-aiding trial using in vitro drug sensitivity assay for stage II primary breast cancer

1. Primary tumor is sent for routine histopathology, estrogen receptor assay and in vitro clonogenic assay. Standard clinical staging workup is completed
2. Tumor is tested in vitro against eight or more standard drugs known to have activity in breast cancer [adriamycin, cyclophosphamide (bioactivated), 5-FU, MTX, tamoxifen, mitomycin, vincristine, prednisone]. Some drugs may be tested in combinations
3. If assay results are ready in less than 2 weeks, initiate adjuvant chemotherapy with optimal two or three drug combination. If assay results require more than 2 weeks, initiate standard adjuvant chemotherapy (e.g., CMF or AC) and switch to optimal combination once results are available
4. Measure duration of relapse-free survival and overall survival as a function of presenting prognostic factors, quantitative results of in vitro sensitivity assay and clinical drug protocol selection and adherence
5. Rebiopsy accessible recurrent tumor from patients who relapse from adjuvant therapy and repeat drug sensitivity measurements for correlation and future drug selection

vitro growth conditions will be required before the assay system can be reoutinely applied to primary neoplasms with a high probability of routinely having useful results for clinical application. Nonetheless, for selected tumor types (e.g., bladder, ovarian), the likelihood of adequate growth already exceeds 75% of specimens plated [1, 5, 11], and more routine application to adjuvant trials could be contemplated. Based on our experience to date, the evidence now suggests that the potential of finding one or more useful drugs increases with the number of drugs tested in vitro. In general, when eight or more standard anticancer drugs are tested in vitro against a given patient's tumor, it is extremely likely that at least one agent will prove to be active in vitro. This is seen by a reduction in survival to less than 30% of control at drug concentrations that are 10–20% of the peak plasma concentration or concentration time product [11, 14, 15, 17].

In the course of validating the applicability of the tumor stem cell assay for adjuvant therapy, prospective correlative trials need to be carried out. In such trials, adjuvant regimens are selected on the basis of standardized clinical protocol and, simultaneously and independently, in vitro drug sensitivity measurements are made but are not used to govern adjuvant therapy selection. Standard adjuvant regimens include cyclophosphamide-methotrexate-fluorouracil (CMF) or adriamycin-cyclophosphamide (AC). In vitro measurement of cyclophosphamide activity requires bioactivation with a hepatic microsomal fraction, however, this is now possible to achieve [6]. Should measurements of in vitro sensitivity or resistance prove to be highly predictive of freedom from relapse or recurrence, respectively, then the final stage in clinical trial application can be contemplated; namely, the prospective decision-aiding trial. This final stage in application of in vitro study to clinical trials for the adjuvant therapy of breast cancer is depicted in Table 4. This decision-aiding study design is analogous to that used in selection of antibiotics for infectious disease. Its implementation is of course, predicated on prior successful predictive correlative trials which validate the approach.

Conclusions

This overview of developments on in vitro assay for clonogenic human tumor stem cells is brief and, therefore, can only touch on several highlights and long-term goals associated with these studies. Nonetheless, developments have been sufficiently rapid (and independent confirmation sufficiently convincing) to suggest that in vitro assay for prediction of results of adjuvant therapy may emerge in this decade as a standard component of prospective clinical trials. Should this prediction prove correct the in vitro assay could lead to rational selection of cytotoxic agents, hormones, and biologic response modifiers for clinical trials. It is, of course, too soon to assess the impact that in vitro study could have on standard patient management. However, the general approach clearly has the promise of reducing morbidity and improving curability of cancer, while simultaneously reducing the costs associated with administration of ineffective drugs. Should the in vitro approach fall short of these goals, it still seems likely that it will have substantial influence on our perspectives on cancer biology and new-drug screening, as well as clinical trials in the adjuvant therapy of cancer.

References

1. Buick RN, Stanisic TH, Jry SE, Salmon SE, Trent JM, Krasovich P (1979) Development of an agar-methyl-cellulose clonogenic assay for cells in transitional cell carcinoma of the human bladder. Cancer Res 39: 5051–5056
2. Bruce WR, Valeriote FA (1966) Comparison of the sensitivity of normal hematopoietic and transplanted lymphoma colony-forming cells to chemotherapeutic agents administered in vivo. J Natl Cancer Inst 37: 233–245
3. Hamburger AW, Salmon SE (1977) Primary bioassay of human tumor stem cells. Science 197: 461–463
4. Hamburger AW, Salmon SE (1977) Primary bioassay of human myeloma stem cells. J Clin Invest 60: 846–854
5. Hamburger AW, Salmon SE, Kim MB, Trent JM, Soehnlen BJ, Alberts DS, Schmidt HJ (1978) Direct cloning of human ovarian carcinoma cells in agar. Cancer Res 38: 3438–3443
6. Kovach JS, Ames MM, Powis GP, Lieber MM (1980) Use of a liver microsome system in testing drug sensitivity of tumor cells in soft agar. Proc Am Assoc Cancer Res Am Soc Clin Oncol 21: 257

7. Meyskens FL, Salmon SE (1979) Inhibition of human melanoma colony formation by retinoids. Cancer Res 39: 4055
8. Ogawa M, Bergsagel DE, McCulloch EA (1973) Chemotherapy of mouse myeloma: Quantitative cell culture predictive or response in vivo. Blood 41: 7–15
9. Salmon SE (1980) Request for proposals # NCI-CM-07327. Application of the human tumor stem cell cloning assay to new drug screening. Natl Cancer Inst, Bethesda, MD
10. Salmon SE (1979) Human tumor stem cells and adjuvant therapy of cancer. In: Salmon SE, Jones SE (eds) Adjuvant therapy of cancer II. Grune & Stratton, New York, pp 27–36
11. Salmon SE (ed) (1980) Cloning of human tumor stem cells. Liss, New York
12. Salmon SE, Buick RN (1979) Preparation of permanent slides of intact soft agar colony cultures of hematopoietic and tumor stem cells. Cancer Res 39: 1133–1136
13. Salmon SE, Von Hoff DD (to be published) In vitro evaluation of anticancer drugs with the human tumor stem cell assay. Semin Oncol
14. Salmon SE, Hamburger AW, Soehnlen BJ, Durie BGM, Alberts DS, Moon TE (1978) Quantitation of differential sensitivity of human tumor stem cells to anticancer drugs. N Engl J Med 298: 1321–1327
15. Salmon SE, Alberts DS, Meyskens FL, Durie GM, Jones SE, Soehnlen BJ, Young L (1980) A new concept: in vitro phase II screening with the human tumor stem cell assay. Proc Am Soc Clin Oncol 21: 329
16. Salmon SE, Soehnlen BJ, Alberts DS (1980) New drugs in ovarian cancer: in vitro phase II screening with the human tumor stem cell assay. In: Van Oosterom AT, Muggia FM, Cleton FJ (eds) Therapeutic progress in ovarian cancer, testicular cancer and the sarcomas. Leiden University Press, Leiden, pp 113–128
17. Salmon SE, Meyskens FL, Alberts DS, Soehnlen BJ, Young L (1981) New drugs in ovarian cancer and malignant melanoma: in vitro phase II screening with the human tumor stem cell assay. Cancer Treat Rep 65 (1–2): 1–12
18. Trent JM, Salmon SE (1980) Human tumor karyology: Marked analytic enhancement via short term agar culture. Br J Cancer 41: 867–874
19. Von Hoff DD (1981) Association between human tumor colony forming assay results and response of an individual patient's tumor to chemotherapy. Am J Med 70: 1027–1032
20. Von Hoff DD (1980) New leads from the laboratory for treating testicular cancer. In: Van Oosterom AT, Muggia FM, Cleton FJ (eds) Therapeutic progress in ovarian cancer, testicular cancer and the sarcomas. Leiden University Press, Leiden, pp 225–234

52. *Current Status of Clinical Trials of m-AMSA, Dihydroxyanthracenedione, and Deoxycoformycin*

J. S. Macdonald, S. Marsoni, S. Bruno, and D. Poster

National Cancer Institute, Division of Cancer Treatment,
Cancer Therapy Evaluation Program, Bethesda, MD 20205, USA

Summary

The current status of three drugs of clinical interest to the National Cancer Institute is reviewed. m-AMSA, a drug with a wide spectrum of activity in murine tumors, is now in phase II trial and has shown itself to have a high order of activity in acute nonlymphocytic leukemia. Dihydroxyanthracenedione, a compound with some of the characteristics of anthracyclines but with no cardiac toxicity in animal toxicology studies, is in phase I evaluation. Deoxycoformycin, an adenosine analog which is a potent inhibitor of adenosine deaminase, has shown moderate activity in acute leukemia patients in phase I trials, and has the potential to produce synergistic antitumor toxicity when used with arabinofuranosyladenine.

Introduction

Drugs for chemotherapy of cancer may be of interest to the clinician for several reasons. A compound which is shown in preclinical screening to have a wide spectrum of activity and/or be active in tumors which are resistant to most other agents would have appeal and mandate efforts toward clinical development. Another conceptual approach that is important in choosing drugs for clinical testing is the search for analogs of proven active compounds. One would be interested in analogs which exhibit increased activity or have the potential of modifying a significant toxicity of the parent compound. A third approach that may be used in drug development is to attempt to design compounds which have the potential for pharmacologic synergism with other drugs. Theoretically, such combinations could be synergistic in antitumor effect with relative sparing of the host.

The NCI drug development program has been following all three of the conceptual pathways just outlined. This paper will discuss the current status of drugs in clinical trial which are examples of these various approaches to drug development. The acridine derivative m-AMSA [16] is an example of a drug chosen for clinical testing because of a wide spectrum of activity in animal tumor systems [16]. This anthraquinone dihydroxyanthracenedione was developed because of theoretical considerations suggesting that this anthracycline-like compound might have less potential for cardiac toxicity than classic anthracycline antibiotics [15]. Finally,

Recent Results in Cancer Research, Vol. 80

2-deoxycoformycin (2′-dCF) was brought into clinical trial in the United States for two reasons. The first was the fact that this adenosine deaminase inhibitor might well be capable of pharmacologic synergism with arabinofuranosyladenine (ara-A) [11] and deoxyadenosine [6]. The second reason for interest in 2′-dCF is that this drug may take advantage of differences in cell biology between tumor cells and normal cells. It is known that lymphoblasts have particularly high levels of adenosine deaminase [13] and it would be predicted that 2′-dCF might be particularly active against these blasts and relatively sparing of nonmalignant cells with lower 2′-dCF levels.

m-AMSA

The acridine derivative methanesulfon-m-anisidide 4′-(9-acridinylamino) is one of a number of bisquaternary salts that were synthesized for structure activity studies in experimental tumor systems [4]. This analog, given the acronym m-AMSA, was found to have significant antitumor activity in the L1210 and P388 leukemia screening system but also had antitumor effect in a wide spectrum of murine tumors [16], including the Lewis lung carcinoma, $CD8F_1$ mammary carcinoma, colon cancer lines 26 and 38, and the B16 melanoma. Because of this marked preclinical activity, the drug was selected for clinical trial.

The preclinical evaluation of m-AMSA has been previously reviewed [16]. The drug is a potent inhibitor of DNA synthesis and can be demonstrated to both intercalate DNA and also bind externally to double standard nucleic acid. Preclinical toxicologic evaluation in mice, dogs, and monkeys showed reversible dose-related marrow

Table 1. m-AMSA in acute nonlymphocytic leukemia (ANLL)

Institution	Dose and schedule	No. patients	CR[c]	Median duration of CR
M.D. Anderson [10]	75–120 mg/m²/day × 3–7	44	16 (36%)	3 months (1–8+)
NCOG [9][a]	100–200 mg/m²/day × 5–7	18	3 (17%)	3 months (3–4)
SEG [17][b]	90 mg/m²/day × 5	30	5 (17%)	2.5 months (1–5+)
NCI Files	75–200 mg/m²/day × 5	24	2 (8%)	–
	250 mg/m² × 1 with escalation if no effect on tumor	18	0	–
	60 mg/m²/day to aplasia	9	3 (33%)	3+ months (2.5+ to 3.5+)
		140	30 (21%)	3 months (1–8+)

[a] Northern California Oncology Group
[b] Southeastern Cancer Study Group
[c] Complete remission

suppression with anemia, leukopenia, and lymphopenia being prominent [16]. The thrombocytopenia was sporadic. Liver function abnormalities were also observed in all species. Other findings included renal insufficiency in dogs and vomiting and lymphoid hypoplasia in dogs and monkeys [16].

Clinical phase I trials have been performed at five institutions and have been previously reviewed [16]. The dose-limiting toxicity with m-AMSA has been leukopenia with nadir blood counts developing 10 days after injection. Other toxicities observed have been phlebitis, local tissue necrosis, alopecia, stomatitis, and nausea and vomiting. Thrombocytopenia has not been as consistently seen as leukopenia and has been less severe than the white blood cell depression. Unusual toxic events reported with m-AMSA include grand mal seizures and cardiac arrhythmias [16], but these events have not conclusively been demonstrated to be secondary to drug administration.

Phase I trials of m-AMSA suggested that the drug might be useful in acute leukemia and breast cancer since responses were seen in heavily pretreated patients with these diseases [16]. Consequently, these diseases have been of most interest in phase II development of m-AMSA.

Table 1 details the experience with m-AMSA in acute nonlymphocytic leukemia (ANLL). It should be emphasized that all of these studies were performed in heavily pretreated patients.Table 1 reveals that m-AMSA has been utilized in a wide variety of doses and schedules in acute leukemia patients. The most useful dose schedule has not yet been demonstrated and will require further investigation. Although only nine patients have been treated with the 60 mg/m^2 dose continued daily until evidence of marrow aplasia, this schedule would seem to be a very reasonable one to investigate in the future since it was associated with a relatively high response rate and allows tailoring of the dose given to obtain ablation of bone marrow tumor. As expected, m-AMSA as used in acute leukemia is significantly toxic. High doses of 75–100 mg/m^2/day for 5–7 days have been associated with significant leukopenia [10] and in a series of 44 patients [10] treated at the M.D. Anderson Hospital, all developed leukopenia and infection. Whether modification of drug dosage in acute leukemia will allow for continued antitumor activity with less severe toxicity will require further investigation. When the single-agent dose and schedule of m-AMSA is optimized, studies of this drug in combination therapy of acute leukemia may begin.

There have been suggestions that m-AMSA may be active against other tumors, most notably breast cancer [16]. In 38 previously treated patients with advanced breast cancer (Table 2), five (13%) responses were seen [16]. Although this response rate is small, the fact that all patients treated had received other chemotherapy agents makes the drug worthy of further investigation in breast cancer. m-AMSA has been found to

Table 2. m-AMSA in solid tumors

Disease	No. patients	No. responses	Reference
Breast cancer	38	5 (13%)	[16]
Non-oat cell lung cancer	62	0	[16]
Colon cancer	97	0	[16]
Melanoma	96	3 (3%)	NCI files

be essentially without activity in patients with non-oat cell lung cancer, colon cancer, and melanoma (Table 2).

m-AMSA represents a drug with a wide spectrum of preclinical activity which has been shown to have definite but limited clinical effectiveness. The high order of antitumor effect in previously treated leukemia patients (Table 1) is impressive and should be pursued. The suggestion of activity in breast cancer will also require further study by adding m-AMSA to combination regimens to evaluate its usefulness as a part of the therapy of advanced breast cancer. Also, it is clear that further studies are required to assess the single-agent activity of this drug in less common tumors.

Dihydroxyanthracenedione

The anthracycline antibiotic adriamycin is a highly active antineoplastic drug in a wide range of human tumors [3]. Unfortunately, this class of drug has a significant dose-limiting cardiac toxicity, which seriously limits its usefulness over long periods of time [3]. An analog of the anthracyclines that retained antitumor activity but did not have the cardiac toxicity associated with the parent drugs would be of great use.

Since some evidence suggests that the cardiac toxicity of anthracyclines results from the presence of the amino sugar in the molecule [1], there has been much interest in examining the antitumor activity and toxicity characteristics of anthraquinone drugs lacking a sugar moiety [15]. Such a drug is the dihydroxy dihydrochloride salt of anthracenedione which has been designated dihydroxyanthracenedione (DHAD) [15]. This drug was developed by collaboration between the NCI and the Medical Research Division of Lederle Laboratories (American Cyanamid Company) and is currently in early clinical trial.

Preclinical studies of DHAD were encouraging for two reasons. First, it was demonstrated that the drug was active in animal tumor systems. Significant antitumor effect and, in some instances, long-term survivals were seen in mice bearing P388 leukemia, L1210 leukemia, B16 melanoma, and colon tumor 26 [15]. The second factor of interest was the total lack of cardiac toxicity in experimental systems exhibited by DHAD. This drug is felt to intercalate DNA in a manner similar to the anthracyclines. However, animal toxicology studies in beagle dogs and cynomolgus monkeys demonstrated that DHAD induced no light- or electronmicrographic changes consistent with cardiac toxicity [15]. The major animal toxicities seen were reversible bone marrow suppression, predominantly of the white and red blood cell series, and anorexia, vomiting, diarrhea, and blue discoloration of the urine [15].

DHAD has now entered phase I trial and currently several phase I trials (Table 3) have been initiated under sponsorship of American Cyanamid Company and NCI. A phase I trial has been completed by Von Hoff et al. [15]. Twenty-five patients received a total of 41 courses of therapy in this study with drug administered single IV injection every 4 weeks. Doses were from 1.2–14 mg/m^2 and the maximally tolerated dose in this schedule was 12 mg/m^2. The dose-limiting toxicity was leukopenia and thrombocytopenia, with the median time to nadir of the white blood cell and platelet counts being 9 days with recovery by day 19. No cardiac toxicity was noted, although patients did experience mild phlebitis, diarrhea, and nausea and vomiting with DHAD treatment. Blue discoloration of the urine occurred at doses of 10 mg/m^2 or more. One

Table 3. Dihydroxyanthracenedione in phase I trials

Institution	Starting dose	Schedule
Sidney Farber Cancer Institute	1 mg/m²/day	i.v. 24-h continuous infusion every 21 days
Baltimore Cancer Research Program (NCI)	2 mg/m²/day	i.v. daily × 3 every 21 days
M.D. Anderson Hospital and Tumor Institute	0.5 mg/m²/day	i.v. daily × 5 every 3 weeks
Vermont Regional Cancer Center	1.5 mg/m²/day	i.v. weekly × 3 every 6 weeks
Ohio State University	6 mg/m²/total dose	Single i.v. bolus, i.v. daily × 5 continuous infusion × 5 pharmacology in 5–40 patients
Milwaukee Childrens' Hospital St. Jude's Hospital University of New Mexico NCI (Children Collaborative Study)	1.2 mg/m²/day	i.v. single dose every 28 days

partial response in a patient with metastatic adenocarcinoma of the lung lasted for 7 months.

DHAD schedules and doses are actively being investigated in other phase I studies (Table 3). If the initial findings [15] of acceptable toxicity and lack of acute cardiac toxicity can be confirmed, phase II studies to define the spectrum of activity of this interesting drug will soon be initiated. It should be emphasized that studies examining the effect of chronic DHAD on cardiac function must be completed before the drug can unequivocally be determined to be free of cardiac toxicity.

2-Deoxycoformycin

2-Deoxycoformycin (2′-dCF) is a naturally occurring nucleoside analog antibiotic isolated from *Streptomyces antibioticus* [18]. This drug is a potent inhibitor of the enzyme adenosine deaminase [7]. Adenosine deaminase is present in many tissues but is particularly highly concentrated in lymphoid tissues. T cells and T cell-derived tumors have the highest levels of adenosine deaminase [13]. The mechanism of cellular cytotoxicity of 2′-dCF is the inhibition of adenosine deaminase which results in elevation of intracellular levels of dATP. This nucleoside triphosphate inhibits the enzyme rebonucleotide reductase and thus inhibits DNA synthesis [7].

2′-dCF was of most interest because it was shown to potentiate the antitumor effects of agents such as deoxyadenosine [6] and ara-A [11]. 2′-dCF as a single agent in

Table 4. Clinical studies of deoxycoformycin

Investigator	No. patients	Disease	Dose	Comments
Smyth et al. [14]	18	7 ALL, 2 lymphoma, 9 other	0.1–1.0 mg/kg single dose + 0.25 mg/kg × 5 days	Lymphopenia, hyperuricemia (3/7 PR ALL)
Grever et al. [5]	5	3 ALL, 2 CML	0.1–1.0 mg/kg × 4–14 days	Renal insufficiency (5/5), hepatic dysfunction (3/5), encephalopathy (1/5), pulmonary infiltrates (3/5), 4/5 PR
Kufe et al. [8]	5	3 T-cell ALL, 1 T-cell lymphoma, 1 myosis fungoides	5–30 mg/m^2 × 3–5 days	Renal insufficiency, hyperuricemia, anemia, pulmonary infiltrates, 2/5 PR
Benjamin et al. [2]	12	7 acute leukemia, 5 solid tumor	0.2–40 mg/m^2 once or twice a week + 20–40 mg/m^2 24-h infusion for 1–4 days	Encephalopathy, renal insufficiency, hepatic dysfunction, conjunctivitis, myalgias, nausea-vomiting (4/7 PR leukemia)
Schneider et al. [12]	12	4 ALL, 1 CML, 1 CLL, 1 lymphocytic lymphoma, 1 histiocytic lymphoma, 1 Hodgkin's disease, 2 mycosis fungoides	0.25 mg/kg × 5 days	Renal insufficiency, myositis, conjunctivitis (1 PR ALL)

experimental murine tumors or human xenographs was inactive. Large-animal toxicology of 2′-dCF revealed that the drug produced marked lymphopenia, no leukopenia, and mild hepatopathy as indicated by elevation of alkaline phosphatase and transaminases. Conjunctivitis and mucus discharge from the eyes were observed in dogs. CNS toxicity was also present, as indicated by mild lethargy.

2′-dCF has entered phase I clinical trial as a single agent. Results of reported trials are illustrated in Table 4. As can be noted, there are small numbers of patients who have been treated with this drug and almost all of the experience has been in patients with lymphocytic malignancy. Although partial responses (reduction of bone marrow and peripheral blood tumor-cell numbers) have been seen in 14 patients with leukemia, this sort of response does not translate into increased survival for these patients. Of note is the marked disparity in the toxicity reported by investigators using 2′-dCF. While the initial study performed by Smyth et al. [14] reported only mild toxicity, all of the subsequent studies [2, 5, 8, 12], using schedules and doses similar to those used by Smyth, have reported significant multiorgan toxicity. Reversible renal insufficiency as indicated by elevated blood urea nitrogen (BUN) and creatinine has been common, as has encephalopathy. Of note are reports from the M.D. Anderson Hospital [2] and Memorial Sloan Kettering [12] in which myalgias, severe myositis, and conjunctivitis were prominent findings. The differences in qualitative toxicities between the studies of Smyth [13] kand the other workers have not been adequately explained.

The phase I trials with 2′-dCF present an unusual problem to clinical investigators. It appears that the trials in the United States were initiated at a toxic dose. Thus, at present, phase I investigations of 2′-dCF must aim at deescalation of dose to arrive at a dose and schedule with acceptable toxicity. It should also be emphasized that the mechanism of 2′-dCF toxicity to normal tissue is not well-understood. It is, however, possible that toxicity may be mediated by a toxic nucleoside metabolite. Benjamin et al. [2] and Schneider et al. [12] have demonstrated that at doses of 2′-dCF which abolish red blood cell adenosine deaminase activity, there are greater than five-fold increases of plasma deoxyadenosine levels. Whether this elevation in deoxyadenosine is the cause of systemic toxicity is under active investigation.

At present, further phase I studies with 2′-dCF will have to be carried out to obtain a tolerated dose and schedule. When a clearer understanding of the dose-response characteristics and toxicity of 2′-dCF has been obtained, it will be possible to perform studies to assess possible pharmacologic synergism between this drug and agents such as 8-azadenosine, deoxyadenosine, and ara-A.

Conclusion

This brief review has indicated the status of three drugs of current interest to the NCI. m-AMSA, which has a wide spectrum of action in animal tumors, has been shown to have more limited activity in human cancers, but to be a particularly useful drug in acute leukemia. DHAD, developed because of its potential to produce antracycline-like antitumor activity without cardiac toxicity, will soon enter broad phase II trials. 2′-dCF, a drug of interest because of its potential to exhibit synergistic antitumor effects with other antimetabolites, continues in phase I trial.

References

1. Adamson RH (1974) Daunomycin (NSC-82151) and adriamycin (NSC-123127): A hypothesis concerning antitumor activity and cardiotoxicity. Cancer Chemother Rep Par 1, 58: 293–294
2. Benjamin RS, Plunkett W, Keatiny MJ et al. (1980) Phase I and biochemical pharmacological studies of deoxycoformycin. Proc Am Soc Clin Oncol Am Assoc Cancer Res 21: 337
3. Blum RH, Carter SK (1974) Adriamycin: A new anticancer drug with significant clinical activity. Ann Intern Med 80: 249–259
4. Cain BF, Atwell GJ, Seelye RN (1969) Potential antitumor agents. X. Bisquarternary salts. J Med Chem 12: 199–206
5. Grever M, Miser J, Balcerak S, Neidhart J (1980) Ablation of adenosine deaminase activity by deoxycoformycin induces cell lysis in refractory leukemia. Proc Am Soc Clin Oncol Am Assoc Cancer Res 21: 335
6. Johns DG, Adamson RH (1976) Enhancement of the biological activity of cordycepin (3′deoxyadenosine) by the adenosine deaminase inhibitor 2′deoxycoformycin. Biochem Pharmacol 25: 1441–1444
7. Koller CA, Mitchel BS, Grever MR, Mejias E, Malspeis L, Metz EN (1979) Treatment of acute lymphoblastic leukemia with 2′-deoxycoformycin and biochemical consequences of adenosine deaminase inhibition. Cancer Treat Rep 63: 1948–1952
8. Kufe D, Major P, Agarwal R, Reinherz E, Frei E (1980) Phase I–II trial of deoxycoformycin in T-cell malignancies. Proc Am Soc Clin Oncol Am Assoc Cancer Res 21: 328
9. Lawrence HJ, Ries CA, Reynolds RD, Lewis JP, Koretz MM (1980) m-AMSA: A promising new agent in refractory acute leukemia. Proc Am Soc Clin Oncol Am Assoc Cancer Res 21: 438
10. Legha S, Keating M, Bodey G, McCredie K, Freireich E (1980) Phase II trial of 4′-(9-acridinylamino) methanesulfon-m-aniside (AMSA) in adults with acute leukemia. Proc Am Soc Clin Oncol Am Assoc Cancer Res 21: 442
11. LePage GA, Worth LS, Kimball AP (1976) Enhancement of antitumor activity of arabinofuranosyladenine by 2′-dCF. Cancer Res 36: 1481–1485
12. Schneider R, Korngold G, Vale K, Woodcock T, Tan C, Young C (1980) Clinical and pharmacologic investigations of deoxycoformycin. Proc Am Soc Clin Oncol Am Assoc Cancer Res 21: 184
13. Smyth JF, Harrap KR (1975) Adenosine deaminase activity in leukemia. Br J Cancer 31: 544
14. Smyth JF, Chassin MM, Harrap KP (1979) 2′-dCF phase I trial and clinical pharmacology. Proc Am Soc Clin Oncol Am Assoc Cancer Res 20: 187
15. Von Hoff DD, Pollard G, Kuhn J, Murray E, Coltman CA (1980) Phase I clinical investigation of dihydroxyanthracenedione, a new anthracenedione. Cancer Res 40: 1516–1518
16. Weiss RB, Charles LM, MacDonald JS (to be published) m-AMSA: An exciting new drug in the National Cancer Institute drug development program. Cancer Clin Trials
17. Winton EF, Vogler WR, Rose KL (1980) Phase II study of acridinylaniside (m-AMSA) in refractory adult acute leukemia. Proc Am Soc Clin Oncol Am Assoc Cancer Res 21: 437
18. Woo PWK, Dion HW, Lange SM (1974) A novel adenosine and ara-A deaminase inhibitor, (R)-3-(2-deoxy-β-d-erythropentofuranosyl)-3,6,7,8-tetrahydroimidazo-(4,5-d) (1,3) diazepin-8-01. J Heterocyl Chem 11: 641–643

53. *Three New Agents for Immunotherapy Trials: Azimexon, Bestatin, and Tuftsin*

G. Mathé, I. Florentin, M. Bruley-Rosset, A. Goutner, and B. Serrou*

Hôpital Paul-Brousse, Institut of Cancerology and Immunogenetics, (INSERM U-50), 14–16 Avenue Paul Vaillant Couturier, F-94800 Villejuif, France

Cancer immunotherapy trials in man have almost exclusively been conducted with BCG, *C. parvum,* and MER (methanol extract residue of BCG)]19]. Not only did the clinical researchers meet difficulties concerning tolerance, which certainly decreased their enthusiasm for immunotherapy trials, but a second inconvenience of these materials is the difficulty in quantifying the active agents. This is a major problem because we have shown experimentally, in nontumor [5, 9, 12] as well as in tumor models [14], that while certain doses of BCG may induce the desired immune modification, others may not induce detectable immune effects, and others may induce an immunosuppressive action.

Hence the practical interest of compounds such as levamisole, which has been used in several significantly favorable trials [19]; Pavlovsky [15] in acute lymphoid leukemia, the Finnish Leukemia Group in acute myeloid leukemia, Salmon (personal communication) in myeloma, and Lacour et al. [11], with poly A-poly U which has given a significant benefit as a breast carcinoma adjuvant therapy, are recent examples.

Our group has systematically submitted new chemically pure compounds to a series of immunologic tests including macrophage-mediated cytostatism, cytolytic T-cell activity, antibody-dependent cell-mediated cytotoxicity, natural killer (NK) cell activity, and suppressor cell activity [8]. We have studied young mice (2 months old) after an acute administration of the agents and older mice treated chronically for 6 months until 18 or 20 months of age. Immunologic tests were performed after the end of the treatment, autopsies were done on those which died during treatment, and the remaining animals at the time of testing were killed for autopsy.

We have shown, in young animals, that Azimexon or 2-[2-cyanaziridinyl-(1)-]-2-[2-carbamoylaziridinyl-(1)] propane, prepared by Boehringer [1], stimulates all T cell functions, B cell antibody production, NK cell activity, and macrophage cytotoxicity at the dose of 500 μg/mouse [87, 13, 16]. Tuftsin, which is a synthetic polypeptide (Thr-Lys-Pro-Arg), prepared by Martinez (Montpellier), stimulates, at the dose of 25 μg/mouse T helper-cells, B cell functions, K cell activity, and macrophage cytotoxicity [6, 8, 13].

Bestatin [(2S, 3F)-3-amino-2-hydroxyl-4-phenyl-butanoyl]-L-leucine is a specific inhibitor of aminopeptidase B and leucine aminopeptidase given by Umezawa et al. [20],

* For the EORTC Cancer Immunology and Immunotherapy Group

Recent Results in Cancer Research, Vol. 80

who isolated it from *Streptomyces olivoreticuli* culture filtrates and synthesized it [18]. It potentiates T-dependent and T-independent humoral responses and activates macrophages [7].

Studies on aged mice [2–4] present double interest: (1) Immunodeficiency due to age allows testing of the capacity of adjuvants to restore immune functions; and (2) it gives an experimental tumor model close to the situation observed in humans, as these tumors are spontaneous and studied in strains of mice not known to have received a vertically transmitted tumor-inducing virus. Moreover, human tumors are also known to appear most often late in life. This study has shown that the three agents share the ability to increase the age-depressed tumoricidal activity of peritoneal macrophages.

T cell cytotoxicity is restored by bestatin (100 μg) and tuftsin (10 μg) treatment, but is not by Azimexon (500 μg). Antibody-dependent cell-mediated cytotoxicity (ADCC) which increases with age, is lowered to the level of that of young mice by bestatin only. NK activity, which is strongly impaired by aging, is further decreased by all three agents. Thus, the functions which are commonly increased by bestatin and tuftsin are T cell functions and macrophage activity.

The incidence of spontaneous tumors, which varies 20–40% in nontreated aged mice at the time of autopsy, was only reduced to 10% in the animals treated by Azimexon. This difference was not significant. It is reduced to 5% in those given bestatin and to 0% in those which received tuftsin, and this is highly significant [2–4].

These results have tempted us to submit immunodepressed cancer patients to phase I trials of these compounds, but only Azimexon and bestatin have been available. Among the observed results, Azimexon [10] (200 mg × 3/week for 2 weeks) shows no evidence of toxicity, is able to restore delayed-type hypersensitivity reactions in anergic patients, and increases the tetradecanoyl phorbol acetate (TPA) mitogenic stimulation of the subpopulation of T cells sensitive to this mitogen. It does not stimulate NK cell activity. Bestatin [17], which is also clinically well-tolerated, significantly increases the delayed-type hypersensitivity responses with the Merieux score, the auto-rosette forming cells, and NK cell activity. This last study has been conducted by the EORTC Cancer Immunology and Immunotherapy Group.

References

1. Bicker U, Ziegler BE, Hebold G (1977) 2-[2-cyanaziridinyl-(1)-]-2-[carbamoyl aziridinyl-(1)]-propane (BM 12531). A new substance with immunostimulating action. IRCS Med Sci 5: 299
2. Bruley-Rosset M, Florentin I, Kiger N, Schulz J, Mathé G (1979) Restoration of impaired immune functions of aged animals by chronic bestatin treatment. Immunology 38: 75–83
3. Bruley-Rosset M, Florentin I, Kiger N, Schulz J, Mathe G (to be published) Correction of immunodeficiency in aged mice by levamisole and bestatin administration. Cancer Treat Rep
4. Bruley-Rosset M, Hercend T, Martinez J, Rappaport H, Mathé G (to be published) Prevention of spontaneous tumors of aged mice by immunopharmacological manipulation: Study of immune antitumor mechanisms. J Natl Cancer Inst
5. Florentin I, Bruley-Rosset M, Davigny M, Mathé G (1978) Comparison of the effects of BCG and a preparation of heat-killed *Pseudomonas aeruginosa* on the immune responses in mice. In: Werner GH, Floc'h F (eds) The pharmacology of immunoregulation. Academic Press, New York, pp 335–352

6. Florentin I, Bruley-Rosset M, Kiger N, Imbach JL, Winternitz F, Mathé G (1978) In vivo immunostimulation by tuftsin. Cancer Immunol Immunother 5: 211–216
7. Florentin I, Kiger N, Bruley-Rosset M, Schulz J, Mathé G (1978) Effect of seven immunomodulators on different types on immune responses in mice. In: Serrou B, Rosenfeld C (eds) Human lymphocyte differentiation: Its application to cancer. Elsevier/North-Holland, Biomedical Press, Amsterdam, pp 299–303
8. Florentin I, Schulz J, Bruley-Rosset M, Kiger N, Mathé G (1980) In vivo immunomodulating properties of two synthetic agents: Azimexon and tuftsin. In: Mathé G, Muggia FM (eds) Cancer chemo- and immunopharmacology. II. Immunopharmacology, relations and general problems. Springer, Berlin Heidelberg New York
9. Geffard M, Orbach-Arbouys S (1976) Enhancement of T-suppressor activity in mice by high doses of BCG. Cancer Immunol Immunother 1: 41–44
10. Goutner A, Schwarzenberg L, Mathé G (to be published) Phase I study of Azimexon in immunodepressed cancer patients. In: Terry WD, Rosenberg S (eds) Immunotherapy of cancer: Present status of trials in man. Elsevier/North Holland, New York
11. Lacour F, Lacour J, Spira A, Michelson M, Delage G, Petit JY, Viguier J (to be published) A new adjuvant treatment with poly A-poly U in operable breast cancer. In: Mathé G, Muggia F (eds) Cancer chemo- and immunopharmacology. II. Immunopharmacology, relations and general problems. Springer, Berlin Heidelberg New York
12. Mathé G (1976) Side effects and possible harmful action of immunomanipulation. In: The prediction of chronic toxicity from short-term studies. Excerpta Medica, Amsterdam, pp 67–82
13. Mathé G, Florentin I, Schulz JI, Bruley-Rosset M, Kiger N (1979) Third generation of systemic adjuvants of immunity: Experimental basis for adjuvant combinations. In: Bonadonna G, Mathé G, Salmon SE (eds) Adjuvant therapies and markers of post-surgical minimal residual disease. II. Adjuvant therapies of the various primary tumors. Springer, Berlin Heidelberg New York, pp 449–457
14. Olsson L, Ebbesen P, Kiger N, Florentin I, Mathé G (1978) The antileukemic effect of systemic nonspecific BCG-immunostimulation versus systemic specific immunostimulation with irradiated isogeneic leukemic cells. Eur J Cancer 14: 355–362
15. Pavlovsky S, Garay G, Sackmann Muriel F, Braier L, Svarch E (1980) Chemo-immunotherapy with levamisole (LEV) during maintenance of remission in acute lymphoblastic leukemia (ALL). A four-year report. Proc Am Soc Clin Oncol 71: 436
16. Schulz JI, Florentin I, Bourut C, Bicker U, Mathé G (1978) Delayed-type hypersensitivity response and humoral antibody formation in mice treated with a new immunostimulant 2-[2-cyanaziridinyl-(1)]-2-[2-carbamoylaziridinyl-(1)]-propane (BM 12531) IRCS Med Sci 6: 215
17. Serrou B, Cupissol D, Flad H, Goutner A, Lang JM, Spirzglas H, Plagne R, Beltzer M, Chollet P, Mathé G (to be published) Phase I evaluation of bestatin in patients bearing advanced solid tumors. In: Terry WD, Rosenberg S (eds) Immunotherapy of cancer: Present status of trials in man. Elsevier/North Holland, New York
18. Suda H, Takita T, Aoyagi T, Umezawa H (1976) The chemical synthesis of bestatin. J Antibiot (Tokyo) 26: 600–601
19. Terry WD, Rosenberg S (1981) Second International Conference Immunotherapy of Cancer: Present status of trials in man. National Cancer Institute, Bethesda. Elsevier/North Holland, New York
20. Umezawa H, Aoyagi T, Suda H, Hamada M, Takeuchi T (1976) Bestatin, a new aminopeptidase B inhibitor produced by actinomycetes. J Antibiot (Tokyo) 29: 97–99

54. *Emerging Immunologic Approaches to Treatment of Neoplastic Diseases*

L. Olsson and G. Mathé

Hôpital Paul-Brousse, Institut of Cancerology and Immunogenetics, (INSERM U-50), 14–16 Avenue Paul Vaillant Couturier, F-94800 Villejuif, France

Summary

Recent research on the immunobiology of the tumor-host relationship has demonstrated that nonspecific cellular immune reactions, like natural killer cells and cytotoxic autoreactive cells, may be far more potent antineoplastic mechanisms than specific T lymphocyte cytotoxicity. The hybridoma technique, making it possible to raise monoclonal antibodies against predefined antigens, has rendered passive immunotherapy more attractive. It is suggested that the combination of nonspecific cellular immune reactions with monoclonal antibodies may be a highly efficient antineoplastic therapy for minimal residual disease.

Introduction

The theoretical background, and as such the biologic basis, for immunologic manipulations in the treatment of malignant diseases has been expanded so extensively in the last 5 years that it seems justified to talk about new rationales for immunotherapy of malignant diseases. It seems realistic to expect that these new experimental data may be a useful basis for clinical application of biologic immune modifiers to explore the antineoplastic effects of various immune manipulations on human neoplastic diseases.

Traditional Concepts

A major part of immunologic research in the 1950s was concentrated on mechanisms involved in recognition and eventual rejection of cell and tissue transplants. It was therefore natural that the observations of Foley [4], Prehn and Main [17], and Klein et al. [10] were from the point of view of the transplantation immunologist. Concomitantly with these experiments, and based on transplantation immunology, Ehrlich's idea [3] of natural defenses against the growth of malignant tumors was given new life by Thomas [19] and expressed formally by Burnet in the immunologic surveillance hypothesis [1].

Recent Results in Cancer Research, Vol. 80

The basis of the immune surveillance hypothesis in experimental transplantation immunology focused on specific cellular immune reactions against tumors, neglecting nonspecific cellular immune reactions and antibody mediation as control mechanisms of neoplastic cell growth. The data from such studies, emphasising murine tumor models, showed that T-lymphocyte-mediated cytotoxic immune reactions may induce rejection of some experimental tumor models [2]. However, the experimental tumors were generally induced by high doses of chemicals or rather well-characterized oncogenic viruses [13, 18]. The validity of deductions based on such data regarding human malignant tumors has been questioned [6] and one criticism has been that the frequency of malignant tumors in T lymphocyte-deficient mice ('nude' mice) is the same as in conventional mice. However, while the invalidity of this argument has been discussed in detail elsewhere [8, 9], it is interesting that the frequency of malignant tumors in nude mice indirectly supports the antineoplastic importance of nonspecific cytotoxic immune mechanisms as discussed below. But it is more important that spontaneous murine tumors seem to be without immunogeneity in syngeneic animals, thus suggesting that spontaneous tumors, in contrast to chemical- or virus-induced tumors, do not raise a T lymphocyte response that may lead to tumor rejection [6]. This observation certainly indicates that spontaneous tumors do not elicit a T-lymphocyte rejection mechanism under the given experimental conditions, but cannot be taken as proof of lack of immunogeneity of such tumors in syngeneic recipients. It has been shown that the complex reactivity pattern of the immune system, with interaction of various cellular subsets of the immune system (like T suppressor cells, T helper cells, T cytotoxic cells, antibody-producing cells, and mononuclear phagocytes) may result in an inert immune response despite priming with a substance that is antigenic to a given immune apparatus. The investigations of Hewitt et al. [6] in spontaneous mouse tumors certainly demonstrated that malignant tumor grafts cannot be compared to allogenic cell grafts, but cannot be used to evaluate the immunogeneity of such spontaneous tumors.

New Experimental Approaches

The unsuccessful demonstration of T-lymphocyte-mediated rejection of spontaneous tumors, as well as an apparent lack of neoantigens on such tumors, resulted in some pessimism as to the possibilities for application of immunologic principles in treatment of human neoplastic diseases. Two important developments in immunology have, however, turned the pessimism to a reasonably founded optimism; the so-called natural killer (NK) cell concept [5] and the monoclonal antibody technique [14]. Klein et al. [11] found that normal animals harbor lymphoid cells that may exert a cytotoxic effect on tumor cells independent of immunogenicity of such tumor cells in relation to NK cells. The characteristics of NK cells are still debated and seem to differ to some extent in humans as compared to mice. The original NK concept was based on cytotoxicity to a highly selected tumor cell line (YAC-1; K562) maintained in serial passages in vitro. This weakened considerably interpretations of a possible role for NK cells in relation to spontaneous tumors. However, we were able to demonstrate that cytotoxic autoreactive cells (CAuC), which have many similarities with NK cells, may inhibit growth of naturally occurring tumors. A detailed study of such CAuC by using CAuC-hybridomas demonstrated that CAuC reactivity is restricted to K- and I-region coded antigens of the H2 complex. This differs considerably from the original NK concept and indicates that the NK cell population consists of more than one subset of lymphoid cells with different reactivity spectrums [15].

Almost concomitantly with the introduction of the NK concept, Milstein's group reported successful production of murine monoclonal antibodies against a predefined antigen by the so-called hybridoma technique [12]. The technique involves fusion of murine myeloma cells with antigen-primed lymphoid cells and results in secretion of a monoclonal antibody. The unique specificity of such antibodies enables very accurate immunobiochemical studies of antigenic substances, determination of gene products that code for the production of such proteins, as well as the expression of a given antigen in a given cell population by using monoclonal antibodies in combination with fluorescence-activated cell sorting [7]. It is thus obvious that this technique allows for a profound analysis of antigens on malignant tumor cells and should make it possible to determine the specificity of such antigens and their relationship to malignant transformation.

We are thus now in the rather curious situation that emphasis is on nonspecific cellular immune mechanism and highly specific antibodies, and thus in complete opposition to the traditional concept that emphasized specific cellular immune mechanisms. It is thus obvious that, with changing concepts, the basic rationales are changing too.

Efforts are therefore to be presented concerning the characteristics of NK cells, especially in respect to cell surface markers which allow the measurement of the effect of various biologic immune modifiers on NK-like cells. Further, studies on the interaction of NK-like cells and other immunocompetent cells are important, as well as a careful analysis of the cytotoxic spectrum of NK-like cells against spontaneous tumors. Concomitantly, monoclonal antibody technique should be employed to map the antigenic pattern of human malignant tumors to search for antigens with the highest specificity to the malignant phenotype.

A complicating phenomenon may be antigenic heterogeneity of malignant tumors as shown in murine lymphomas [16], which will require establishment of hybridomas secreting complementary antibodies against tumor-associated antigens within a given tumor cell population. However, even with such a battery of complementary, cytotoxic, monoclonal antibodies, it seems fairly probable that some clonogenic tumor cells within a given tumor cell population are without tumor-associated antigens. In addition to monoclonal antibody therapy, immunologic mechanisms independent of tumor-associated antigens are therefore important. The most obvious candidate is the NK-like cell, especially if the activity of such cells can be appropriately monitored by biologic immune modifiers.

In conclusion it seems reasonable to talk about old and new immunologic approaches to treatment of malignant diseases. Traditionally, emphasis has been on specific cellular immune mechanisms, particularly T-cytotoxic lymphocytes, but recent studies strongly indicate that NK-like cells and monoclonal antibodies may be more potent weapons in immunologic approaches to treatment of neoplastic diseases.

References

1. Burnet FM (1970) The concept of immunological surveillance. Prog Exp Tumor Res 13: 1–27
2. Cerottini JC, Brunner KT (1974) Cell-mediated cytotoxicity, allograft rejection, and tumor immunity. Adv Immunol 18: 67–132

3. Ehrlich P (1909) Über den jetzigen Stand der Karzinomforschung. Ned Tijds Chr Geneeskd 1: 273–290
4. Foley EJ (1953) Antigenic properties of methylcholanthrene-induced tumors in mice of the strain of origin. Cancer Res 13: 835–837
5. Herberman R, Holden HT (1978) Natural cell-mediated immunity. Adv Cancer Res 27: 305–377
6. Hewitt HB (1978) The choice of animal tumors for experimental studies of cancer therapy. Adv Cancer Res 27: 149–200
7. Hulett HR, Bonner WA, Barrett J, Herzenberg LA (1969) Cell sorting: Automated separation of mammalian cells as a function of intracellular fluorescence. Science 166: 747–749
8. Klein G (1980) Immune and non-immune control of neoplastic development. Contrasting effects of host and tumor evolution. Cancer 45: 2486–2499
9. Klein G, Klein E (1979) Immune surveillance against virus-induced tumors and non-rejectability of spontaneous tumors: Contrasting consequences of host-versus-evolution. Proc Natl Acad Sci 74: 2121–2125
10. Klein G, Sjögren HO, Klein E, Hellström KE (1960) Demonstration of resistance against methylcholanthrene-induced sarcomas in the primary autochthnous host. Cancer Res 20: 1561–1572
11. Klein E, Masucci MG, Masucci G, Vauley F (to be published) Natural and activated lymphocyte killers, which affect tumor cells. In: Natural cell-mediated immunity against tumors. Academic Press, New York
12. Köhler G, Milstein C (1975) Continuous cultures of fused cells secreting antibody of predefined specificity. Nature 256: 495–497
13. Law LW (1970) Studies of tumour antigens and tumour specific immune mechanisms in experimental systems. Transpl Proc 2: 117–132
14. Melcher F, Potter M, Warner N (1978) Lymphocyte hybridomas. Mod Top Immunol Microbiol 81: 1–246
15. Olsson L (to be published) Immunity and malignant tumors. Cancer Biol Rev
16. Olsson L, Ebbesen P (1979) Natural polyclonality of spontaneous AKR leukemia and its impact on so-called specific immunotherapy. J Natl Cancer Inst 62: 623–627
17. Prehn RT, Main JM (1957) Immunity to methylcholanthrene-induced sarcomas. J Natl Cancer Inst 18: 769–778
18. Sjögren HO (1965) Transplantation methods as a tool for detection of tumor-specific antigens. Prog Exp Tumor Res 6: 289–322
19. Thomas L (1959) Discussion. In: Lawrence HS (ed) Cellular aspects of the hypersensitive state. Hoeber, New York, p 530

55. *Cellular Interactions Modulating Host Resistance to Tumours**

R. W. Baldwin, V. S. Byers, D. Hannant, J. A. Jones, M. V. Pimm, and M. R. Price

University of Nottingham, Cancer Research Campaign Laboratories, University Park, Nottingham NG7 2RD, United Kingdom

Summary

Active specific immunotherapy of carcinogen-induced rat tumours can be effected using vaccines containing tumour cells admixed with bacterial vaccines such as BCG and *C. parvum*. The nature of the tumour antigen preparation is important, the most effective immunogen being viable tumour cells whose growth is controlled by responses generated by the bacterial agent in the vaccine. Soluble tumour antigen preparations are usually ineffective due to the preferential induction of suppressor lymphocyte responses in normal hosts. In comparison, removal of suppressor precursors by cyclophosphamide treatment of animals leads to the development of tumour immunity following immunization with soluble antigen preparations. One component of the immune rejection response involves the generation of non-specific effector cells. This type of response can also be induced by administering chemical hypersensitizing agents so as to localize tumour deposits. This approach has proved highly effective in treating the guinea pig line 10 hepatoma by intralesional injection of alkylcatechols. These compounds are highly potent hypersensitizers, being the active constituents of the poison ivy/oak (urushiol oil), and localize in tumour cell membranes.

Introduction

Immune responses elicited against tumour cells are highly complex, involving the induction and proliferation of specifically sensitized T lymphocytes following recognition of tumour-associated antigens, stimulation of natural-killer cells and activated macrophages as well as induction of antibody. These responses may be viewed as part of an intricate immunological network which is subject to a series of specific and non-specific feedback mechanisms involving the generation of suppressor T cells and macrophages [2]. In addition, tumour-host interactions lead to the development of both specific and non-specific humoral factors which may interfere with cell-mediated

* These studies were supported by a grant from the Cancer Research Campaign. Dr. Vera S. Byers, Department of Dermatology, University of California, San Francisco, USA, is supported by NIH grant 501 AI-12947

immunity. This includes the release of tumour antigen and/or immune complexes into the circulation and tumour cells either directly or, through interactions with host factors, release immunosuppressive products. It is most likely that tumour rejection involves multiple effector mechanisms and this offers several potential possibilities for manipulation of the tumour-host relationship for therapy.

Generation of Tumour-Specific Immune Responses

There are several criteria which must be fulfilled for the generation of tumour-directed immune rejection responses. Of these the most obvious requirement is for the tumour to express an appropriate cell-surface antigen which can elicit anti-tumour immunity. This condition is fulfilled by many, but not all, experimental animal tumours induced by chemical carcinogens or oncogenic viruses [4, 12]. This is not so, however, with the great majority of naturally arising animal tumours [5], as emphasized by a series of studies with naturally arising rat tumours, mainly sarcomas and mammary adenocarcinomas, where only 7 of 44 proved to be immunogenic.

Role of Effector Cell Populations

The role of specifically sensitized lymphocytes and natural immunity, as in natural killer (NK) cells and macrophages, in tumour rejection responses has been evaluated using a series of aminoazo dye [4-dimethylaminoazobenzene (DAB)]-induced rat hepatocellular carcinomas and 3-methyl-cholanthrene (MCA)-induced fibrosarcomas. These tumours, like most carcinogen-induced tumours [4], express individually distinct tumour rejection antigens, and enhancement of the specific arm of the tumour immune response can lead to an effective tumour rejection reaction. This is illustrated by the experiments summarized in Fig. 1 from recent investigations on the immunotherapy of rat hepatoma D192A. Injection i.m. of hepatoma D192A cells produces progressive tumour growth, but as illustrated, a contralateral i.m. injection of viable tumour cells admixed with BCG (Glaxo Percutaneous vaccine) suppresses tumour growth. In the three experiments summarized, administration of the tumour cell-BCG vaccine at the

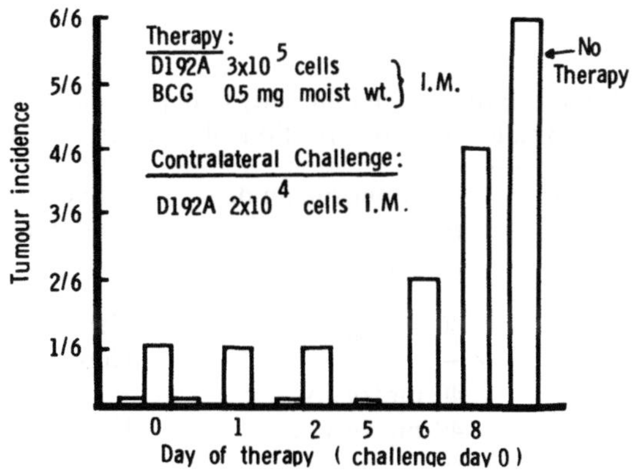

Fig. 1. Active specific immunotherapy of i.m. implants of rat hepatoma D192A. Hepatoma D192A cells injected i.m. were treated up to 8 days later by a contralateral i.m. injection of hepatoma D192A cells admixed with BCG. This immunostimulating inoculum does not produce a progressive tumour and the systemic host response inhibits the contralateral tumour challenge

time of tumour challenge completely suppressed tumours in 17 of 18 treated rats. Tumour growth was also suppressed when treatment was delayed until 6–8 days after tumour implantation, signifying that this was a real therapeutic response rather than another example of immunoprophylaxis.

In accord with previous findings with other carcinogen-induced hepatomas and sarcomas [6, 13], the nature of the tumour antigen preparation used in the vaccine was critically important. Hence, vaccines containing viable tumour cells, prevented from progressive growth by contact with BCG organisms, consistently produced tumour immunity whereas radiation-attenuated tumour cells were ineffective.

Of more importance in the design of immunotherapeutic procedures was the finding that vaccines containing 3 M KCl extracts of hepatoma D192A together with BCG were also completely ineffective in generating anti-tumour immunity. This is consistent with extensive studies showing that membrane preparations and soluble (3 M KCl) extracts of DAB-induced hepatomas and MCA-induced sarcomas lacked significant immunogenicity, defined by the capacity to elicit tumour rejection responses [6, 13]. The current view is that the failure of these tumour preparations, especially soluble extracts, to elicit tumour immunity reflects inappropriate antigen processing. This is emphasized by the experiments summarized in Table 1 showing that immunization with 3 M KCl extracts of hepatoma D23 following pretreatment of the rats with cyclophosphamide (CY) (40 mg/kg body weight) leads to the induction of immunity to the tumour. This effect was not achieved in normal CY-treated rats and the tumour-immune response in CY-treated animals was specific, since no resistance to challenge with hepatoma D192A was induced. CY treatment is known to suppress the development of suppressor lymphocytes controlling the generation of delayed hypersensitivity responses to contact hypersensitizing agents [1] and the induction of immunity to tumour cells [10]. This conclusion is further supported by related studies showing that thymus-derived cells from rats immunized with 3 M KCl tumour extracts or from tumour-bearers suppress tumour immunity [14].

Effector Cells Involved in Tumour Rejection

It is generally accepted that the host responses stimulated by immunization with tumour cell-containing vaccines include the generation of specifically sensitized T lymphocytes. This is emphasized by the experiments summarized in Fig. 2, showing that lumbar lymph node cells draining an i.m. implant of viable hepatoma D192A cells

Table 1. Induction of immunity to hepatoma D23 with soluble 3 M KCl extracts of tumour. Rats were treated by i.p. injection of 1, 2, 3, and 4 mg extract on days 3, 5, 7, and 9

Group	Cyclophosphamide treatment (day 0)	Tumor extract treatment	Tumour incidence (challenges: -10^3 hepatoma D23 cells S.C. day 13)
1	40 mg/kg i.v.	Hepatoma D23	3/11
2	–	Hepatoma D23	10/10
3	40 mg/kg i.v.	–	5/5
4	40 mg/kg i.v.	Hepatoma D192A	6/6

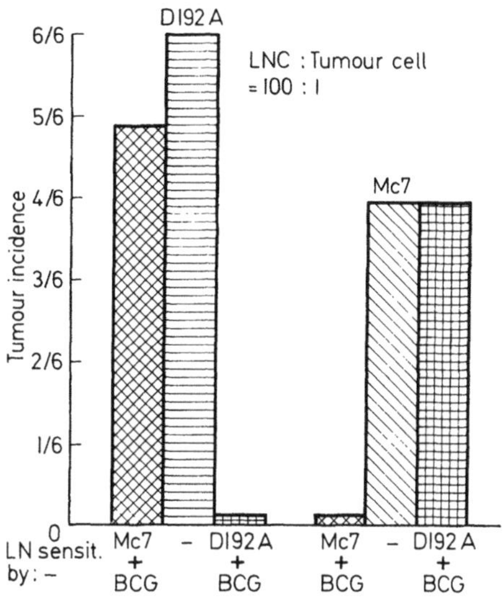

Fig. 2. Inhibition of growth of rat hepatoma D192A and sarcoma Mc7 by lumbar lymph node cells obtained from rats immunized by i.m. challenge with tumour cells admixed with BCG (Glaxo Percutaneous Vaccine). Lymph node cells from tumour-immune donors mixed with tumour cells at a ratio of 100 : 1 were injected into normal rats and assayed for inhibitory activity (Winn test)

together with BCG suppress growth of hepatoma D192A when assayed in the Winn test. These D192A-stimulated lymph node cells were ineffective against another tumour (sarcoma Mc7). Conversely, in the specificity control, lymph node cells sensitized to sarcoma Mc7 suppressed growth of this tumour but not hepatoma D192A (Fig. 2). As already commented upon, the immune response generated systemically by vaccines containing hepatoma D192A together with BCG is also directed specifically against hepatoma D192A, since a contralateral challenge with hepatoma D192A is suppressed but not with other tumour vaccines. The conclusion from these studies is that specifically sensitized lymphocytes generated by immunization with tumour cell-containing vaccines form part of the systemic response with the capacity to localize in tumour deposits at sites distant from the immunizing inoculum. This is supported by related studies on the influence of lymphadenectomy, where excision of the lymph node draining the i.m. hepatoma D192A-BCG vaccine site abrogated the response-suppressing tumour growth at a contralateral site, whereas removal of the lymph node draining the challenge site had no effect. The cellular interactions leading to destruction of tumour cells are less clearly understood, since it has been found that immunization with tumour cell vaccines, especially where bacterial agents such as BCG are incorporated, also generates NK cell activity and/or activated macrophages [3]. Therefore, whilst tumour challenge tests, as well as Winn-type assays, establish the requirement for specifically sensitized lymphocytes, there is no unequivocal evidence, at least with solid tumours, that these are the final effector cells mediating cytotoxic or cytostatic reactions. This point is emphasized by several studies using both short- and long-term in vitro cytotoxicity tests, where it could not be demonstrated conclusively that immunization of syngeneic rats with DAB-hepatomas and MCA-sarcomas generated cytotoxic lymphocytes with the characteristic individual specificity, as revealed by in vivo tumour rejection [4, 9]. Furthermore, analysis of host cells infiltrating MCA-induced sarcomas led to the identification of a highly reactive lymphocyte population preventing tumour growth in Winn assays using effector to tumour cell ratio as low as 1.5 : 1 [15]. Again, however, these lymphocyte populations did not display the characteristic specificity as revealed by tumour challenge tests.

Non-Specific Anti-Tumour Responses

The finding that anti-tumour responses generated at the site of tumour deposits, following specific generation of immunity to tumour-associated antigens, may involve non-specific effector cells [2, 4, 9] suggests that stimulation of natural immunity may have therapeutic potential. In most instances, however, systemic stimulation of NK cells and/or activated macrophages by treatment with bacterial agents such as BCG or *C. parvum* does not effectively suppress tumour growth [3]. This is illustrated in a series of studies with rat hepatoma D192A, where i.m. injection of BCG enhances NK cell activity in the draining lymph node, but does not influence growth of a contralateral i.m. challenge with the tumour [6]. As already noted (Fig. 1), treatment with vaccines containing tumour cells admixed with BCG is highly effective in preventing tumour growth and there is a clear requirement for specifically sensitized lymphocytes. One interpretation of these findings is that sensitized lymphocytes may localize in tumour deposits and, whilst not directly cytotoxic, may lead to the stimulation and/or infiltration of NK cells and macrophages through the release of soluble factors [2, 3]. This is compatible with the well-established finding that immunomodulating agents, especially bacterial preparations, are most effective when administered so as to localize in tumour deposits, this being defined as regional immunotherapy [2, 5]. Many of the agents tested for regional immunotherapy, such as BCG organisms and subcellular products, have multiple functions such as the capacity to elicit delayed type hypersensitivity (DTH). In this case, recent studies indicate that BCG-mediated suppression of naturally arising rat mammary carcinomas is more effective in tuberculin-sensitized animals. It is also possible to elicit antitumour responses by intratumoral injection of hypersensitizing agents into recipients already

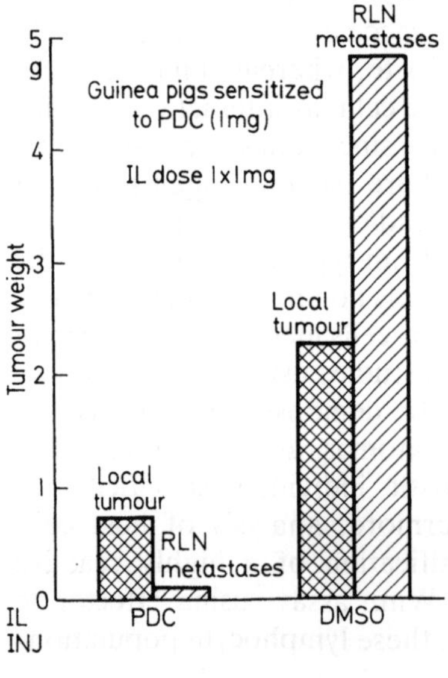

Fig. 3. Effect of intralesional injection of 3-n-pentadecylcatechol (PDC) in dimethylsulphoxide (DMSO) on intradermal growth of line 10 hepatoma and the development of regional lymph node metastases in PDC-sensitized guinea pigs

pre-sensitized to the compound, thus producing local DTH responses. This is illustrated by recent studie on the treatment of guinea pig line 10 hepatoma by intralesional injection of alkylcatechols in animals presensitized to the hapten (Fig. 3). These compounds are highly potent hypersensitizing agents, being the active products of poison ivy/oak urushiol [7]. As illustrated (Fig. 3), injection of 3-n-pentadecyl-catechol (PDC) into intradermal grafts of line 10 hepatoma in PDC-sensitized guinea pigs suppressed growth of the local tumour and markedly inhibited the development of regional lymph node metastases. Since these initial studies using PDC in dimethyl-sulphoxide, it has been found that squalene is a more suitable vehicle, enhancing the therapeutic response to intralesional injection of PDC or a urushiol oil [9].

Conclusions

One of the most effective approaches in manipulating the tumour-host relationship for therapy involves augmentation of immunity to tumour-associated antigens. This requires the generation of specifically sensitized T lymphocytes, although the function of these effector cells is still unclear. With some tumours, especially virus-induced lymphomas, they may be directly cytotoxic. However, this is less likely to be the pathway leading to anti-tumour responses with solid tumours, since in tests with a range of rat tumours in vitro cytotoxicity responses with sensitized lymphocytes could not be demonstrated. It may be, therefore, that anti-tumour responses are mediated by other cell types which are triggered by factors produced following interaction of sensitized lymphocytes and tumour cells. This hypothesis would reconcile the contradictory findings that whilst cell-mediated responses to the individually distinct antigens on carcinogen-induced rat tumours are required for tumour rejection, the host cells derived from regressing tumours lack specificity [2, 5, 9, 15].

Development of this approach in human cancer depends upon the identification of tumour-associated antigens on human tumours. Formal identification of these cell membrane products has still to be presented. Whilst there is a large body of evidence derived from both in vivo and in vitro tests for cell-mediated immunity [2], much of this is still viewed as equivocal. An alternative approach of preparing monoclonal antibodies following fusion of antibody-producing B lymphocytes, from BALB/c mice immunized with tumour cells and murine myeloma cells, has led to the identification of tumour-associated antigens on several tumour types including malignant melanoma [11, 17] and osteogenic sarcoma [8]. At the present state of development of these studies it does appear, however, that some of the antigens detected are not truly tumour-specific and so it remains to be established whether they elicit immune responses in patients.

Another approach to immune manipulation involves stimulation of natural immunity, this being mediated by NK cells and/or activated macrophages. Whilst this type of response can be induced with several immunomodulating agents, the therapeutic effect is generally low. In contrast, promotion of local responses by administrating immunomodulating agents so as to localize in tumour deposits frequently produces an effective antitumour effect, even with tumours lacking immunogenicity [2, 3]. One approach here is to stimulate local delayed-type hypersensitivity responses using hypersensitizing agents. This type of response has been used to treat rat mammary carcinomas with PPD in tuberculin-sensitized animals. As discussed, however, chemically defined agents such as alkylcatechols which are highly potent hypersensitizing agents, may be more effective. These compounds can be administered in a variety of non-toxic solvents and rapidly become incorporated into the lipid phase of tumour cell membranes [7]. It is also possible to enhance the hypersensitizing potential since, in humans, compounds with unsaturated bonds in the alkyl side chain are more potent than the fully saturated compounds such as PDC [7, 7a].

References

1. Asherson GL, Perera MACC, Thomas WR (1979) Contact sensitivity and the DNA response in mice to high and low doses of oxazolone: Low-dose unresponsiveness following painting and feeding and its prevention by pretreatment with cyclophosphamide. Immunology 36: 449–452
2. Baldwin RW (to be published) Immunotherapy of tumours. Cancer Chemother Ann 2
3. Baldwin RW, Byers VS (1979) Immunoregulation by bacterial organisms and their role in the immunotherapy of cancer. Springer Semin Immunopathol 2: 79–100
4. Baldwin RW, Price MR (to be published) Neoantigen expression in chemical carcinogenesis. In: Cancer: A comprehensive treatise, 2nd ed, vol 1. Plenum Press, New York
5. Baldwin RW, Embleton MJ, Pimm MV (1979) Host responses to spontaneous rat tumours. In: Chandra P (ed) Antiviral mechanisms in the control of neoplasia. Plenum Press, New York, pp 333–353
6. Baldwin RW, Pimm MV, Robins RA (1979) Active specific immunotherapy. Ad Med Oncol Res Educ 6: 67–75
7. Byers VS, Baldwin RW (to be published) Modulation of tumor cell membranes with lipophilic haptens: An approach to modifying tumor immunogenicity. In: Bach FH, Bonavida B, Vitetta ES, Fox CF (eds) T and B lymphocyte, recognition and function. Academic Press, New York

7a. Byers VS, Epstein WL, Castagnoli N, Baer H (1979) In vitro studies of poison oak immunity. I. In vitro reaction of human lymphocytes to urushiol. J Clin Invest 64: 1437–1448

8. Embleton MJ, Gunn B, Byers VS, Baldwin RW (to be published) Antitumor reactions of monoclonal antibody against a human osteogenic sarcoma cell. Br J Cancer
9. Flannery GR, Robins RA, Baldwin RW (to be published) Cell. Quantitative studies of natural immunity to solid tumours in rats. Natural killer cells infiltrate transplanted chemically-induced sarcomas. Cell Immunol
10. Glaser M (1979) Regulation of specific cell-mediated cytotoxic response against SV40-induced tumor-associated antigens by depletion of suppressor T cells with cyclophosphamide in mice. J Exp Med 149: 774–777
11. Koprowski H, Steplewski Z, Herlyn D, Herlyn M (1978) Study of antibodies against human melanoma produced by somatic cell hybrids. Proc Natl Acad Sci USA 75: 3405–3409
12. Moore M (1978) Antigen of experimentally induced neoplasms: A conspectus in immunological aspects of cancer. In: Castro JE (ed) Immunological aspects of cancer. MTP Press, Lancaster, pp 15–39
13. Price MR, Preston VE, Robins RA, Zöller M, Baldwin RW (1978) Induction of immunity to chemically-induced rat tumours. Cancer Immunol Immunother 3: 247–252
14. Price MR, Hannant D, Bowen JG, Baldwin RW (to be published) Suppressor cells in rats immunized against solubilized hepatoma-specific antigens. Br J Cancer
15. Robins RA, Flannery GR, Baldwin RW (1979) Tumour-derived lymphoid cells are able to prevent tumour growth in Winn assays. Br J Cancer 40: 946–949

16. Robins RA, Rees RC, Brooks CG, Baldwin RW (1979) Spontaneous development of cytotoxic activity in cultured lymph node cells from tumour-bearing rats. Br J Cancer 39: 659–666
17. Yeh M-Y, Hellström I, Brown JP, Warner CA, Hansen JA, Hellström KE (1979) Cell surface antigens of human melanoma identified by monoclonal antibody. Proc Natl Acad Sci USA 76: 2927–2931

56. *Preliminary Clinical Results with Norgamem (Thioproline) and Revercan (2-Amino-2-Thiazoline): The First Inducers of Reverse Transformation*

A. Brugarolas and M. Gosálvez

Hospital General de Asturias, Department of Oncology, Oviedo, Spain

Introduction

Puck [6] defined the term reverse transformation as the recovery of normal morphology and normal membrane functions by transformed cells in tissue culture treated with high concentrations of dibutyryl adenosine 3′:5′-cyclic phosphate (cAMP). Gosálvez [3, 5] sought for compounds able to induce reverse transformation at pharmacologic concentrations using three screening systems; the capping of lymphocytes, the differentiation of the mold *Dyctostelium discoideum,* and the restoration of contact inhibition of HeLa cells in tissue culture. One compound, thiazoline-4-carboxylic acid, also called thioproline, passed the screening. This compound showed no toxicity in animals and no activity in transplantable animal tumors. It was brought to a phase I clinical trial in Spain in patients with advanced cancer of several types with encouraging results [1], especially in head and neck epidermoid carcinoma. The compound was called norgamem for use in clinical trails. Gosálvez [5] sought for analogs of thioproline, and only 2-amino-2-thiazoline passed the three screening systems. This compound, called revercan for clinical trials, was used in a clinical trial in Spain with bladder carcinoma and showed encouraging results [2]. Although norgamem and revercan could have activity in a wide series of tumors, we summarize here the current data on norgamem (epidermoid carcinoma of the head and neck) and on revercan (bladder carcinoma). Both compounds show antitumor activity without toxicity and, although the rate of response could not be defined due to excessive selection of patients and low number of patients, our results encourage the study of these two compounds in a wide phase II study of all tumor types. Whether norgamem and revercan will be demonstrated to be with or without utility in cancer clinics, they represent the first two inducers of reverse transformation or "transrecers," a new group of substances in anticancer therapy which should be further explored.

Patients and Methods

Thioproline (Norgamem) in Head and Neck Carcinoma

Norgamem was supplied as a lyophilized powder in 250 mg ampules. It was dissolved in water prior to injection. Two different schedules were used. In the first schedule,

Recent Results in Cancer Research, Vol. 80

norgamem was given as a continuous infusion of 20 mg/kg daily for 5 consecutive days repeated every 2–3 weeks. Subsequently, it was given i.m. in four equal doses daily for 4 months.

The criteria used in the selection of patients were: pathologic diagnosis of locally advanced or metastasic cancer resistant to treatment; physical condition allowing outpatient care; measurable tumor for the assessment of the response; no other anticancer treatment in the 4 weeks before or during norgamem treatment; and informed consent from the patients.

Clinical assessment included complete history and examination, measurement of tumors, chest X-ray, ECG, complete blood counts, liver profile, and urine analysis. These assessments were made before treatment began and every 1–3 weeks during treatment.

The evaluation of response was made according to the following criteria: Complete response was considered to be the disappearance of all signs and symptoms of the disease for at least 1 month, and partial response was a 50% or more decrease in tumor size (sum of the products of the two largest perpendicular diameters of all measurable lesions) for more than 1 month. All other reactions including less than 50% decrease in tumor size for periods of less than 1 month, mixed response, stabilization of tumor grouwth, and continuous tumor growth were considered to be progression of the disease.

Thirty-eight patients (32 males and six females) were treated with thioproline, and their ages were 33–85 years (median 59). Karnofsky scale status was 50–100 (median 70). Twenty-eight patients had received prior surgical excision of the tumor and 31 patients received previous radiotherapy. Only eight patients received previous cytotoxic chemotherapy.

Tumor characteristics according to primary site, tumor differentiation, and site of evaluable disease for the assessment of the response are indicated in Table 1.

Table 1. Response to thioproline (norgamem) according to tumor site, pathologic differentiation, and site of measurable disease

Characteristics of tumors	Patients	Complete response	Partial response	Progression
Tumor site				
Oral cavity	14	2	1	11
Oropharynx	10	2	1	7
Hypopharynx	6	–	–	6
Larynx	6	2	2	2
Skin	3	–	2	1
Tumor differentiation				
Well	12	6	2	4
Moderately	12	–	4	8
Poorly	14	–	–	14
Measurable disease				
Primary site	13	–	4	9
Lymph nodes	19	–	3	16
Lung	13	6	–	7

2-Amino-2-Thiazoline (Revercan) in Bladder Carcinoma

Revercan was supplied as a lyophilized powder in vials containing 250 mg pure compound. It was dissolved in sterile water at the time of administration.

Two different dose escalation schedules were used. In the first schedule (Hospital Clínico San Carlos, Madrid), revercan (1.5–10 mg/kg body weight) was given daily i.v. for 5 consecutive days and repeated every 3 weeks. In the second schedule (Hospital General de Asturias, Oviedo) revercan (3–12 mg/kg body weight) was given daily i.v. for 6 months. Some patients later in the study received the same amount of drug i.m.

Selected patients had pathologically proven advanced carcinoma of the urinary bladder, with tumor clearly visualized by cystoscopy, computerized tomography (CT scan), and cystogram, had no previous local or systemic anticancer therapy other than surgery, adequate performance status for outpatient care and follow-up, and gave informed consent.

Different patients were treated at each dose level and schedule, and the response was assessed by cystoscopy and biopsy, CT scan, and cystogram every 1–3 months.

In evaluating the response, complete remission was considered to be the disappearance of all clinical and radiologic evidences of disease when a confirmatory biopsy of the previous tumor site indicated absence of tumor. A partial response was considered to be a 50% or more decrease in the tumor size as measured by the product of the two largest perpendicular diameters. All other reactions were considered progression of the disease.

Thirty-one patients (24 males and seven females) with recurrent or advanced transitional carcinoma of the urinary bladder were treated with revercan. The age range was 52–84 (median 69) years of age and performance status was 40–100 (median 70) in the Karnofsky scale. Seventeen patients received previous surgery and four patients received previous radiotherapy.

The stage of the tumor according to the UICC classification was I in two patients, II in 17 patients, III in seven patients, and IV in six patients.

Results

Thioproline (Norgamem)

Six patients received 4 months of daily thioproline and 17 patients received daily thioproline for more than 2 months. One patient had an episode of flu-like syndrome and thioproline was discontinued temporarily. Another two patients indicated mental fatigue and mild confusion, but both were continued on thioproline. There was no clinical alteration in mental status, orientation, and memory. No other side effects were noticed.

Among 11 patients receiving thioproline (20 mg/kg) three patients showed a partial response (27%, lasting 1, 2, and 7 months, respectively). The latter patients presented slow progression of the disease after discontinuation of therapy and thioproline failed to reinduce a second remission.

Among 27 patients receiving thioproline (40 mg/kg daily), six patients had a complete response and three patients a partial response (33%). Partial responses lasted 1.5, 2, and 2.5 months, respectively. The six patients (five males and one female) with a

complete response had tumor of the oral cavity in two patients, oropharynx in two patients, and larynx in two patients. All had well-differentiated epidermoid carcinoma; three of these were composed of small cells and the other three were made up of intermediate keratinizing cells. Complete responses were observed 2–3 months after initiation of therapy. All six patients received 4 months of thioproline before discontinuation. Tumor recurrences in previously known tumor sites occurred in five of the complete-response patients at 1, 2, 2, 4, and 6 months after cessation of thioproline treatment, respectively. In spite of reinitiation of thioproline therapy, none of these patients responded. Three patients received subsequent chemotherapy with conventional agents and to presented a transient partial response. In four patients, a fine-needle aspiration biopsy was obtained at the time of progression, and indicated poorly differentiated epidermoid carcinoma.
Sequential biopsies of the tumor site in two patients treated at 20 mg/kg indicated maturation of tissues, while at 40 mg/kg, sequential biopsies indicated focal cellular necrosis and increased capillary formation. Response and the different tumor characteristics are analyzed in Table 1.

2-Amino-2-Thiazoline Revercan

At 1.5–6 mg/kg, no toxicity was observed. At 6 mg/kg, one elderly patient presented oral ulcerations after 1 month of therapy, which improved in spite of the continuation of therapy. At 10–12 mg/kg, two patients of five had nausea and occasional vomiting, and another two patients had complaints of mental confusion. These symptoms disappeared when the drug dose was reduced to 6 mg/kg daily. There was no other general or local toxicity. Evaluation indicated absence of myelodepression and no alteration in pulmonary, cardiac, hepatic, or renal function.
Three biopsy-proven complete responses and five partial responses were observed. Responses occurred with different doses and schedules, with a total response rate of 31% of 22 evaluable patients at the time of this report (Table 2). Responses occurred

Table 2. Results of 2-amino-2-thiazoline (revercan) therapy according to dose, schedule, and category of response

Drug dose	Evaluable/-total patients	Complete response	Partial response	Progression
1.5 mg/kg[a]	1/1	–	–	1
3.0 mg/kg[a]	4/5	1	1	2
3.0 mg/kg[b]	2/2	1	1	–
6.0 mg/kg[a]	3/5	–	1	2
6.0 mg/kg[b]	9/13	1	1	7
10.0 mg/kg[a]	1/2	–	–	1
12.0 mg/kg[a]	2/3	–	1	1
Total	22/31	3	5	14
		(31%)		

[a] Intermittent schedule, treatment given daily × 5 every 3 weeks
[b] Daily continuous therapy

2–3 months after initiation of therapy. The median duration of response for patients with partial response was 1.5 months. All three patients with a complete response maintained the response for 7, 4, and 2 months, respectively, at the time of this report. As shown in Table 1, responses were observed in the two different hospitals and at and all doses used.

Twelve patients among 18 of one institution were evaluable for tumor differentiation studies. According to this analysis, both of the two patients with well-differentiated transitional cell carcinoma had a complete response. Another two patients of five with moderately differentiated transitional cell carcinoma had a partial response. On the other hand, none of the five patients with poorly differentiated transitional cell carcinoma responded.

Discussion

Thioproline was active in epidermoid carcinoma of the head and neck, but only in well-differentiated tumors. Similarly, only well-differentiated transitional cell carcinoma of the urinary bladder appeared to respond to 2-amino-2-thiazoline. The responses with both drugs occurred rather slowly over a prolonged period of time (2–3 months). Both compounds were free of toxicity. The dose of 6 mg/kg is recommended for 2-amino-2-thiazoline.

Broad phase II clinical trials with a great number of tumor types are recommended for both compounds.

References

1. Brugarolas A, Gosálvez M (1980) Treatment of cancer by an inducer of reverse transformation. Lancet 1: 68–70
2. Brugarolas A, Uson A, Junguera Villa JM, Subiza C, Ribas A, Gosálvez M (to be published) 2-Amino-2-thiazoline, an analog of thioproline in anticancer therapy. Initial clinical evaluation in carcinoma of the urinary bladder. Lancet
3. Gosálvez M (1979) The plasma membrane as the target in anticancer chemotherapy. Proc. Am Assoc Cancer Res Am Soc Clin Oncol 20: 17
4. Gosálvez M (1980) Norgamem and revercan, the first two inducers of reverse transformation (transrecers) in anticancer therapy. Proc Am Assoc Cancer Res Am Soc Clin Oncol 21: 132
5. Gosálvez M, Vivero C, Alvarez I (1979) Restoration of contact inhibition of tumor cells in tissue culture by treatment with thiazolidin-4-carboxylic acid. Biochem Soc Trans 7: 191–192
6. Puck TT (1977) Cyclic AMP, the microtubule microfilament system and cancer. Proc Natl Acad Sci USA 74: 4491–4495

57. *Biologic-Response Modifiers and Adjuvant Chemotherapy: Consideration of Selected Preclinical Investigations in Relation to Clinical Potential*

A. Goldin, M. A. Chirigos, J. S. Macdonald, A. Fefer, and E. Mihich*

National Cancer Institute, Division of Cancer Treatment, Cancer Therapy Evaluation Program, Bethesda, MD 20205, USA

In cancer therapeutics, attention has been focused increasingly on the interrelationship between host responses to tumor, tumor effects on the host, and effects of the antitumor treatment being studied. Biologic-response modifiers include agents or approaches that are capable of modifying the tumor-host relationships in such manner that there is an alteration in host response to tumor cells. Since such an alteration may be beneficial, it is of interest to consider the potentiality of biologic- response modifiers in the management of cancer.

Biologic-response modifiers may be somewhat arbitrarily classified according to the different types of action they may have on host-tumor relationships:

1) Immunoaugmenting agents may increase host defense response to tumor through stimulation of macrophage and reticuloendothelial system functions. Examples of agents acting primarily through such mechanisms include the bacterial products BCG, BCG fractions, and *C. parvum;* extracts, such as lentinan, bestatin, and glucan; and synthetic compounds such as pyran copolymers and azimexone.
2) Immunomodulating treatments with anticancer and other agents may alter the balance of the immune response through effects on specific components of the immune system such as T cell subsets, B cells, or natural killer (NK) cells. These treatments may decrease undesired components of the host response. For example, suppressor-cell function may be depressed by drugs, such as indomethacin or cimetidine.
3) Chemicals with immunorestorative properties may restore the immunologic capabilities of the host where immunologic reactivity has been decreased as a result of progressive tumor growth, age, or other factors. Levamisole is an agent which may act in this fashion.

---

* The authors wish to acknowledge the source material in the "Interim report. Subcommittee on Biological Response Modifiers (BRM) of the Division of Cancer Treatment, NCI, Board of Scientific Counselors" September 30, 1979, which is in preparation for publication. The BRM Subcommittee was founded by V. T. DeVita, Jr., Director of the Division of Cancer Treatment (currently Director of the National Cancer Institute) and the Board of Scientific Counselors, to provide program recommendations. The subcommittee membership includes E. Mihich (Chairman), A. Fefer (Vice Chairman), J. Bertram, A. Goldstein, E. Hersh, M. Krim, M. Mastrangelo, M. Mitchell, H. Oettgen, J, Whisnant, A. Goldin (Special NCI Advisor), and M. Chirigos (NCI Liaison)

Recent Results in Cancer Research, Vol. 80

4) Inducers of response mediators are exemplified by interferon inducers, such as poly IC and pyrimidinole derivatives.
5) Among the cytokines, the interferons are the agents of greatest current interest as they appear to exert measurable antitumor effects. Tumor necrosis factor is another example of a cytokine which may exert action through the host.
6) Thymic hormones and factors may increase host resistance through effects on the maturation of T cells from precursor cells and thus possibly result in immunorestoration in cancer patients with T cell function deficiencies.
7) Tumor prevention or retardation of the expression of neoplastic transformation may be affected by agents, such as the retinoids. Interference with the development of primary tumors in high-risk patients, or possibly prevention of reinduction of secondary malignancies in successfully treated patients, may be achieved through the use of such agents.
8) Maturation-differentiation factors have been defined in experimental systems which may induce maturation of tumor cells to a more differentiated state. The potential use of such agents in the clinics should be pursued through careful studies directed towards a clarification of their role in humans.
9. Identification and characterization of tumor antigens and the use of tumor cell surface modifiers may provide ways to increase the immunogenicity of tumor cells and thereby stimulate host antitumor immune mechanisms. The susceptibility of tumor cells to immunologic destruction may also be increased and there may be an alteration of cellular interactions, including those involved in cell to cell contact and in certain phases of the metastatic process.
10) Adoptive transfer of lymphoid cells sensitized against tumor cells may exert therapeutic effects in tumor-bearing animals, in conjunction with noncurative chemotherapy. However, the development of graft-versus-host reactions (GVH) in the adoptive transfer of immune lymphocytes may constitute a serious complication which must be overcome.
11) The utilization of antitumor antibodies is receiving renewed attention due to the possibility of preparing hybridomas as factories for production of monoclonal antibodies directed against tumor-associated antigens.

Biologic-response modifiers may be employed alone or in conjunction with one or more antitumor agents or other treatment modalities. For the biologic-response modifier it is important, as with the investigation of individual drugs, to establish dose-response relationships for both host toxicity and antitumor effects. In addition, such relationships must also be determined with reference to the biologic-response which is expected to be modified. Characteristically, with an active drug, as the dosage is increased the survival time of the animals is increased and reaches a maximum at an optimal dose, following which the toxicity for the host becomes dominant and the survival time diminishes. With the biologic-response modifiers, however, the maximum tolerated dose may not necessarily be the optimal dose. The utilization of biologic-response modifiers in conjunction with chemotherapy may, in some cases, be based on the established concept that combination chemotherapy with two or more drugs can be more effective than the drugs employed individually in providing an enhanced therapeutic outcome (therapeutic synergism). However, in most cases, the utilization of biologic-response modifiers along with individual drugs or drug combinations may lead to additional advantages stemming from augmented host response-conditioning enhancement. With combination drug therapy there may be a greater possibility for sufficient reduction of the tumor cell population so that by the addition of biologic-response modifiers, host participation may contribute to the destruction of residual tumor cells and, thereby, result in total eradication of tumor.

With the employment of biologic-response modifiers in conjunction with antitumor agents, just as for combination chemotherapy, studies of dose-response relationships for determination of optimal ratios and optimal dosages, should be stressed. Whether the biologic-response modifier is employed alone or in combination, it is important to establish optimal schedules and routes of administration and to clarify their relationship to the nature and extent of disease.

An example is provided with a combination of BCNU and the biologic-response modifier levamisole in the treatment of Moloney LSTRA leukemia in mice [3]. In this study levamisole was ineffective, and BCNU was only moderately effective in increasing the number of survivors. However, the combination of levamisole-BCNU increased markedly the number of survivors.

In another study the combination of methyl CCNU-levamisole was used to tread relatively advanced Lewis lung carcinoma [3]. Levamisole was ineffective in increasing the median survival time of the animals, although there was a moderate decrease in the primary tumor weight and in the number of lung lesions. Methyl CCNU resulted in a moderate increase in the survival time of the animals, and also in some reduction of both primary tumor weight and number of lung lesions. However, with the combination of methyl CCNU-levamisole, there was a marked increase in survival time and further reduction of both primary tumor weight and the number of lung lesions.

An investigation with Graffi leukemia illustrates the influence of dosage with an antitumor drug plus levamisole (Chirigos, unpublished observations). At lower dosages of cyclophosphamide (50 or 100 mg/kg), although the drug produced a definite increase in the survival time of the animals, levamisole (2.5–10 mg/kg) made no further beneficial contribution. However, at a higher dosage of cyclophosphamide (200 mg/kg) administered on day 8 after tumor inoculation, followed by levamisole on day 11, there were extensive increases in survival time and a high incidence of 100-day survivors.

Similar studies were performed with the C3H mammary adenocarcinoma C16. Chemotherapy with adriamycin plus 5-fluorouracil (5-FU) administered when the tumor was 4–9 mm in size, resulted in 36% inhibition of tumor growth, 41% increase in life span, and 34% survivors (Chirigos, unpublished observations). Further reduction in tumor growth, and additional increases in survival time and percentage of survivors were observed with chemotherapy with adriamycin plus 5-FU in combination with brupel, interferon, or pyran copolymer.

It has been demonstrated that an alteration of the immunogenicity of tumor cells may accompany the origin of resistance to chemotherapeutic agents and that the immunologic response of the host to the altered tumor cells, when coupled with chemotherapy with an agent that is active against the resistant tumor, may result in an increased therapeutic response (collateral sensitivity) [1, 8, 12, 13].

Adoptively transferred antitumor lymphocytes as an adjunct to chemotherapy have also been used effectively in many animal models. A variety of viral and nonviral tumors in mice have been eradicated by noncurative chemotherapy and/or radiation plus infusion of appropriate syngeneic or allogeneic lymphocytes [5]. In one example [4], with Moloney lymphoma, cyclophosphamide plus specifically sensitized allogeneic or syngeneic spleen cells resulted in marked increases in survival time and a definitive percentage of long-term survivors. In another type of study, chemoimmunotherapy of L1210 Cr leukemia in CDF_1 mice with cyclophosphamide or BCNU plus adoptive transfer of lymphocytes sensitized to DTIC, resulted in an increase in the survival time of the animals [6].

Thus, there are various ways in which drugs and biologic-response modification may be employed in combination therapy, and the full potential of this approach remains to be determined.

The utilization of biologic-response modifiers in conjunction with surgery or with chemotherapy plus surgery is based on the preclinical and clinical evidence that surgery plus chemotherapy may result in marked enhancement of therapeutic response.

A number of advantages may accrue as a result of treatment with the combined modality of surgery plus chemotherapeutic agents. Such advantages may include: (1) Surgery by reduction in body burden of tumor cells may increase survival sufficiently to permit further drug therapy; (2) surgery may lead to improved host tolerance so that higher dosage can be employed; (3) surgery may reduce the immunosuppressive effect of drug treatment; (4) surgery may diminish the immunosuppression associated with progressive tumor growth; (5) surgery may reduce the absolute number of spontaneous and drug-induced resistant mutants and the degree of metastatic spread and attendant tumor cell sequestration; (6) surgery may be followed by an increase in the proliferative fraction of tumor cells, and thereby result in increased drug sensitivity; (7) reduction in tumor challenge by surgery may result in sufficient increase in drug effectiveness against metastatic disease so that total tumor eradication can become a more readily attainable objective.

There have not been extensive investigations of combinations of biologic-response modifiers in conjunction with surgery or in conjunction with combination chemotherapy plus surgery. In one study by Karrer et al. [9], an increase in the number of survivors was achieved in treatment of moderately advanced Lewis lung carcinoma with a combination of *C. parvum* and surgery. With *C. parvum* administered either before or following surgery on day 5 following tumor inoculation, there were increases in the number of survivors. However, with more advanced disease at the time of surgery, the combined modality of *C. parvum* plus surgery was diminished in effectiveness.

In related studies, Schabel et al. [15] demonstrated that when *C. parvum* was administered 1 day following inoculation of Lewis lung carcinoma and surgery was conducted on day 7, there was an increase in the percentage of 90-day survivors. The importance of timing is emphasized by the further observation that when *C. parvum* was given on day 8, following surgery on day 7, the increase in percentage of 90-day survivors was less evident.

The importance of quantitative methodological approaches in clinical investigations with biologic-response modifiers is exemplified by the results of recent studies with interferon. The clinical experience to date has been primarily with human leukocyte interferon [2, 7, 10, 11, 14]. Table 1 outlines the more recent studies performed with interferon. Most studies have been performed in patients with advanced measurable cancers in whom it was possible to objectively assess tumor response. As can be seen from Table 1, the experience with human leukocyte interferon represents 94 patients with different diseases and different dose schedules. There is some disparity between the results of different workers. For example, Gutterman et al. [7] reported a response rate of 41% in breast cancer, while Borden et al. [2] reported a response rate of 22%.

Table 1. Human leukocyte interferon: clinical trials in advanced cancer

Investigator	Disease	Interferon dose	Partial response
Borden et al. [2]	Untreated breast carcinoma	$3-9 \times 10^6$ units/day $\times$ 42 days	5 of 23 (22%)
Osserman et al. [14]	Multiple myeloma (9 of 11 untreated)	$3-6 \times 10^6$ units/day $\times$ 6 months	4 of 11 (29%)
Krown et al. [10]	Non-oat cell lung cancer (2 of 16 untreated)	3×10^6 units/day $\times$ 30 days	0 of 16
Gutterman et al. [7]	Breast carcinoma Non-Hodgkin's lymphoma	$3-9 \times 10^6$ units/day $\times$ 30 days	7 of 17 (41%) 6 of 11 (55%), complete response 2 of 11 (18%)
	Multiple myeloma	Same	6 of 10 (60%)
Merigan et al. [11]	Non-Hodgkin's lymphoma	10^7 units/day $\times$ 30 days	3 of 6 (50%), 3 of 3 in nodular lymphocytic lymphoma

Osserman et al. [14] reported a response rate of 29% in 11 myeloma patients, while Gutterman [7] reported a 60% response rate in this disease.

Of note in these early clinical trials is the toxicity reported in patients treated with interferon. Both Gutterman et al. [7] and Borden et al. [2] reported significant but manageable toxicity with human leukocyte interferon. All patients developed low-grade fever during therapy and most patients had mild leukopenia, malaise, and anorexia. Alopecia was occasionally noted. Thus, it appears that the crude human interferon preparation (0.1% pure) used in these studies produces a spectrum of toxicity in some aspects similar to that of cytotoxic chemotherapeutic agents.

Two facts should be clear from these initial studies of human leukocyte interferon. First, most studies have shown that the material does have some antitumor activity in man. Secondly, it is clear that carefully planned and executed studies of this material must continue so that the specific activity, optimal dosage schedules, and an understanding of possible synergistic effects with antitumor drugs and other combined modalities of cancer therapy can be obtained. Only following systematic approaches will it be possible to define the role of current interferon preparations and other biologic-response modifiers in cancer therapy.

In conclusion, there is clearly significant potential for the biologic-response modifiers to achieve improved antineoplastic therapy. Because of the encouraging prospect, it was considered desirable in the Division of Cancer Treatment, NCI (USA), to initiate an organized program to expedite the study and development of already available and new biologic-response modifiers.

References

1. Bonmassar E, Bonmassar A, Vadlamudi S, Goldin A (1970) Immunological alteration of leukemic cells in vivo after treatment with an antitumor drug. Proc Natl Acad Sci USA 66: 1089
2. Borden E, Dao T, Holland J, Gutterman J, Merigan T (1980) Interferon in recurrent breast carcinoma: Preliminary report of the American Cancer Society Clinical Trials Program. Proc Am Assoc Cancer Res Am Soc Clin Oncol 21: 187
3. Chirigos MA, Amery WK (1978) Combined levamisole therapy: An overview of its protective effects. In: Immunotherapy of human cancer. The University of Texas System Cancer Center. M.D. Anderson Hospital und Tumor Institute. Raven Press, New York, pp 181–195
4. Fefer A (1971) Adoptive chemoimmunotherapy of a Moloney lymphoma. Int J Cancer 8: 364
5. Fefer A, Einstein AB Jr, Cheever MA (1976) Adoptive chemotherapy of cancer in animals: A review of results, principles and problems. Ann NY Acad Sci 277: 492
6. Goldin A, Nicolin A, Bonmassar E (1979) Interrelationship between chemotherapy and immunotherapy in the treatment of disseminated disease. In: Bonadonna G, Mathé G, Salmon SE (eds) Recent results in cancer research, vol 68. Springer, Berlin Heidelberg New York, p 458–464
7. Gutterman J, Yap Y, Buzdar A, Alexanian A, Hersh E, Cabanillas F (1979) Leukocyte interferon induces tumor regression in patients with breast cancer and B-cell neoplasms. J Clin Hematol Oncol 9(4): 295
8. Hutchison DJ (1963) Cross-resistance and collateral sensitivity studies in cancer chemotherapy. Adv Cancer Res 7: 235
9. Karrer K, Rella W, Goldin A (1979) Surgery plus *Corynebacterium parvum* immunotherapy for Lewis lung carcinoma in mice. Eur J Cancer 15: 867
10. Krown S, Stoopler M, Gralla R, Cunningham-Rundles S, Stewart W, Pollack M, Oettgen H (1980) Phase II trial of human leukocyte interferon (HuLeIF) in non-small cell lung cancer (NSCLC): Proc of 2nd International Conference on Immunotherapy of Cancer: Present status of trials in man. NCI 32
11. Merigan TC, Sikora K, Breeden JH, Levy R, Rosenberg SA (1978) Preliminary observations on the effect of human leukocyte interferon in non-Hodgkin's lymphoma. N Engl J Med 299: 1449
12. Mihich E (1969) Modification of tumor regression by immunologic means. Cancer Res 29: 2345
13. Nicolin A, Vadlamudi S, Goldin A (1972) Antigenicity of L 1210 leukemic sublines induced by drugs. Cancer Res 32: 653–657
14. Osserman EF, Sherman WH, Alexanian R, Gutterman JU (1980) Preliminary results of the American Cancer Society (ACS)-sponsored trial of human leukocyte interferon (IF) in multiple myeloma (MM). Proc Am Assoc Cancer Res Am Soc Clin Oncol 21: 161
15. Schabel FM Jr, Griswold DP Jr, Corbett TH, Laster WR Jr, Dykes DJ, Rose WC (1979) Recent studies with surgical adjuvant chemotherapy or immunotherapy of metastatic solid tumors of mice. In: Jones SE, Salmon SE (eds) Adjuvant therapy of cancer, vol II. Grune & Stratton, New York, pp 3–17

Recent Results in Cancer Research

Sponsored by the Swiss League against Cancer. Editor in Chief: P. Rentchnick, Genève

For information about Vols. 1–9, please contact your bookseller of Springer-Verlag

10 NELSON, R. S.: Radioactive Phosphorus in the Diagnosis of Gastrointestinal Cancer.
11 FREEMAN, R. G. and J. M. KNOX: Treatment of Skin Cancer.
12 LYNCH, H. T.: Hereditary Factors in Carcinoma.
13 Tumours in Children, 2nd Edition. Edited by H. B. MARSDEN and J. K. STEWARD.
14 ODARTCHENKO, N.: Production Cellulaire Erythropoïétique.
15 SOKOLOFF, B.: Carcinoid and Serotonin.
16 JACOBS, M. L.: Malignant Lymphomas and Their Management.
17 Normal and Malignant Cell Growth. Edited by R. J. M. FRY, M. L. GRIEM, and W. H. KIRSTEN (Symposium).
18 ANGLESIO, E.: The Treatment of Hodgkin's Disease.
19 BANNASCH, P.: The Cytoplasm of Hepatocytes during Carcinogenesis. Electron- and Lightmicroscopical Investigations of the Nitrosomorpholineintoxicated Rat Liver.
20 Rubidomycin. A new Agent against Cancer. Edited by J. BERNARD, R. PAUL, M. BOIRON, C. JACQUILLAT, and R. MARAL.
21 Scientific Basis of Cancer Chemotherapy. Edited by G. MATHÉ (Symposium).
22 KOLDOVSKÝ, P.: Tumor Specific Transplantation Antigen.
23 FUCHS, W. A., J. W. DAVIDSON, and H. W. FISCHER: Lymphography in Cancer. With contributions by G. JANTET AND H. RÖSLER.
24 HAYWARD, J.: Hormones und Human Breast Cancer. An Account of 15 Years Study.
25 ROY-BURMAN, P.: Analogues of Nucleic Acid Components. Mechanisms of Action.
26 Tumors of the Liver. Edited by G. T. PACK and A. H. ISLAMI.
27 SZYMENDERA, J.: Bone Mineral Metabolism in Cancer.
28 MEEK, E. S.: Antitumour and Antiviral Substances of Natural Origin.
29 Aseptic Environments and Cancer Treatment. Edited by G. MATHÉ (Symposium).
30 Advances in the Treatment of Acute (Blastic) Leukemias. Edited by G. MATHÉ (Symposium).
31 DENOIX, P.: Treatment of Malignant Breast Tumors. Indications and Results.
32 NELSON, R. S.: Endoscopy in Gastric Cancer.
33 Experimental and Clinical Effects of L-Asparaginase. Edited by E. GRUNDMANN and H. F. OETTGEN (Symposium).
34 Chemistry and Biological Actions of 4-Nitroquinolin 1-Oxide. Edited by H. ENDO, T. ONO, and T. SUGIMURA.
35 PENN, I.: Malignant Tumors in Organ Transplant Recipients.
36 Current Concepts in the Management of Lymphoma and Leukemia. Edited by J. E. ULTMANN, M. L. GRIEM, W. H. KIRSTEN, and R. W. WISSLER (Symposium).
37 CHIAPPA, S., R. MUSUMECI, and C. USLENGHI: Endolymphatic Radiotherapy in Malignant Lymphomas. With contributions by G. BONADONNA, B. DAMASCELLI, G. FAVA, F. PIZZETTI, U. VERONESI.
38 KOLLER, P. C.: The Role of Chromosomes in Cancer Biology.
39 Current Problems in the Epidemiology of Cancer and Lymphomas. Edited by E. GRUNDMANN and H. TULINIUS (Symposium).
40 LANGLEY, F. A. and A. C. CROMPTON: Epithelial Abnormalities of the Cervix Uteri.
41 Tumours in a Tropical Country. A Survey of Uganda (1964–1968). Edited by A. C. TEMPLETON.
42 Breast Cancer: A Challenging Problem. Edited by M. L. GRIEM, E. V. JENSEN, J. E. ULTMANN, and R. W. WISSLER (Symposium).
43 Nomenclature, Methodology and Results of Clinical Trials in Acute Leukemias. Edited by G. MATHÉ, P. POUILLART, L. SCHWARZENBERG (Symposium).
44 Special Topics in Carcinogenesis. Edited by E. GRUNDMANN (Symposium).
45 KOLDOVSKÝ, P.: Carcinoembryonic Antigens.
46 Diagnosis and Therapy of Malignant Lymphoma. Edited by K. MUSSHOFF (Symposium).
47 Investigation and Stimulation of Immunity in Cancer Patients. Edited by G. MATHÉ and R. WEINER (Symposium).
48 Platinum Coordination Complexes in Cancer Chemotherapy. Edited by T. A. CONNORS and J. J. ROBERTS (Symposium).
49 Complications of Cancer Chemotherapy. Edited by G. MATHÉ and R. K. OLDHAM (Symposium).
50 Cancer Registry, Edited by E. GRUNDMANN and E. PEDERSEN (Symposium).
51 Gliomas. Current Concepts in Biology, Diagnosis and Therapy. Edited by J. HEKMATPANAH (Symposium).

52 The Ambivalence of Cytostatic Therapy. Edited by E. GRUNDMANN and R. GROSS (Symposium).

53 A. CLARYSSE, Y. KENIS, and G. MATHÉ: Cancer Chemotherapy.

54 Malignant Bone Tumors. Edited by E. GRUNDMANN.

55 MATHÉ, G.: Cancer Active Immunotherapy, Immunoprophylaxis, and Immunorestoration.

56 Lymphocytes, Macrophages, and Cancer. Edited by G. MATHÉ, I. FLORENTIN, and M.-C. SIMMLER (Symposium).

57 Breast Cancer: A Multidisciplinary Approach. Edited by G. ST. ARNEAULT, P. BAND, and L. ISRAËL (Symposium).

58 B. S. SCHOENBERG: Multiple Primary Malignant Neoplasms.

59 Selective Heat Sensitivity of Cancer Cells. Edited by A. ROSSI-FANELLI, R. CAVALIERE, B. MONDOVI, and G. MORICCA.

60 Tumors of the Male Genital System. Edited by E. GRUNDMANN and W. VAHLENSIECK (Symposium).

61 D. METCALF: Hemopoietic Colonies.

62 Tactics and Strategy in Cancer Treatment. Edited by G. MATHÉ (Symposium).

63 Antitumor Antibiotics. Edited by S. K. CARTER, H. UMEZAWA, J. DOUROS, and Y. SAKURAI (Symposium).

64 Lymphoid Neoplasias I: Classification, Categorization, Natural History.

65 Lymphoid Neoplasias II: Clinical and Therapeutic Aspects.
Lymphoid Neoplasias I & II. Proceedings of the 1977 CNRS-EORTC International Colloquium. Editors: G. MATHÉ, M. SELIGMANN, M. TUBIANA. Devided into two volumes.

66 Carcinogenic Hormones. Edited by C. H. LINGEMAN.

67/68 Adjuvant Therapies and Markers of Post-Surgical Minimal Residual Disease I & II. Proceedings of the 1978 Annual Plenary Meeting of the EORTC. Editors: G. BONADONNA, G. MATHÉ, S. E. SALMON. Divided into two volumes.

67 Markers and General Problems of Cancer Adjuvant Therapies.

68 Adjuvant Therapies of the Various Primary Tumors.

69 Strategies in Clinical Hematology. Edited by R. GROSS and K.-P. HELLRIEGEL.

70 New Anticancer Drugs. Edited by S. K. CARTER

71 Endocrine Treatment of Breast Cancer. Edited by B. HENNINGSEN, F. LINDER, C. STREICHELE.

72 CAWLEY, J. C., BURNS, G. F., HAYHOE, F. G. J.: Hairy-Cell Leukaemia.

73 Thyroid Cancer. Edited by W. DUNCAN.

74 Cancer Chemo- and Immunopharmacology. 1. Chemopharmacology. Edited by G. MATHÉ and F. M. MUGGIA.

75 Cancer Chemo- and Immunopharmacology. 2. Immunopharmacology, Relations and General Problems. Edited by G. MATHÉ and F. M. MUGGIA.

76 New Drugs in Cancer Chemotherapy. Edited by S. K. CARTER, Y. SAKURAI, H. UMEZAWA

77 K. STANLEY, J. STJERNSWÄRD, M. ISLEY: The Conduct of a Cooperative Clinical Trial.

78 Prostate Cancer. Edited by W. DUNCAN.

79 Chemotherapy and Radiotherapy of Gastrointestinal Tumors. Edited by H. O. KLEIN.

80 Adjuvant Therapies of Cancer. Edited by G. MATHÉ, G. BONADONNA, S. SALMON.

MIX
Papier aus verantwortungsvollen Quellen
Paper from responsible sources
FSC® C105338

If you have any concerns about our products,
you can contact us on
ProductSafety@springernature.com

In case Publisher is established outside the EU,
the EU authorized representative is:
Springer Nature Customer Service Center GmbH
Europaplatz 3, 69115 Heidelberg, Germany

Printed by Libri Plureos GmbH
in Hamburg, Germany